TOP TRAILS™

Sacramento

Exploring Valley, Foothills, and Mountains in the Sacramento Region

Written by

Steven L. Evans

 WILDERNESS PRESS ...*on the trail since 1967*

*To Barbara, for all her love, support, and patience,
and to all my trail companions, past, present, and future:
Happy Trails!*

**Top Trails Sacramento: Exploring Valley, Foothills, and Mountains
in the Sacramento Region**

1st EDITION 2008
   6th printing 2017

Copyright © 2008 by Steven L. Evans

All photos copyright by Steven L. Evans, except where noted
Maps: Lohnes + Wright
Cover design: Frances Baca Design and Larry Van Dyke
Interior design: Frances Baca Design
Book production: Larry B. Van Dyke
Book editor: Elaine Merrill

ISBN 978-0-89997-991-5

Published by: **Wilderness Press**
                An imprint of AdventureKEEN
                2204 First Ave. S., Suite 102
                Birmingham, AL 35233
                (800) 443-7227; FAX (205) 326-1012
                info@wildernesspress.com
                www.wildernesspress.com
Visit our website for a complete listing of our books and for ordering information.

Cover photos: The American River Parkway, Sacramento, by Lee Foster;
              deer (inset), by Steven L. Evans

All rights reserved. No part of this book may be reproduced in any form, or by any means electronic, mechanical, recording, or otherwise, without written permission from the publisher, except for brief quotations used in reviews.

SAFETY NOTICE: Although Wilderness Press and the author have made every attempt to ensure that the information in this book is accurate at press time, they are not responsible for any loss, damage, injury, or inconvenience that may occur to anyone while using this book. You are responsible for your own safety and health while in the wilderness. The fact that a trail is described in this book does not mean that it will be safe for you. Be aware that trail conditions can change from day to day. Always check local conditions and know your own limitations.

The Top Trails™ Series

Wilderness Press

When Wilderness Press published *Sierra North* in 1967, no other trail guide like it existed for the Sierra backcountry. The first run of 2800 copies sold out in less than two months and its success heralded the beginning of Wilderness Press. In the past 40 years, we have expanded our territories to cover California, Alaska, Hawaii, the U.S. Southwest, the Pacific Northwest, New England, Canada, and Baja California.

Wilderness Press continues to publish comprehensive, accurate, and readable outdoor books. Hikers, backpackers, kayakers, skiers, snowshoers, climbers, cyclists, and trail runners rely on Wilderness Press for accurate outdoor adventure information.

Top Trails

In its Top Trails guides, Wilderness Press has paid special attention to organization so that you can find the perfect hike each and every time. Whether you're looking for a steep trail to test yourself on or a walk in the park, a romantic waterfall or a city view, Top Trails will lead you there.

Each Top Trails guide contains trails for everyone. The trails selected provide a sampling of the best that the region has to offer. These are the "must-do" hikes, walks, runs, and bike rides, with every feature of the area represented.

Every book in the Top Trails series offers:

- The Wilderness Press commitment to accuracy and reliability
- Ratings and rankings for each trail
- Distances and approximate times
- Easy-to-follow trail notes
- Maps & permit information

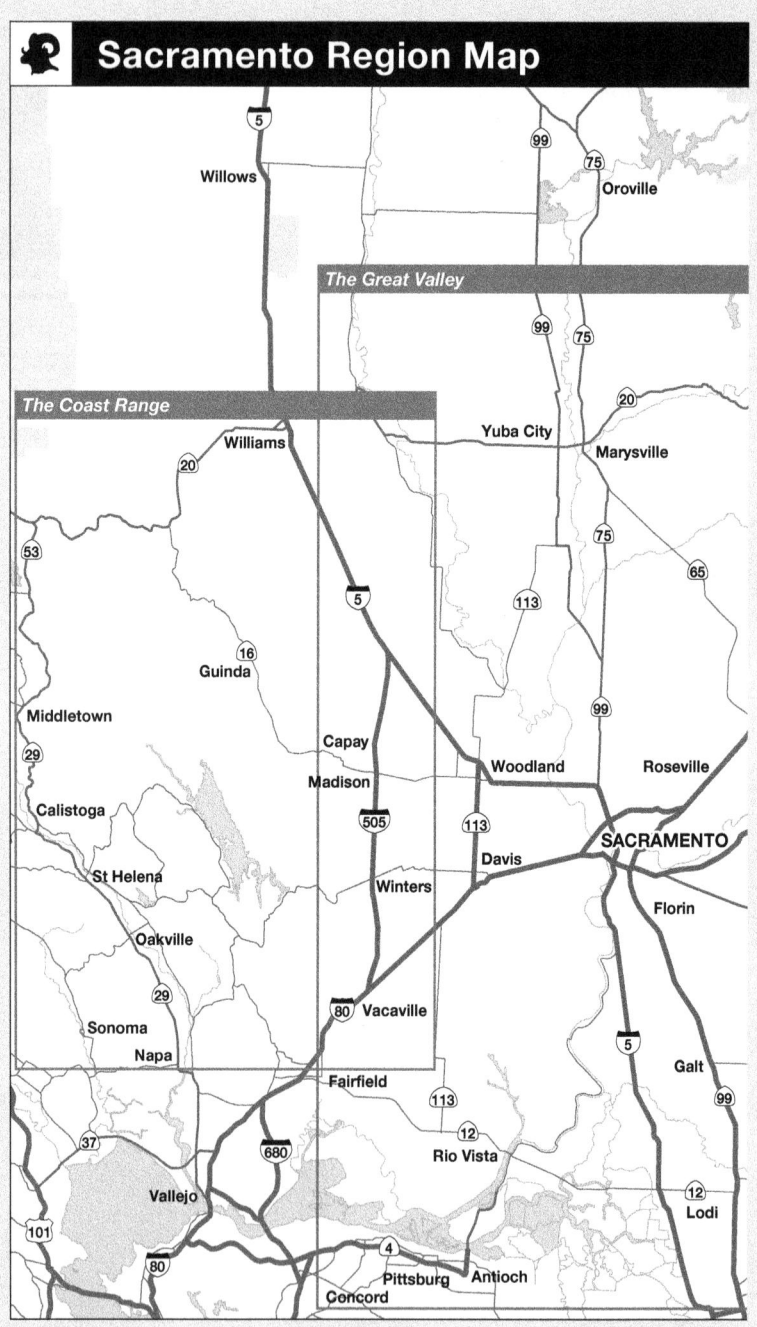

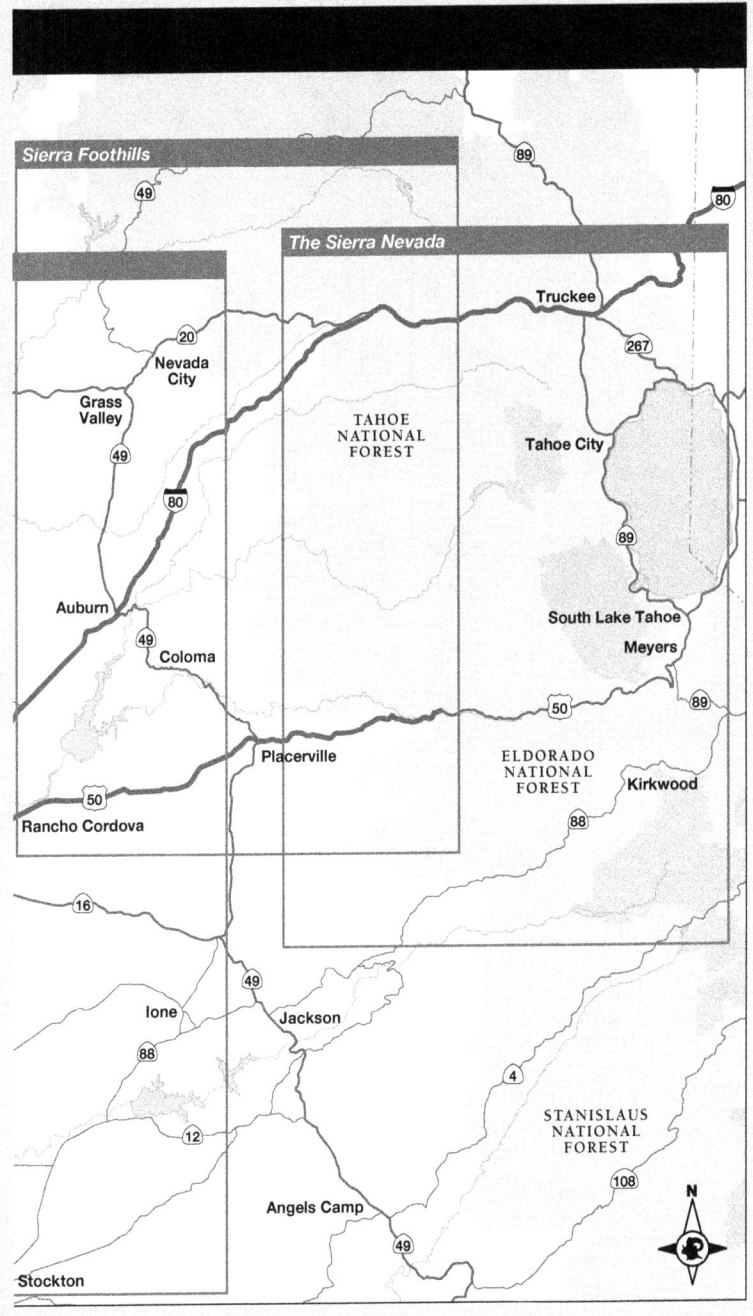

Sacramento Trails

Trail Number and Name	Page	Difficulty -12345+	Length in Miles	Type	Hiking	Horses	Running	Biking	Child Friendly	Handicap Access	Fee
1. The Great Valley											
1. Bobelaine Sanctuary Trails	29	3	5.3	Loop	🚶				👪		
2. River Walk Trail	35	2	3.0	Loop	🚶				👪		
3. Deer Creek Hills Preserve Trails	41	2/3	2.0–7.0	Variable	🚶	🐎			👪		$
4. Delta Meadows State Park and Historic Locke	47	1	2.44	Out & Back	🚶				👪		
5. Effie Yeaw Natural Area Loop Trail	53	1	1.0	Loop	🚶				👪		$
6. Gibson Ranch Regional Park Loop Trail	59	2	2.86	Loop	🚶	🐎	🏃		👪		$
7. Wetlands Discovery and Loop Trails	65	1/2	.83/2.64	Loop	🚶				👪	♿	$
8. Sutter Buttes Trails	73	2/3/4	3.0–8.0	Variable	🚶				👪		$
9. Howard Ranch Trail	79	4	6.83	Loop	🚶				👪		$
10. Jedediah Smith Memorial Trail Loop	85	3	4.2	Loop	🚶		🏃	🚴	👪	♿	$
11. Lake Natoma Loop	91	4	10.3	Loop	🚶	🐎	🏃	🚴	👪	♿	$
12. Sacramento Northern Bikeway	99	4	10.0	Variable	🚶		🏃	🚴		♿	
13. Sacramento Waterfront Loop	107	2	3.5	Variable	🚶		🏃	🚴		♿	
14. Wren Wetlands Trail	115	2	3.68	Out & Back	🚶				👪		
2. The Coast Range											
15. Blue Ridge Trail	127	5	5.56	Out & Back	🚶						
16. Cache Creek Ridge Trail	133	4	9.9	Variable	🚶	🐎	🏃	🚴			
17. Redbud Trail	141	3	4.02	Out & Back	🚶	🐎					
18. Cold Canyon–Blue Ridge Loop Trail	147	5	4.9	Variable	🚶		🏃		👪		
3. Sierra Foothills											
19. North Yuba River Trail	163	4	7.5	Point-to-Point	🚶		🏃	🚴			
20. Humbug Creek–South Yuba Trails	169	4	6.82	Point-to-Point	🚶		🏃	🚴			
21. Empire Mine State Historic Park Loop Trails	177	3	4.47	Loop	🚶	🐎	🏃	🚴	👪		$

USES & ACCESS
- 🚶 Hiking
- 🐎 Horses
- 🏃 Running
- 🚴 Biking
- 👪 Child Friendly
- ♿ Handicap Access
- $ Fee
- Permit Required
- Dogs Allowed

TYPE
- Loop
- Out & Back
- Point-to-Point
- V Variable

DIFFICULTY
-12345+
less   more

TERRAIN
- River or Stream
- Waterfall
- Lake
- Wetland
- Meadow
- Canyon
- Mountain

FLORA & FAUNA
- Wildflowers
- Fall Colors
- Birds
- Wildlife

FEATURES
- Historic Interest
- Geologic Interest
- Great Views
- Steep
- Secluded
- Camping

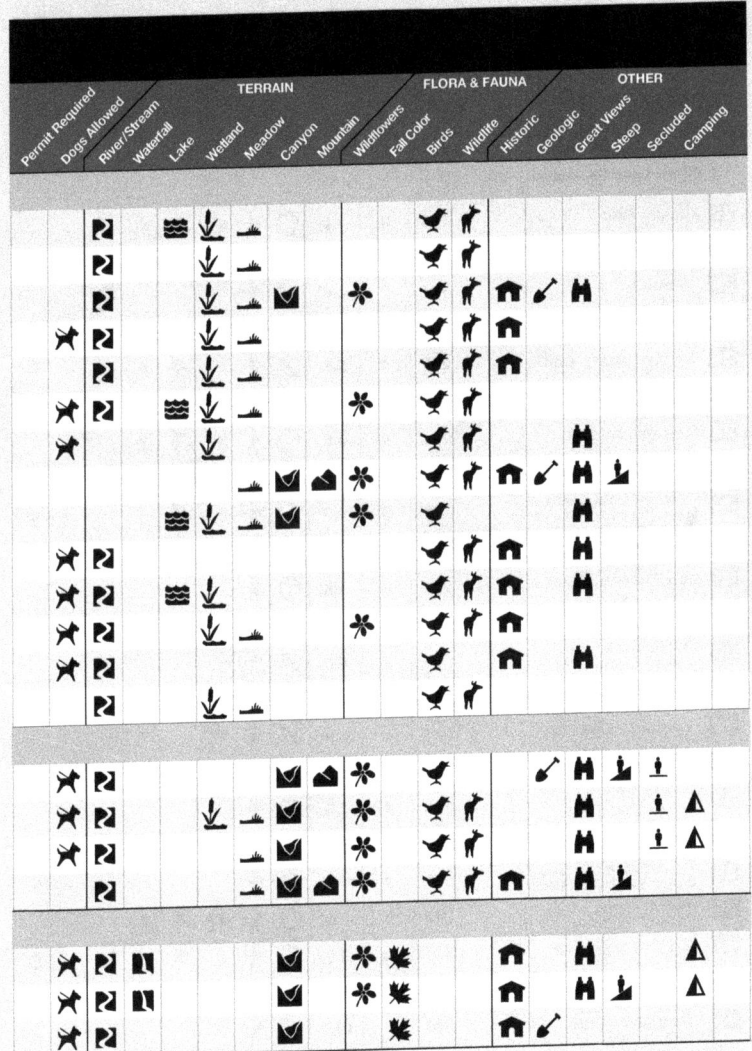

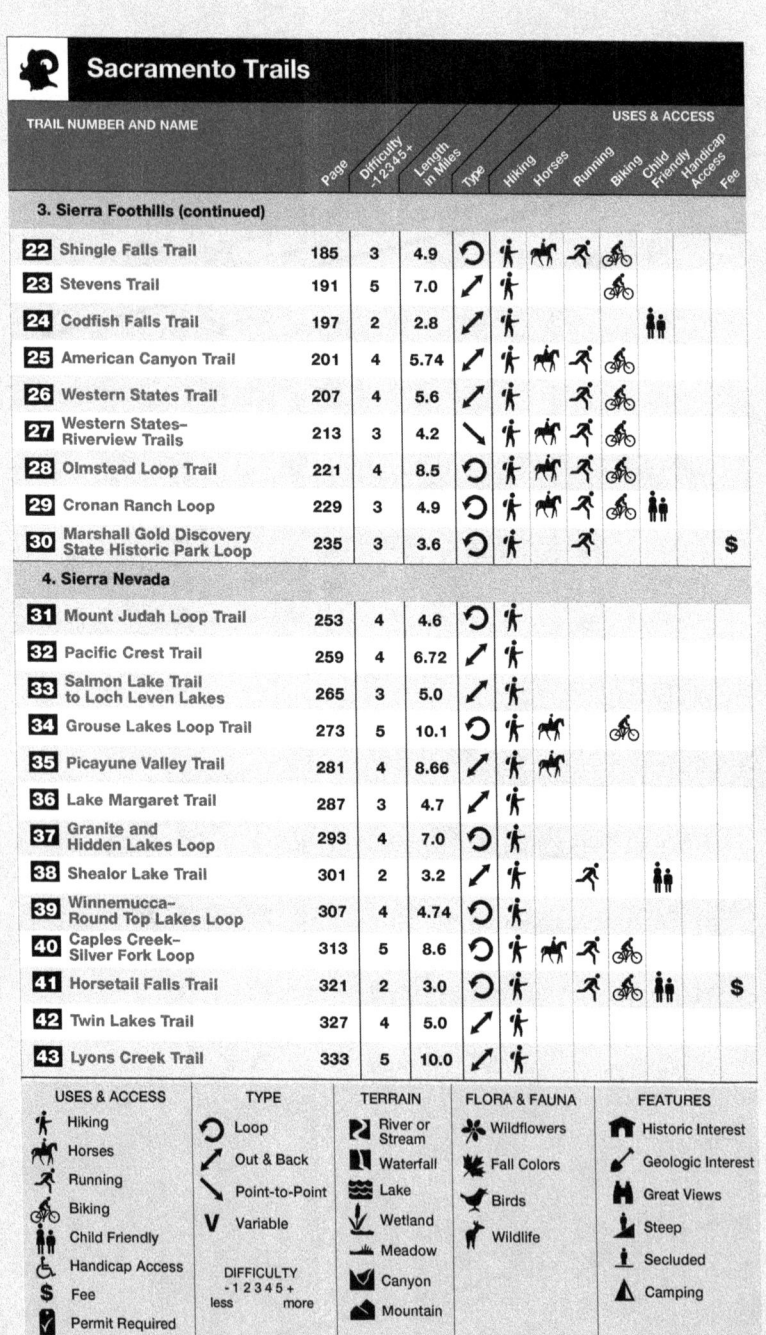

Permit Required	Dogs Allowed	River/Stream	Waterfall	Lake	Wetland	Meadow	Canyon	Mountain	Wildflowers	Fall Color	Birds	Wildlife	Historic	Geologic	Great Views	Steep	Secluded	Camping
			TERRAIN						**FLORA & FAUNA**				**OTHER**					
✈	▶	▮▮			▬	▼			✽		🐦	🦌	🏠		M	▲		
✈	▶	▮▮				▼			✽	🍁	🐦		🏠		M			△
✈	▶	▮▮				▼			✽						M			
✈	▶	▮▮			▬	▼			✽	🍁			🏠		M		▲	
✈	▶					▼							🏠		M	▲	▲	△
✈	▶	▮▮				▼			✽	🍁	🐦	🦌	🏠		M			
✈	▶	▮▮			▬	▼			✽	🍁	🐦	🦌		🪚	M			
✈	▶				▬	▼			✽		🐦	🦌			M			
	▶					▼				🍁		🦌	🏠		M	▲		
	✈					▬		▲	✽		🐦			🏠	M	▲		
	✈	▶				▬		▲	✽	🍁				🪚	M	▲		△
	✈			≈											M			△
	✈	▶	▮▮	≈	▬	▼	▲		✽						M			△
✓	✈	▶	▮▮		▬	▼			✽	🍁					M			△
	✈	▶		≈	▬				✽		🐦				M			△
	✈			≈	▬										M			△
	✈			≈			▼		✽					🪚	M			△
✓	✈	▶		≈	▬			▲	✽	🍁			🏠		M	▲		
	✈	▶	▮▮		▬	▼			✽	🍁	🐦	🦌			M	▲	▲	△
	✈	▶	▮▮			▼								🪚	M	▲		
✓	✈	▶	▮▮	≈				▲	✽						M	▲		△
✓	✈	▶	▮▮	≈	▬				✽						M	▲		△

Contents

Sacramento Region Map iv
Sacramento Region Trails Table vi

Using Top Trails xiv
   Organization of Top Trails xiv
   Choosing a Trail xvii

Introduction to the Sacramento Region 1
   Geology, Topography, Hydrology, and Climate 1
   Ecoregions of the Sacramento Area 3
      California Central Valley Grasslands Ecoregion (Great Valley) 3
      California Woodlands and Interior Chaparral Ecoregion
      (the Coast Range and Sierra Foothills) 5
      Sierra Nevada Forests Ecoregion (Sierra Nevada) 7

On the Trail 9
   Have a Plan 9
   Carry the Essentials 10
   Less than Essential, but Useful 13
   Trail Etiquette 14

CHAPTER 1
The Great Valley 17

1. Bobelaine Sanctuary Trails: Feather River 29
2. River Walk Trail: Cosumnes River Preserve 35
3. Deer Creek Hills Preserve Trails 41
4. Delta Meadows State Park and Historic Locke 47
5. Effie Yeaw Natural Area Loop Trail 53
6. Gibson Ranch Regional Park Loop Trail 59
7. Wetlands Discovery & Loop Trails: Gray Lodge Wildlife Area ... 65
8. Sutter Buttes Trails 73
9. Howard Ranch Trail 79
10. Jedediah Smith Memorial Trail Loop: American River Parkway .. 85

- 11. Lake Natoma Loop: Folsom Lake State Recreation Area 91
- 12. Sacramento Northern Bikeway 99
- 13. Sacramento Waterfront Loop................................. 107
- 14. Wren Wetlands Trail: Stone Lakes National Wildlife Refuge 115

CHAPTER 2
The Coast Range ... 119
- 15. Blue Ridge Trail: Cache Creek Natural Area 127
- 16. Cache Creek Ridge Trail: Cache Creek Natural Area............ 133
- 17. Redbud Trail: Cache Creek Wilderness 141
- 18. Cold Canyon–Blue Ridge Loop Trail: Stebbins UC Reserve...... 147

CHAPTER 3
Sierra Foothills ... 153
- 19. North Yuba River Trail 163
- 20. Humbug Creek–South Yuba Trails:
  South Yuba Wild & Scenic River............................. 169
- 21. Empire Mine State Historic Park Loop Trails................. 177
- 22. Shingle Falls Trail: Spenceville Wildlife Area............... 185
- 23. Stevens Trail: North Fork American Wild & Scenic River....... 191
- 24. Codfish Falls Trail: Auburn State Recreation Area............ 197
- 25. American Canyon Trail: Auburn State Recreation Area 201
- 26. Western States Trail: El Dorado Canyon 207
- 27. Western States–Riverview Trails: Auburn State Recreation Area ... 213
- 28. Olmstead Loop Trail: Auburn State Recreation Area 221
- 29. Cronan Ranch Loop: South Fork American River 229
- 30. Marshall Gold Discovery State Historic Park Loop 235

CHAPTER 4
The Sierra Nevada ... 241
- 31. Mount Judah Loop Trail 253
- 32. Pacific Crest Trail: Castle Peak Area 259
- 33. Salmon Lake Trail to Loch Leven Lakes...................... 265
- 34. Grouse Lakes Loop Trail 273
- 35. Picayune Valley Trail: Granite Chief Wilderness 281
- 36. Lake Margaret Trail: Caples Creek Proposed Wilderness........ 287
- 37. Granite and Hidden Lakes Loop 293
- 38. Shealor Lake Trail: Caples Creek Proposed Wilderness......... 301
- 39. Winnemucca–Round Top Lakes Loop: Mokelumne Wilderness ... 307

40. Caples Creek–Silver Fork Loop:
   Caples Creek Proposed Wilderness 313
41. Horsetail Falls Trail 321
42. Twin Lakes Trail: Desolation Wilderness 327
43. Lyons Creek Trail: Desolation Wilderness 333

Appendices 338
   Top Rated Trails 338
   Weekend Getaways 339
   Governing Agencies 342
   Major Organizations 344
   Useful Resources 348
   Maps 349

Index 354
Author 361

Map Legend

Trail	River
Other Trail	Stream
Freeway	Seasonal Stream
Major Road	
Minor Road	Body of Water
Tunnel	Marsh/Swamp
Bridge	Dam
Building	Peak
Trailhead Parking	Park/Forest Boundary
Picnic	
Camping	
Gate	
Start/Finish	North Arrow

Using Top Trails™

Organization of Top Trails

Top Trails is designed to make identifying the perfect trail easy and enjoyable, and to make every outing a success and a pleasure. With this book you'll find it's a snap to find the right trail, whether you're planning a major hike or just a sociable stroll with friends.

The Region

Top Trails begins with the **Sacramento Region Map** (pages iv-v), displaying the entire region covered by the guide and providing a geographic overview. The map is clearly marked to show which area is covered by each chapter.

After the Regional Map comes the **Sacramento Region Trails Table** (pages vi-ix), which lists every trail covered in the guide along with attributes for each trail. A quick reading of the Regional Map and the Trails Table will give a good overview of the entire region covered by the book.

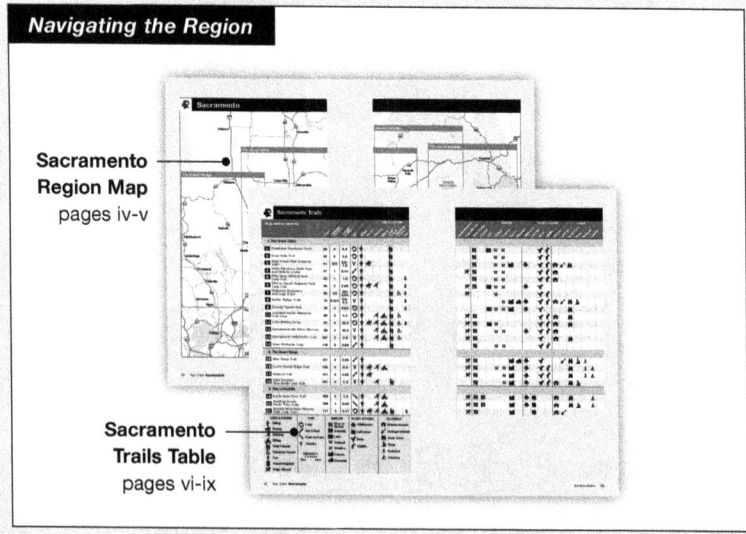

Navigating the Region

Sacramento Region Map
pages iv-v

Sacramento Trails Table
pages vi-ix

The Areas

The region covered in each book is divided into Areas, with each chapter corresponding to one area in the region.

Each Area chapter starts with information to help you choose and enjoy a trail every time out. Use the Table of Contents or the Regional Map to identify an area of interest, then turn to the Area chapter to find the following:

- An Overview of the Area, including park and permit information
- An Area Map with all trails clearly marked
- A Trail Feature Table providing trail-by-trail details
- Trail Summaries, written in a lively, accessible style

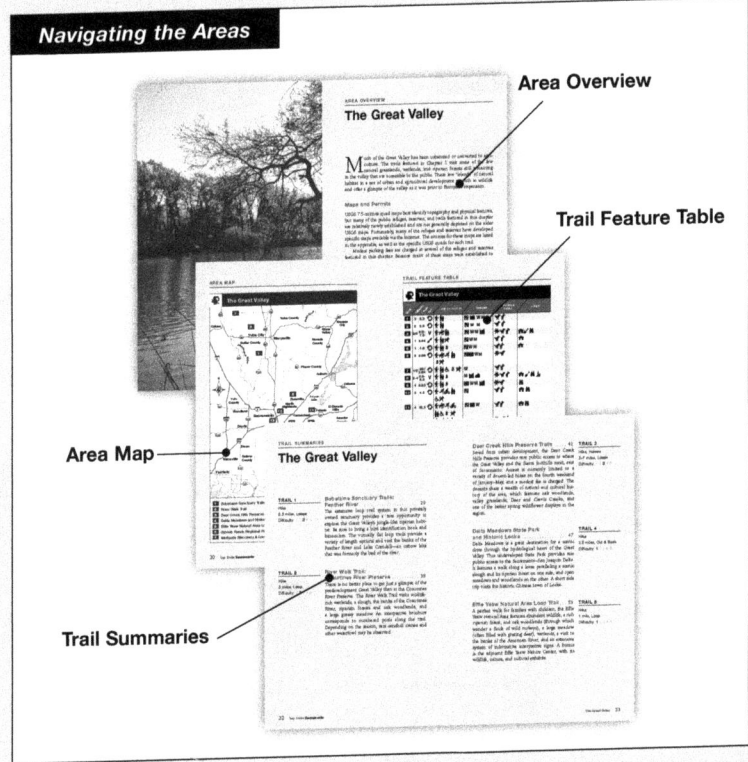

Using Top Trails XV

The Trails

The basic building block of the Top Trails guide is the Trail Entry. Each one is arranged to make finding and following the trail as simple as possible, with all pertinent information presented in this easy-to-follow format:

- A Trail Map
- Trail Descriptors covering difficulty, length, and other essential data
- A written Trail Description
- Trail Milestones providing easy-to-follow, turn-by-turn trail directions

Some Trail Descriptions offer additional information:

- An Elevation Profile
- Trail Options
- Trail Highlights

In the margins of the Trail Entries, keep your eyes open for graphic icons that signal passages in the text.

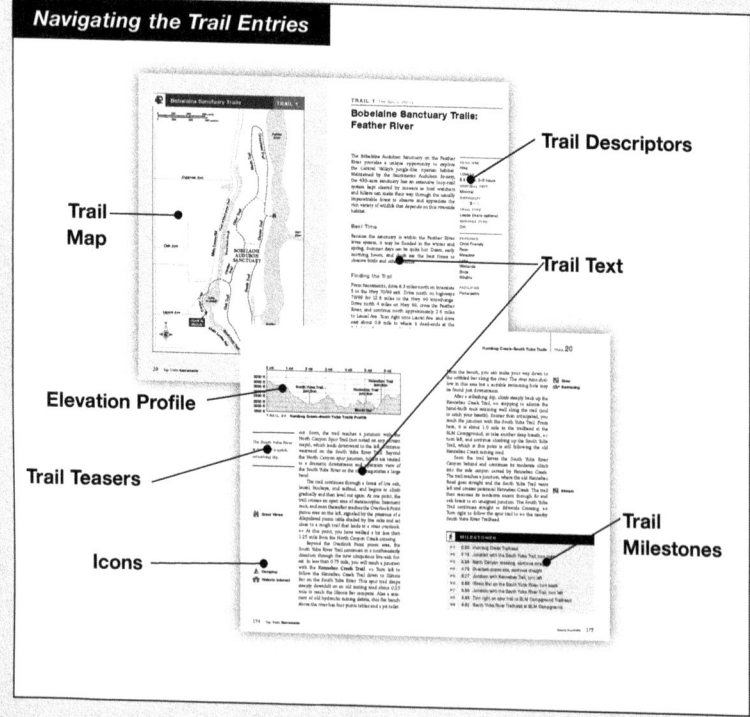

Choosing a Trail

Top Trails provides several different ways of choosing a trail, all presented in easy-to-read tables, charts, and maps.

Location

If you know in general where you want to go, Top Trails makes it easy to find the right trail in the right place. Each chapter begins with a large-scale map showing the starting point of every trail in that area.

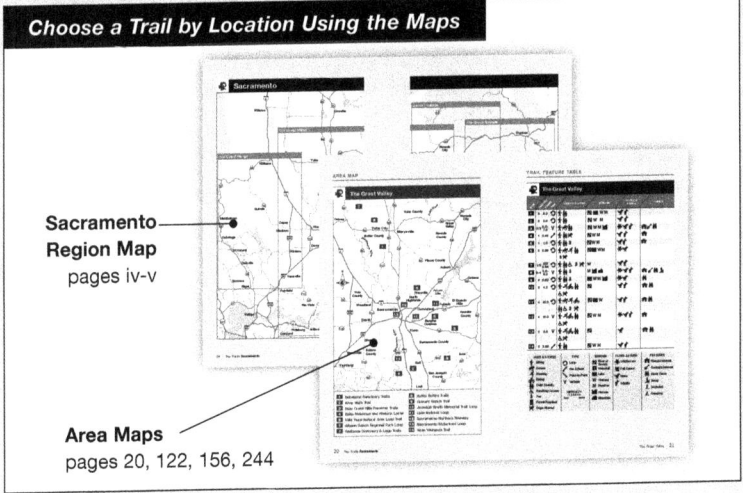

Choose a Trail by Location Using the Maps

Sacramento Region Map pages iv-v

Area Maps pages 20, 122, 156, 244

Features

This guide describes the Top Trails of the Sacramento region. Each trail is chosen because it offers one or more features that make it interesting. Using the trail descriptors, summaries, and tables, you can quickly examine all the trails for the features they offer, or seek a particular feature among the list of trails.

Season and Condition

Time of year and current conditions can be important factors in selecting the best trail. For example, an exposed grassland trail may be a riot of color in early spring, but an oven-baked taste of hell in mid-summer. Wherever relevant, Top Trails identifies the best and worst conditions for the trails you plan to hike.

Difficulty

Each trail has an overall difficulty rating on a scale of 1 to 5, which takes into consideration length, elevation change, exposure, trail quality, etc., to create one (admittedly subjective) rating.

The ratings assume you are an able-bodied adult in reasonably good shape using the trail for hiking. The ratings also assume normal weather conditions—clear and dry.

Readers should make an honest assessment of their own abilities and adjust time estimates accordingly. Also, rain, snow, heat, and poor visibility can all affect the pace on even the easiest of trails.

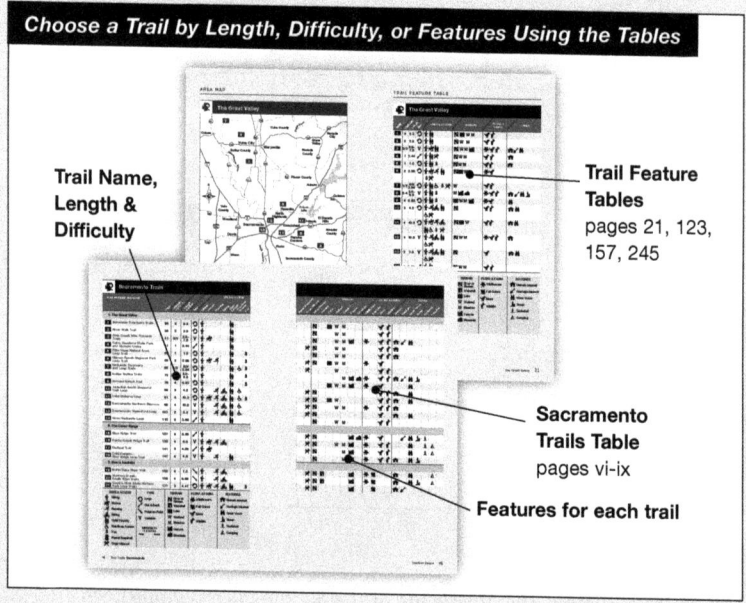

Choose a Trail by Length, Difficulty, or Features Using the Tables

Trail Name, Length & Difficulty

Trail Feature Tables
pages 21, 123, 157, 245

Sacramento Trails Table
pages vi–ix

Features for each trail

Vertical Feet

This important measurement is often underestimated by hikers and bikers when gauging the difficulty of a trail. The Top Trails measurement accounts for all elevation change, not simply the difference between the highest and lowest points, so that rolling terrain with lots of up and down will be identifiable.

The calculation of Vertical Feet in the Top Trails series is accomplished by a combination of trail measurement and computer-aided estimation. For routes that begin and end at the same spot—i.e., Loop or Out & Back—the vertical gain exactly matches the vertical descent. With a point-to-point route the vertical gain and loss will most likely differ, and both figures will be provided in the text.

Finally, some of Trail Entries in the Top Trails series have an Elevation Profile, an easy means for visualizing the topography of the route. These profiles graphically depict the elevation throughout the length of the trail.

Top Trails Difficulty Ratings

1. A short trail, generally level, which can be completed in 1 hour or less.
2. A route of 1 to 3 miles, with some up and down, which can be completed in 1 to 2 hours.
3. A longer route, up to 5 miles, with uphill and/or downhill sections.
4. A long or steep route, perhaps more than 5 miles or climbs of more than 1000 vertical feet.
5. The most severe, both long and steep, more than 5 miles long with climbs of more than 1000 vertical feet.

Surface Type

Each Trail Entry provides information about the surface of the trail. This is useful in determining what type of footwear or bicycle is appropriate. Surface Type should also be considered when checking the weather—on a rainy day a dirt surface can be a muddy slog; an asphalt surface might be a better choice (although asphalt can be slick when wet).

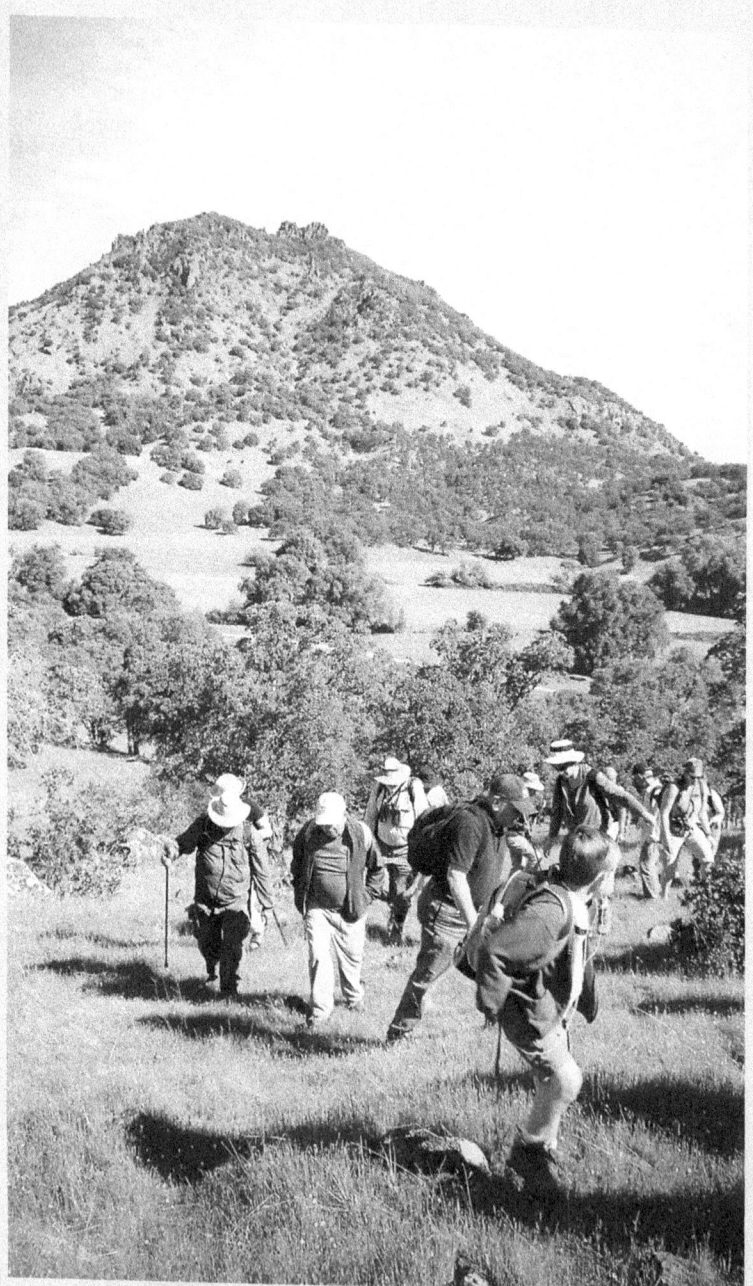

North Butte dominates the view *as hikers make their way into the Sutter Buttes (Trail 8).*

Introduction to the Sacramento Region

There is a long-running joke about Sacramento being "that place" conveniently located between San Francisco and Lake Tahoe. All regional biases aside, even loyal Sacramentans love the fact that they are equidistant from the culture and cool fog of the Bay Area and the high mountain lakes and green forests of the Sierra. Sacramento is, in fact, ideally located for people who would like to explore the Coast Range to the west, the Sierra Nevada to the east, and the Great Valley (a.k.a. the Central Valley) in between. Whether you want to swim in a high Sierra lake, climb a remote Coast Range ridge, watch thousands of geese rise from the remnant marshes of the Great Valley, explore vernal pools spangled with a dazzling display of wildflowers, or experience a bit of Gold Rush history in the Sierra foothills, the Sacramento region provides all of this, as well as many opportunities for year-round hiking and other outdoor pursuits as diverse as the surrounding countryside.

Geology, Topography, Hydrology, and Climate

About 500 million years ago, California didn't exist. It was all under an ancient sea and the west coast of North America was somewhere in Nevada. Erosion of very old mountains to the east layered mud, sand, and gravel on the ocean floor, which consisted of ophiolite, a mixture of serpentine and lava extruded from underwater volcanoes. What was to become California was created by a number of geologic processes, including plate tectonics (formerly known as continental drift), volcanism above and below ground, uplifting, erosion, faulting, and glacial movement.

About 250 million years ago, the iconic granite of the Sierra Nevada began forming as molten rock underground. The molten rock cooled into granite. Hot liquid and gases carried gold upward into cracks in the ancient rocks and cooled granite. A chain of lava-extruding volcanoes rose from the surface of the sea in the vicinity of what is today the Sierra, but most of California was still underwater.

About 150 million years ago, a huge slab of oceanic crust and mantle was thrust over the edge of the North American continent, putting in place the ophiolite basement that underlies much of the Great Valley and the Coast Range today.

About 65 million years ago, the Farallon Plate dove below the North American Plate and began to uplift the ancestral Sierra, forming a low mountain range a couple of thousand feet high. Erosion stripped the upper layers off the mountain range, exposing the granite and gold veins. The entire range tilted westward and became a broad upland. This tectonic movement also created an offshore depression that filled with sediments eroded from the ancestral Sierra. These sediments later become the sandstones and shales that make up the Great Valley sequence that covers much of the Coast Range today.

About 30 million years ago, the Pacific Plate crashed (geologically speaking) into the Farallon Plate, dividing it in two and pushing it to the north and south. The pressure compressed the edge of the North American Plate, further uplifting both the Sierra and the Coast Range. Volcanic eruptions buried the northern Sierra under lava and mudflows, filling canyons and passes. An inland sea filled the depression that would later become the Great Valley we know today.

Less than 5 million years ago, uplift and downward movement along fault systems to the west and east began creating the modern Sierra, which eventually grew to more than 10,000 feet in the northern part of the range. About 3 million years after the modern Sierra uplift began, the earth cooled and the Great Ice Age (actually a series of ice ages) caused glaciers to grow and shrink. This glacial movement carved and smoothed the Sierra granite, scattered and deposited large boulders, and created ridges made of rock, soil, and other debris.

About 650,000 years ago, faulting allowed the rising water of the inland sea to break through the Coast Range and flow out through what eventually became the modern San Francisco Bay to the Pacific Ocean. As tectonic forces continued to push the Coast Range and Sierra upward, the Great Valley continued to act like a giant bathtub, capturing eroded sediments that were transported by rivers from the mountains to the valley's relatively flat alluvial plain.

About 10,000 years ago, the Great Ice Age ended (or at least took a break) in the Sierra. By then, the Sacramento region looked pretty much as it does today, minus all the cities, freeways, farms, etc.—a large, central valley ringed by mountains to the west (the Coast Range) and higher mountains to the east (the Sierra Nevada), with rivers and streams flowing down from the mountain ranges, combining into larger rivers in the valley, meeting at the Delta, and then flowing west to the San Francisco Bay and out the Golden Gate.

Topography and geology play an important role in the weather, climate, and vegetation found in the Sacramento area. California's Mediterranean climate provides cool, wet winters and hot, dry summers. The 3000–4000-foot-high peaks and ridges of the Coast Range and the 10,000 foot-high peaks and crest of the northern Sierra squeeze moisture in the form of rain and snow from the winter storm clouds that roll in from the Pacific Ocean. Precipitation averages 35 inches a year in the portion of the Coast Range west of Sacramento and more than 60 inches a year (much of it snow) in the higher elevations of the northern Sierra. But in the foothills and valley, precipitation is dramatically less, averaging just 15–20 inches per year.

Except for flood times, much of the valley and foothills is accessible year-round, but summertime temperatures can often be uncomfortable by mid-day and into the afternoon. Spring and fall and the occasionally sunny winter day offer the best time to recreate in these regions. Snow often covers the ground in the upper elevations of the Sierra until June or July, which makes the period from mid-summer to mid-fall the best time to visit. You can literally follow the seasonal wildflower bloom by ascending in elevation, beginning in early March and extending typically through April in the Great Valley, moving into the foothills in April through May, and into the higher elevations of the Sierra, in June and even into August.

Ecoregions of the Sacramento Area

The hikes featured in *Top Trails Sacramento* visit three major ecoregions, each with its unique ecology, flora, and fauna. These include the California Central Valley Grasslands Ecoregion, which dominates the Great Valley; the California Woodlands and Interior Chaparral Ecoregion, which encompasses the Coast Range and Sierra foothills; and the Sierra Nevada Forests Ecoregion, found in the mid- to higher-elevation portions of the Sierra.

California Central Valley Grasslands Ecoregion (Great Valley)

The Great Valley was once California's Serengeti. A unique mosaic of marshes, wetlands, savannas, prairies, riparian woodlands, shrublands, and near-desert areas, the valley teemed with deer, antelope, elk, and grizzly bears. Ducks and geese blocked out the sky, and it was said that you could walk across rivers on the backs of thousands of migrating salmon. But much of the valley today has been either converted to agriculture or urbanized. More than 90 percent of its wetlands and marshlands have been filled or drained and 95 percent of its riparian woodlands have been cleared. There are very few "natural" areas of the California Central Valley Grasslands

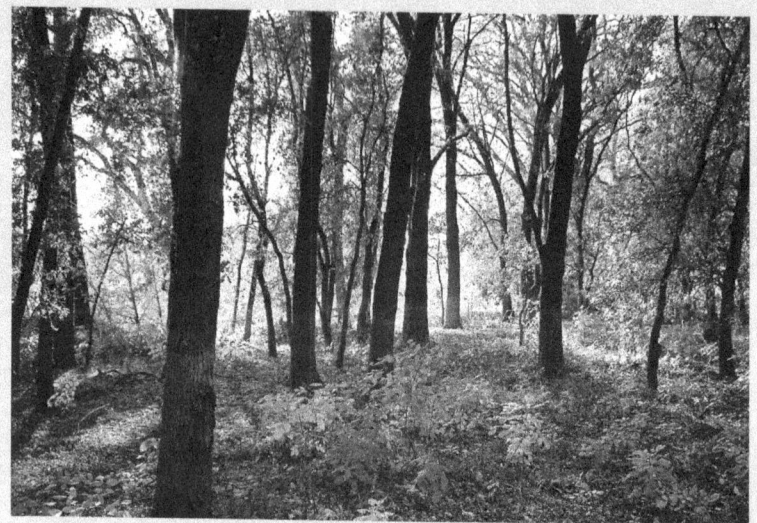

Riparian forest *is an important habitat in the Cosumnes Preserve.*

Ecoregion left, but those remaining areas give you an idea of just how rich the Great Valley once was.

Concerted efforts over the last 50 years to preserve and restore marshlands in the Great Valley have resulted in a major comeback for waterfowl. The Great Valley is a major stopover on the Pacific Flyway for millions of ducks, geese, and other waterfowl. Today, the call of migrating geese in the fall and spring is common, and even the formerly elusive and unique trill of the rare sandhill crane is heard. Still, only 6 percent of the valley's former marshlands remain today. The Sacramento region has a rich diversity of wetlands and marshlands in federal, state, and private waterfowl refuges, many of which offer public access so that we can appreciate this endangered habitat and its seasonal occupants.

Unfortunately, other habitats that make up the region are rare and remain threatened. The rivers of the Great Valley were once lined with extensive riparian forests made up of box elder, coyote bush, buttonwillow, wild grape, black walnut, cottonwood, sycamore, and valley oak. But the riverside forests have largely been cleared, and many of the rivers and streams have been lined with levees, rock, and concrete. Sacramento is fortunate to have led the way in the United States in the preservation of river-based parks, with the establishment of the American River Parkway nearly 50 years ago. The Parkway offers a glimpse of the primeval riparian forests that once clothed the valley's mighty rivers, and supports runs of migrating steelhead and salmon. Some species of waterfowl, including mallards, mergansers, and Canada geese are permanent residents of the few remaining natural river and wetland habitats, which also provide important migration corridors for many wildlife species.

Another habitat that has almost disappeared from the ecoregion is the valley's once-extensive native grasslands. What hasn't been plowed under by agriculture or paved over by urban development has been largely taken over by non-native grasses and other weedy species. The native grasslands of the Great Valley were once dotted with small seasonal pools, called vernal pools. Approximately 66 percent of the vernal pool habitat in the Great Valley has been destroyed. These seasonal pools provide important habitat for threatened and endangered wildlife and plants, and produce an amazing display of spring wildflowers. Only a few examples of undeveloped grasslands with vernal pools exist today in the Great Valley.

Humans have lived in the Great Valley Ecoregion for thousands of years. Permanent Indian villages were located in the few high spots of the valley terrain that avoided the valley's seasonal flooding. Some tribes migrated seasonally between the foothills and the marshes and flood-prone rivers in the valley to harvest the water's rich bounty of fish, waterfowl, and other food.

Today, Sacramento and its neighboring cities lie in the heart of the Great Valley. Here and there, a few examples of the natural wetlands, grasslands, and riverside riparian forests remain, and some have been acquired to protect habitat for rare species and to provide us with an inkling of the former natural glory of the Great Valley. Nevertheless, public lands available for outdoor recreation remain a relative rarity in the Great Valley. Many of the hikes featured in *Top Trails Sacramento* focus on these rare areas.

California Woodlands and Interior Chaparral Ecoregion (the Coast Range and Sierra Foothills)

Ranging in elevation from 300 to 3000 feet, the California Woodlands and Interior Chaparral Ecoregion encompasses the entire southern section of the Coast Range and also the foothills of the Sierra Nevada. The icon of this ecoregion is the blue oak. It tends to dominate the woodlands found in the lower elevations of the Coast Range and Sierra foothills, mixed in with its cousins, the coast, canyon, and interior live oaks, as well as the increasingly rare valley (or white) oak. Gray (or foothill) pines are well known companions of the oak woodlands. As elevations increase, pockets of pine grow, including Ponderosa in the Sierra and knobcone and big cone Douglas fir in the Coast Range.

The understory of the oak woodlands consists of the ubiquitous scrub oak, fragrant-smelling laurel, redbud, dogwood, buckeye, skunkbush, and the seasonally showy Christmasberry toyon. The oak woodlands are often mixed in with open grassland and with large swaths of sometimes nearly impenetrable chaparral, including manzanita, buckbrush, and chamise. The native perennial bunchgrasses that formerly dominated California's

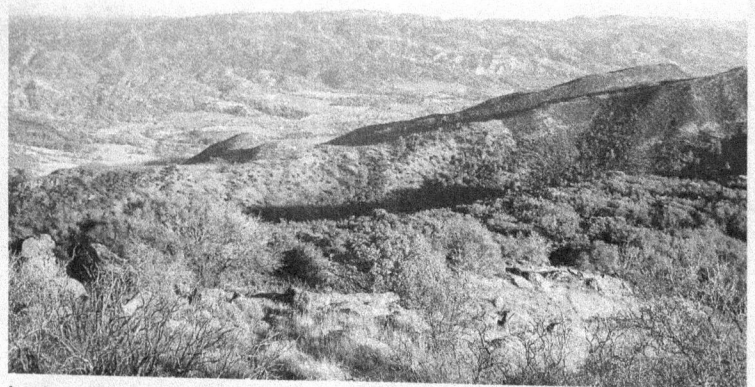

Looking east to the Capay Valley *from Blue Ridge*

grasslands have been largely replaced by non-native seasonal Mediterranean grasses and weeds, but can still be found in some undisturbed areas.

As in virtually every ecoregion found in seasonally dry California, riparian vegetation along streams and rivers, including willow, alder, maple, sycamore, cottonwood, blackberry, and various streamside sedges, provides critical habitat for wildlife and attractive recreation destinations for visitors, as well. Unique soils, such as serpentine in the Coast Range, are home to the rare McNabb and Sargent's cypress. Gabbro soils in the Sierra foothills of El Dorado County support several rare plant species, including three found nowhere else in the world: the Pine Hill flannelbush, the El Dorado bedstraw, and the El Dorado mule-ear.

The California Woodlands and Interior Chaparral Ecoregion as a whole supports more endemic mammals than any other ecoregion in the United States or Canada, including more than 100 species of birds and more than 2000 species of plants other than trees. Unfortunately, the ecoregion has been invaded by more than 2100 non-native plant species, representing 30 percent of the total plants found here—again, the most of any ecoregion in the United States and Canada.

Although wildlife is abundant in the undeveloped portions of this ecoregion, the only California grizzly you can find today is on the state flag. Antelope have retreated to far northeastern California. Elk are found only in a few well-nurtured herds. Deer, bear, coyote, and cougar are still fairly common. Neotropical songbirds migrate to the woodlands and riparian habitats of this ecoregion every summer to nest and forage. The once endangered bald eagle has become increasingly common in this ecoregion, along with the turkey vulture and red-tailed hawk.

Humans have lived in this ecoregion for thousands of years. The foothill habitats provided plentiful deer, salmon, and acorns, as well as vegetation used to make clothes, baskets, and houses. Today, the ecoregion is the focus of intense development on private lands, particularly in the Sierra foothills. Public lands in the ecoregion were formerly sparse, but recent acquisitions by land trusts and government agencies have increased the number of public lands, parks, and preserves in some parts of the Coast Range and in the Sierra foothills. These lands provide important public access and diverse opportunities for outdoor recreation.

Many of the hikes in *Top Trails Sacramento* feature outings in the oak woodlands, savanna, and chaparral of the Coast Range and the Sierra foothills. These areas not only offer year-round opportunities for outdoor recreation, they also provide insights into California's rich natural and human history.

Sierra Nevada Forests Ecoregion (Sierra Nevada)

From its yellow pine belt to the subalpine regions just above treeline, the northern portion of the Sierra Nevada Ecoregion possesses a diverse array of habitats. More than 400 vascular plant species are found only in the Sierra and nowhere else in the world. The steep canyons and river valleys, high ridges and alpine (and sometimes volcanic) peaks, mountain lakes, large meadows, and rich forests provide not only ideal habitat but attractive outdoor recreation for millions of people.

The oaks, grasslands, and chaparral of the foothills transition into the Sierra Nevada Forests Ecoregion at about 3000 feet in elevation. This is where the mixed conifer forest begins to dominate, with the ponderosa (yellow) pine mixed in with sugar pine, incense cedar, white fir, and Douglas fir. Black oaks are found in groves in the mixed conifer forest up to an elevation of 5000 feet or so. Manzanita, buckbrush, and other chaparral species are also an important component of this ecoregion, particularly in areas recently burned. Open meadows provide important habitat for grazing species and as always, riparian areas along streams and rivers consisting of willow, alder, cottonwood, and aspen at the higher elevations diversify the habitat for numerous wildlife species.

Tree species in the mixed conifer forest transition to Jeffrey pine and white and red fir at higher elevations. Aspens provide seasonal color along streams and around meadows. As elevation increases in the Sierra, old-growth red-fir forests tend to dominate, with hemlock, and whitebark pine, juniper, and sagebrush appearing as you approach the Sierra crest (and the Great Basin Ecoregion to the east). Meadows at the higher elevations provide an exceptional wildflower display, sometimes well into August.

Deer, bears, coyotes, bobcats, and cougars are still relatively common in the foothills. Seasonal waterfowl, bald eagles, and beavers can often be found at ponds, wetlands, and along rivers and streams, while streamside riparian habitat attracts dozens of species of seasonally migrating neotropical songbirds. Old-growth forests are home to several sensitive, threatened, and endangered species, including the California spotted owl, goshawk, pine marten, and Pacific fisher. Every major river in the Sierra formerly supported migrating salmon and steelhead. But today, dams have blocked more than 90 percent of the historical habitats for these fish in the Sierra. The native rainbow trout remains, as well as several other native and nonnative fish species.

Fire is a major component of the natural Sierra Ecosystem. Large old-growth trees tend to be fire resistant. Seasonal fires set by Native Americans tended to remove the brushy undergrowth and preserve park-like stands of old growths. But catastrophic, forest-replacing fires were also common. Burned areas naturally revegetated with chaparral species that fix nitrogen. Oaks and pines eventually replaced the brush, with large sun-seeking species like the ponderosa pine ultimately dominating the forest overstory. But without continued intervention by fire, undergrowth and shade tolerant species like fir grow under the pines and create fuel ladders that fuel the burning of entire forests. A debate rages today on how to reintroduce and manage fire in the forests of the Sierra Nevada. This debate has intensified as new development in the fire-prone Sierra has put structures, houses, and entire communities in harm's way.

Humans have also lived in the Sierra Nevada Ecoregion for thousands of years, but mostly at the lower elevations. Native Americans typically migrated to higher elevations in the summer season and then retreated to the foothills in the winter. This way of life ended when gold was discovered in 1849. The influx of miners, entrepreneurs, and adventurers decimated the Indian tribes through the introduction of new diseases, the loss of land needed for hunting and living, and outright slaughter—a truly dark chapter in California history. Ultimately, mining gave way to logging and ranching. Large forest reserves (now known as the National Forest System) were established at the mid to higher elevations by the federal government at the turn of the nineteenth century. Although mining and logging continue on public and private lands in the Sierra, resource development is now giving way to tourism and to expanding communities that attract people seeking the kind of high-quality lifestyle fostered by easy public access to the great outdoors.

Today, the Sierra Nevada is a mecca for people who enjoy living in a beautiful setting, as well as the destination of choice for those who want to escape California's summer heat and partake of the cool, clean air of the high country. *Top Trails Sacramento* features some of the best high-country trails within a short drive of the state's capital.

On The Trail

Every outing should begin with proper preparation, which usually takes just minutes. Even the easiest trail can turn up unexpected surprises. Hikers never think that they will get lost or suffer an injury, but accidents do happen. Simple precautions can make the difference between a good story and a dangerous situation.

Use the Top Trails ratings and descriptions to determine if a particular trail is a good match with your fitness and energy level, given current conditions and time of year. Pay particular attention to the Best Time description given for each trail. As a general rule, summer heat may be a challenge on trails in the Great Valley, Sierra Foothills, and Coast Range. On the other hand, these regions offer hiking opportunities generally unavailable in the higher elevations during late fall, winter, and spring. The higher-elevation trails in the Sierra Nevada offer a great way to escape the summer heat, but care should be taken at all times, as high country weather may change quickly, and mountain thunderstorms can be a particular concern.

Have a Plan

Choose Wisely The first step to enjoying any trail is to match the trail to your abilities. It's no use overestimating your experience or fitness—know your abilities and limitations, and use the **Top Trails Difficulty Rating** that accompanies each trail (see pg xix).

Leave Word The most basic of precautions is leaving word of your intentions with family or friends. Many people will hike the backcountry their entire lives without ever relying on this safety net, but establishing this simple habit is free insurance.

It's best to leave specific information—location, trail name, intended time of travel—with a responsible person. However, if this is not possible or if plans change at the last minute, you should still leave word. If there is a registration process available, make use of it. If there is a ranger station or park office, check in.

Review the Route Before embarking on any trail, be sure to read the entire description and study the map. It isn't necessary to memorize every detail, but it is worthwhile to have a clear mental picture of the trail and the general area.

If the trail and terrain are complex, augment the trail guide with a topographic map. Maps as well as current weather and trail condition information are often available from local ranger and park stations.

Check Before Going It's a good idea to check in with the local ranger or land management agency to determine the status of the trail and the roads to the trailhead, particularly just after the winter storm season. Roads and trails may be washed out by floods, or covered in late-season snow.

Prepare and Plan

- Know your abilities and limitations
- Leave word about your plans
- Know your route and the area

Carry the Essentials

Proper preparation for any type of trail use includes gathering certain essential items to carry. Trip checklists will vary tremendously by trail and conditions.

Clothing When the weather is good, light, comfortable clothing is the obvious choice. It's easy to believe that very little spare clothing is needed, but a prepared hiker has something tucked away for any emergency from a surprise shower to an unexpected overnight in a remote area.

Clothing includes proper footwear, essential for hiking and running trails. As a trail becomes more demanding, you will need footwear that performs. Running shoes are fine for many trails. If you will be carrying substantial weight or encountering sustained rugged terrain, step up to hiking boots.

In hot, sunny weather, proper clothing includes a hat, sunglasses, long-sleeved shirt and sunscreen. In cooler weather, particularly when it's wet, carry waterproof outer garments and quick-drying undergarments (avoid cotton). As general rule, whatever the conditions, bring layers that can be combined or removed to provide comfort and protection from the elements in a wide variety of conditions.

Also, long pants and long-sleeved shirts are useful against poison oak, ticks, and mosquitoes (see Pests and Hazards, on page 11).

Water Never embark on a trail without carrying water. At all times, particularly in warm weather, adequate water is of key importance. Experts recommend at least 2 quarts of water per day, and when hiking in heat a gallon or more may be more appropriate. At the extreme, dehydration can be life threatening. More commonly, inadequate water brings fatigue and muscle aches.

For most outings, unless the day is very hot or the trail very long, you should plan to carry sufficient water for the entire trail. Unfortunately, natural water sources in the three regions featured in *Top Trails Sacramento* are questionable, and may be polluted with bacteria, viruses, and even heavy metals from old mines.

Water Treatment If it's necessary to make use of trailside water, you should filter or treat it. There are three methods for treating water: boiling, chemical treatment, and filtering. Boiling is best, but often impractical—it requires a heat source, a pot, and time. Chemical treatments, available in sporting goods stores, handle some problems, including the troublesome Giardia parasite, but will not combat many human-made chemical pollutants. The preferred method is filtration, which removes Giardia and other contaminants and doesn't leave any unpleasant aftertaste.

If this hasn't convinced you to carry all the water you need, one final admonishment: be prepared for surprises. Water sources described in the text or on maps can change course or dry up completely. Never run your water bottle dry in expectation of the next source; fill up when water is available and always keep a little in reserve.

Food

While not as critical as water, food is energy and its importance shouldn't be underestimated. Avoid foods that are hard to digest, such as candy bars and potato chips. Carry high energy, fast-digesting foods: nutrition bars, dehydrated fruit, gorp, jerky. Bring a little extra food—it's good protection against an outing that turns unexpectedly long, perhaps due to weather or losing your way.

Pests and Hazards As much as we like to think of the outdoors as our home, it can surprise us with some annoying pests like poison oak, ticks, mosquitoes, and rattlesnakes.

Many of the trails in chapters 1 and 2 below 4000 feet in elevation may support thickets of trailside poison oak. People susceptible to poison oak should wear long pants and long-sleeved shirts to avoid poison oak rash.

If you suspect that poison oak has touched your skin, rinse off in a nearby stream or lake and be sure to shower as soon as you get home. Consult your doctor about medications to avoid and treat poison oak rash.

Lower-elevation trails may also have ticks lurking in the trailside vegetation. As a precaution against Lyme disease, which is spread by ticks, it is a good idea to avoid getting a tick bite by wearing long pants and a long-sleeved shirt. Tuck your pant legs into your boots. Check your appendages frequently for ticks. Wear light-colored clothing to spot ticks more easily. If you are bitten by a tick, clutch it firmly between two fingers and pull it out. Even though most ticks are not disease carriers, it is best to save the tick in a bag or film canister. If your tick bite becomes inflamed, acquires a suspicious bulls-eye-like ring around it, or if you come down soon after the bite with flu-like symptoms, consult you doctor immediately and be sure to bring the tick for identification. The long-term affects of Lyme disease can be both permanent and debilitating. Better safe than sorry!

Depending on the time of the year, all three regions featured in *Top Trails Sacramento* may host mosquitoes. In the valley, mosquitoes may, in rare instances, carry encephalitis or the West Nile virus. But typically, you simply have to be concerned about the obnoxious itching bite of these pests. Again, long pants and long-sleeved shirts are a good first line of defense, along with mosquito repellant.

Rattlesnakes are common at elevations as high as 5000 feet. Despite these snakes' bad rap, rattlesnake bites are rare in California, and rattlers and other snakes perform an important ecosystem function by eating rats, mice, and other small mammals that would soon strip most of the vegetation from our outdoor areas if they were not kept in check. Snakes are cold-blooded and may be found in the middle of a trail or in other open spaces sunning themselves. Just be sure to look ahead as you walk along a trail and be alert for the telltale rattling. Also, be sure to look on the other side before stepping over or sitting on logs and rocks. Rattlesnakes want nothing more than to be left alone, so avoid harassing, following, or poking at a rattler.

Attacks by mountain lions and bears on humans are very rare in California. The smaller and usually non-aggressive California black bear is more of a threat to your camping food than to anything else. Although decades often go by in California without reports of mountain lion attacks on humans, there have been at least 12 attacks since 1992. The increase is probably due to more humans living and recreating in what was formerly mountain lion habitat. In 1994, a woman trail running alone late in the afternoon was killed by a mountain lion not far from the American Canyon Trail (Trail 25 in this book). Some mountain lion avoidance tips: Avoid hiking on trails at dawn or dusk (preferred mountain lion hunting periods) and avoid hiking alone. If accosted by a mountain lion, make yourself look big, wave your arms, yell and scream. Ironically, I have longed to glimpse but have never seen a mountain lion in my more than 30 years of hiking on hundreds of miles of trails in California.

Thunderstorm-derived lightning is a concern at higher elevations. Peaks, ridgetops, and tall trees may attract lightning strikes. It's best to get to lower elevations and avoid being the highest object in your area (like you are if you're standing in a meadow) during thunderstorms.

Trail Essentials

- Spare cold-weather clothing
- Plenty of water
- Adequate food (plus a little more).

Less than Essential, but Useful

Map & Compass (and the know-how to use them) Many trails don't require much navigation, meaning a map and compass aren't always as essential as water or food—but it can be a close call. If the trail is remote or infrequently visited, a map and compass should be considered necessities. As the budgets of federal and state land management agencies have declined, so have the frequency and reliability of trail signs, as well as maintenance of the trails themselves.

A hand-held GPS is also a useful trail companion, but is really no substitute for a map and compass; knowing your longitude and latitude is not much help without a map.

Cell Phone Most parts of the country, even remote destinations, have some level of cellular coverage, particularly peaks and ridgetops. In extreme circumstances, a cell phone can be a lifesaver. But don't depend on it; coverage is unpredictable and batteries fail. And be sure that the occasion warrants the phone call—a blister doesn't justify a call to search and rescue, nor should the cell phone be used for routine calls. Although you may enjoy calling your friend to brag about bagging a peak, the others sharing the peak-bagging experience may not enjoy the intrusion into what should be a real wilderness experience.

Gear Depending on the remoteness and rigor of the trail, there are many additional useful items to consider: pocketknife, flashlight, fire source (water-proof matches, lighter, or flint), and a first-aid kit. Always carry some toilet paper and a light plastic trowel in case there is a need to go in the woods. Bury your waste at least six inches deep and more than 300 feet away from all water sources. Also, bring extra plastic bags to carry your used toilet paper out for proper disposal. A hiking staff or walking poles may enhance your experience by reducing the load on your feet and legs. Small binoculars are useful for viewing and identifying wildlife.

Every member of your party should carry the appropriate essential items described above; groups often split up or get separated along the trail. Solo hikers should be even more disciplined about preparation, and carry more gear. Traveling solo is inherently more risky. This isn't meant to discourage solo travel, simply to emphasize the need for extra preparation.

Trail Etiquette

The overriding rule on the trail is "Leave No Trace." Interest in visiting natural areas continues to increase in North America, even as the quantity of unspoiled natural areas continues to shrink. These pressures make it ever more critical that we leave no trace.

Never Litter If you carried it in, it's easy enough to carry it out. Leave the trail in the same, if not better condition than you find it. Try picking up any litter you encounter and packing it out—it's a great feeling! Just one piece of garbage and you've made a difference.

Stay on the Trail Paths have been created, sometimes over many years, for many purposes: to protect the surrounding natural areas, to avoid dangers, and to provide the best route. Leaving the trail can cause damage that takes years to undo. Never cut switchbacks. Shortcutting rarely saves energy or time, and it takes a terrible toll on the land, trampling plant life and hastening erosion. Moreover, safety and consideration intersect on the trail. It's hard to get truly lost if you stay on the trail.

Share the Trail The best trails attract many visitors, and you should be prepared to share the trail with others. Do your part to minimize impact.

Many of the trails in this book are used by hikers, mountain bikers, and equestrians. Some of the non-wilderness trails are even open to motorized use. Commonly accepted trail etiquette dictates that motor vehicles and bike riders yield to both hikers and equestrians, hikers yield to horseback riders, downhill hikers yield to uphill hikers, and everyone stays to the right. Not everyone knows these rules of the road, so let common sense and good humor be the final guide.

Leave It There Destruction or removal of plants and animals, or historical, prehistoric or geological items, is certainly unethical and almost always illegal.

Follow Campfire Rules Many of the higher-elevation areas are off-limits to campfires due to high use and impacts on local vegetation from wood gathering. Lower-elevation areas may have seasonal campfire prohibitions during dry periods to reduce the chance of starting a wildfire. Check with the management agency before your outing for permanent and seasonal rules.

Trail Etiquette

- Leave no trace—Never litter
- Stay on the trail—Never cut switchbacks
- Share the trail—Use courtesy and common sense
- Leave it there—Don't disturb wildlife

Getting Lost If you become lost on the trail, stay on the trail. Stop and take stock of the situation. In many cases, a few minutes of calm reflection will yield a solution. Consider all the clues available; use the sun to identify directions if you don't have a compass. If you determine that you are indeed lost, stay on the main trail and stay put. You are more likely to encounter other people if you stay in one place.

CHAPTER 1

The Great Valley

1. Bobelaine Sanctuary Trails: Feather River
2. River Walk Trail: Cosumnes River Preserve
3. Deer Creek Hills Preserve Trails
4. Delta Meadows State Park and Historic Locke
5. Effie Yeaw Natural Area Loop Trail
6. Gibson Ranch Regional Park Loop Trail
7. Wetlands Discovery & Loop Trails: Gray Lodge Wildlife Area
8. Sutter Buttes Trails
9. Howard Ranch Trail
10. Jedediah Smith Memorial Trail Loop: American River Parkway
11. Lake Natoma Loop: Folsom Lake State Recreation Area
12. Sacramento Northern Bikeway
13. Sacramento Waterfront Loop
14. Wren Wetlands Trail: Stone Lakes National Wildlife Refuge

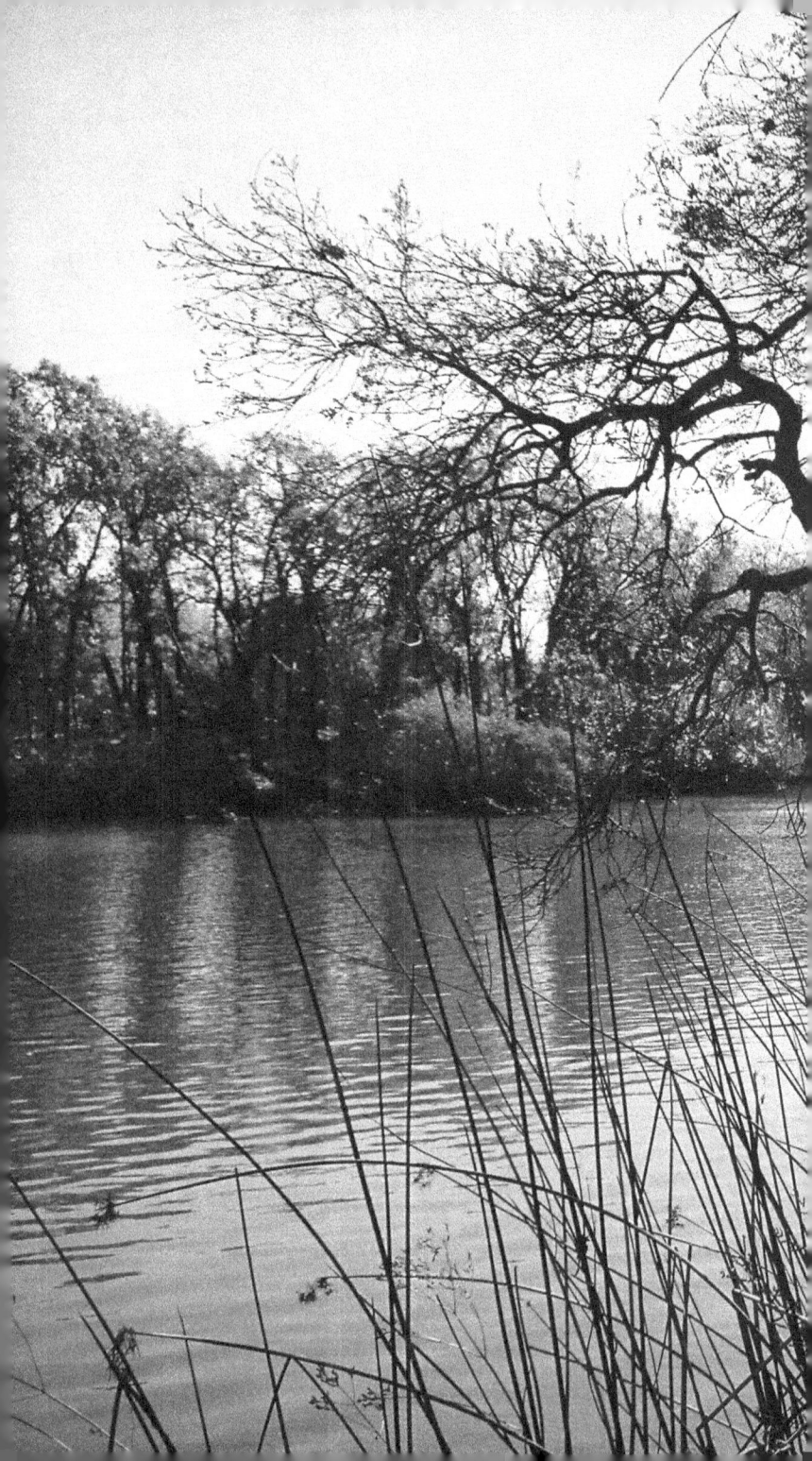

AREA OVERVIEW

The Great Valley

Much of the Great Valley has been urbanized or converted to agriculture. The trails featured in Chapter 1 visit some of the few natural grasslands, wetlands, and riparian forests still remaining in the valley that are accessible to the public. These few "islands" of natural habitat in a sea of urban and agricultural development are rich in wildlife and offer a glimpse of the valley as it was prior to European expansion.

Maps and Permits

USGS 7.5-minute quad maps best identify topography and physical features, but many of the public refuges, reserves, and trails featured in this chapter are relatively newly established and are not generally depicted on the older USGS maps. Fortunately, many of the refuges and reserves have developed specific maps available via the Internet. The sources for these maps are listed in the appendix, as well as the specific USGS quads for each trail.

Modest parking fees are charged at several of the refuges and reserves featured in this chapter. Because many of these areas were established to preserve wildlife and their habitat, dogs are prohibited or are required to be on leash.

Overleaf and opposite: *The Sacramento–San Joaquin Delta is one of the most fragile and endangered ecosystems in California (Trail 4).*

AREA MAP

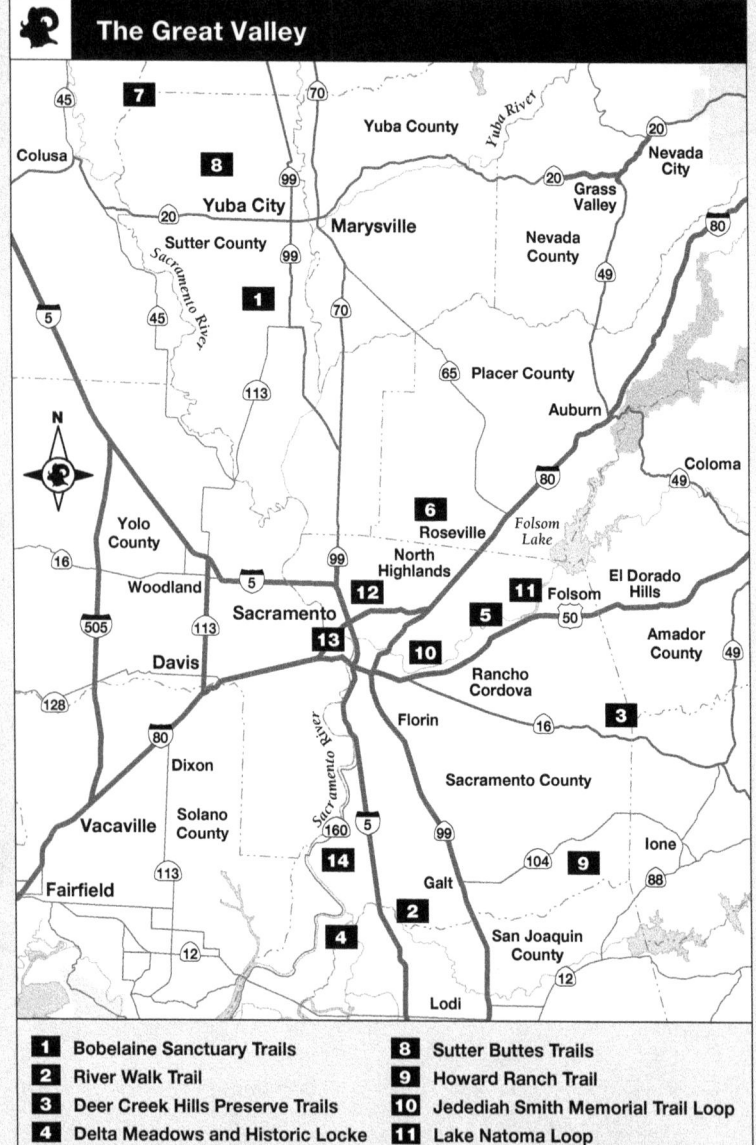

TRAIL FEATURE TABLE

The Great Valley

Trail	Difficulty	Length	Type	Uses & Access	Terrain	Flora & Fauna	Other
1	3	5.3	Loop	Hiking, Child Friendly	River/Stream, Lake, Wetland, Meadow	Birds, Wildlife	
2	2	3.0	Loop	Hiking, Child Friendly	River/Stream, Wetland, Meadow	Birds, Wildlife	Photo Opportunity
3	2/3	2.0–7.0	Variable	Hiking, Horses, Child Friendly, Fee	River/Stream, Wetland, Meadow	Wildflowers, Birds, Wildlife	Historic Interest, Geologic Interest, Great Views, Photo Opportunity
4	1	2.44	Point-to-Point	Hiking, Child Friendly, Dogs Allowed	River/Stream, Wetland, Meadow	Birds, Wildlife	Historic Interest, Photo Opportunity
5	1	1.0	Loop	Hiking, Child Friendly, Fee	River/Stream, Wetland, Meadow	Birds, Wildlife	Historic Interest, Photo Opportunity
6	2	2.86	Loop	Hiking, Horses, Running, Child Friendly, Fee, Dogs Allowed	River/Stream, Lake, Wetland, Meadow	Wildflowers, Birds, Wildlife	
7	1/2	.83/2.64	Loop	Hiking, Child Friendly, Handicap Access, Fee, Dogs Allowed	Wetland	Birds, Wildlife	Great Views
8	2–4	3.0–8.0	Variable	Hiking, Child Friendly, Fee	Meadow, Canyon, Mountain	Wildflowers, Birds, Wildlife	Historic Interest, Geologic Interest, Great Views, Steep, Photo Opportunity
9	4	6.83	Loop	Hiking, Child Friendly, Fee	Lake, Wetland, Meadow, Canyon	Wildflowers, Birds, Wildlife	Great Views, Photo Opportunity
10	3	4.2	Loop	Hiking, Running, Biking, Child Friendly, Handicap Access, Dogs Allowed, Fee	River/Stream	Birds, Wildlife	Historic Interest, Great Views, Photo Opportunity
11	4	10.3	Loop	Hiking, Horses, Running, Biking, Child Friendly, Handicap Access, Fee, Dogs Allowed	River/Stream, Lake, Wetland	Birds, Wildlife	Historic Interest, Great Views, Photo Opportunity
12	4	10.0	Variable	Hiking, Running, Biking, Child Friendly, Handicap Access	River/Stream, Wetland, Meadow	Wildflowers, Birds, Wildlife	Historic Interest
13	2	3.5	Variable	Hiking, Running, Biking, Child Friendly, Handicap Access, Dogs Allowed	River/Stream	Birds	Historic Interest, Great Views, Photo Opportunity
14	2	3.68	Point-to-Point	Hiking, Child Friendly	River/Stream, Wetland, Meadow	Birds, Wildlife	

Legend

USES & ACCESS: Hiking, Horses, Running, Biking, Child Friendly, Handicap Access, Fee ($), Permit Required, Dogs Allowed

TYPE: Loop, Out & Back, Point-to-Point, Variable (V)

DIFFICULTY: −1 2 3 4 5+ (less ↔ more)

TERRAIN: River or Stream, Waterfall, Lake, Wetland, Meadow, Canyon, Mountain

FLORA & FAUNA: Wildflowers, Fall Colors, Birds, Wildlife

FEATURES: Historic Interest, Geologic Interest, Great Views, Steep, Secluded, Camping, Photo Opportunity

TRAIL SUMMARIES

The Great Valley

TRAIL 1
Hike
5.3 miles, Loops
Difficulty: 1 2 **3** 4 5

Bobelaine Sanctuary Trails:
Feather River 29
The extensive loop trail system in this privately owned sanctuary provides a rare opportunity to explore the Great Valley's jungle-like riparian habitat. Be sure to bring a bird identification book and binoculars. The virtually flat loop trails provide a variety of length options and visit the banks of the Feather River and Lake Crandall—an oxbow lake that was formerly the bed of the river.

TRAIL 2
Hike
3.0 miles, Loop
Difficulty: 1 **2** 3 4 5

River Walk Trail:
Cosumnes River Preserve 35
There is no better place to get just a glimpse of the predevelopment Great Valley than at the Cosumnes River Preserve. The River Walk Trail visits wildlife-rich wetlands, a slough, the banks of the Cosumnes River, riparian forests and oak woodlands, and a large, grassy meadow. An interpretive brochure corresponds to numbered posts along the trail. Depending on the season, rare sandhill cranes and other waterfowl may be observed.

Deer Creek Hills Preserve Trails 41
Saved from urban development, the Deer Creek Hills Preserve provides rare public access to where the Great Valley and the Sierra foothills meet, east of Sacramento. Access is currently limited to a variety of docent-led hikes on the fourth weekend of January–May, and a modest fee is charged. The docents share a wealth of natural and cultural history of the area, which features oak woodlands, valley grasslands, Deer and Crevis creeks, and one of the better spring wildflower displays in the region.

TRAIL 3

Hike, Horses
2.0–7.0 miles, Loops
Difficulty: 1 2 **3** 4 5

Delta Meadows State Park and Historic Locke 47
Delta Meadows is a great destination for a scenic drive through the hydrological heart of the Great Valley. This undeveloped State Park provides rare public access to the Sacramento–San Joaquin Delta. It features a walk along a levee paralleling a scenic slough and its riparian forest on one side, and open meadows and woodlands on the other. A short side trip visits the historic Chinese town of Locke.

TRAIL 4

Hike
2.5 miles, Out & Back
Difficulty: **1** 2 3 4 5

Effie Yeaw Natural Area Loop Trail ... 53
A perfect walk for families with children, the Effie Yeaw Natural Area features abundant wildlife, a rich riparian forest, and oak woodlands (through which wander a flock of wild turkeys), a large meadow (often filled with grazing deer), wetlands, a visit to the banks of the American River, and an extensive system of informative interpretive signs. A bonus is the adjacent Effie Yeaw Nature Center, with its wildlife, nature, and cultural exhibits.

TRAIL 5

Hike
1.0 mile, Loop
Difficulty: **1** 2 3 4 5

TRAIL 6

Hike
2.9 miles, Loop
Difficulty: 1 **2** 3 4 5

Gibson Ranch Regional Park Loop Trail 59

The Gibson Ranch Regional Park preserves a slice of Sacramento County's agrarian heritage. This easy loop trail features a segment of the as yet incomplete Dry Creek Parkway, livestock pastures (feel free to pat the noses of horses and other friendly livestock), wetlands, and a nice view of the nearby Sierra Nevada. Gibson Lake provides fishing and family picnicking.

TRAIL 7

Hike
3.5 miles, Loops
Difficulty: 1 **2** 3 4 5

Wetlands Discovery & Loop Trails: Gray Lodge Wildlife Area 65

More waterfowl visit the Gray Lodge Wildlife Area than any other region of the Pacific Flyway. During the fall and early winter, visitors may observe hundreds of thousands of geese and ducks, and enjoy a stunning view of the nearby Sutter Buttes. Various blinds, platforms, and hides along the way enhance the viewing experience. The Wetlands Discovery Trail is paved, is accessible to the handicapped, and has an interpretive brochure.

TRAIL 8

Hike
2.0–8.0 miles,
Loops, Out & Back
Difficulty: 1 **2 3 4** 5

Sutter Buttes Trails 73

Rising dramatically out of the Great Valley floor, the volcanic Sutter Buttes are largely privately owned. The nonprofit Middle Mountain Foundation works with the private landowners and offers docent-led hikes to this tiny mountain range (reputed to be the smallest in the United States) for a fee. A wide variety of hikes, ranging from easy to difficult, explore the Butte's scenic valleys, ridges, and mountaintops.

Howard Ranch Trail 79
Vernal pools seasonally spangled with wildflowers are the primary feature of this hike. It also offers one of the few opportunities to walk in the Great Valley's formerly extensive grasslands. Hikers will enjoy tantalizing views of the nearby Sierra foothills and scenic Rancho Seco Lake. Bring your wildflower identification book and a hand lens so you can get up close and personal with the flower display.

TRAIL 9

Hike
6.8 miles, Loop
Difficulty: 1 2 3 **4** 5

Jedediah Smith Memorial Trail Loop: American River Parkway 85
Here's an opportunity to enjoy a section of the 37-mile-long Jedediah Smith Memorial Trail in the American River Parkway. This paved loop, which spans the American River between the Watt Ave. Bridge and the Guy West Bridge, makes its way through rich riparian forest on the north side of the river and open oak woodlands on the south side. The south side also offers an equestrian trail option and visits the former site of one of the largest Indian villages on the river.

TRAIL 10

Hike, Run, Bike, Horse
4.2 miles, Loop
Difficulty: 1 2 **3** 4 5

Lake Natoma Loop: Folsom Lake State Recreation Area 91
Pretty Lake Natoma is the feature of this entirely paved loop trail. Wooded bluffs on each side provide a scenic backdrop to the lake, waterfowl are abundant along the lake edge, and trailside interpretive signs provide insights into the natural and cultural history of the area. This trail is accessible from Sacramento's light rail system, so you can leave your car behind.

TRAIL 11

Hike, Run, Bike, Horse
10.3 miles, Loop
Difficulty: 1 2 3 **4** 5

TRAIL 12

Hike, Run, Bike
10 miles, Point to Point
or Out & Back
Difficulty: 1 2 3 **4** 5

Sacramento Northern Bikeway 99

This bikeway connects downtown Sacramento with the semirural community of Elverta to the north. It follows the route of the historic Sacramento Northern Railroad and winds its way through the heart of several northern Sacramento neighborhoods and communities, including Norada, Del Paso Heights, Robla, Rio Linda, and Elverta. The Bikeway also provides access to portions of the American River and Dry Creek Parkways, as it follows its own linear park all the way to Elverta.

TRAIL 13

Hike, Run, Bike
3.4 miles, Loop
Difficulty: 1 **2** 3 4 5

Sacramento Waterfront Loop 107

Enjoy the historic Old Sacramento waterfront, three riverside parks, and two historic bridges on this urban walk that follows paved paths and boardwalks around and parallel to the Sacramento River. The loop features West Sacramento's new River Walk between the Tower and I St. bridges, as well as an out-and-back side trip to Sacramento's architecturally unique water intake structure and to Discovery Park at the confluence of the American and Sacramento rivers. Top the walk off with visits to the State Railroad Museum and other tourist attractions in Old Sacramento.

Wren Wetlands Trail: Stone Lakes National Wildlife Refuge 115

Open on the second and fourth Saturday of the month (except July–August), this trail provides the only public access to one of the most recently established national wildlife refuges. Stone Lakes is a rich mosaic of lakes, sloughs, wetlands, riparian woodlands, and grasslands. Bring your bird book and binoculars so your family can enjoy the seasonal visitations of rare sandhill cranes, white pelicans, Canada geese, and other waterfowl.

TRAIL 14

Hike
3.7 miles, Out & Back
Difficulty: 1 **2** 3 4 5

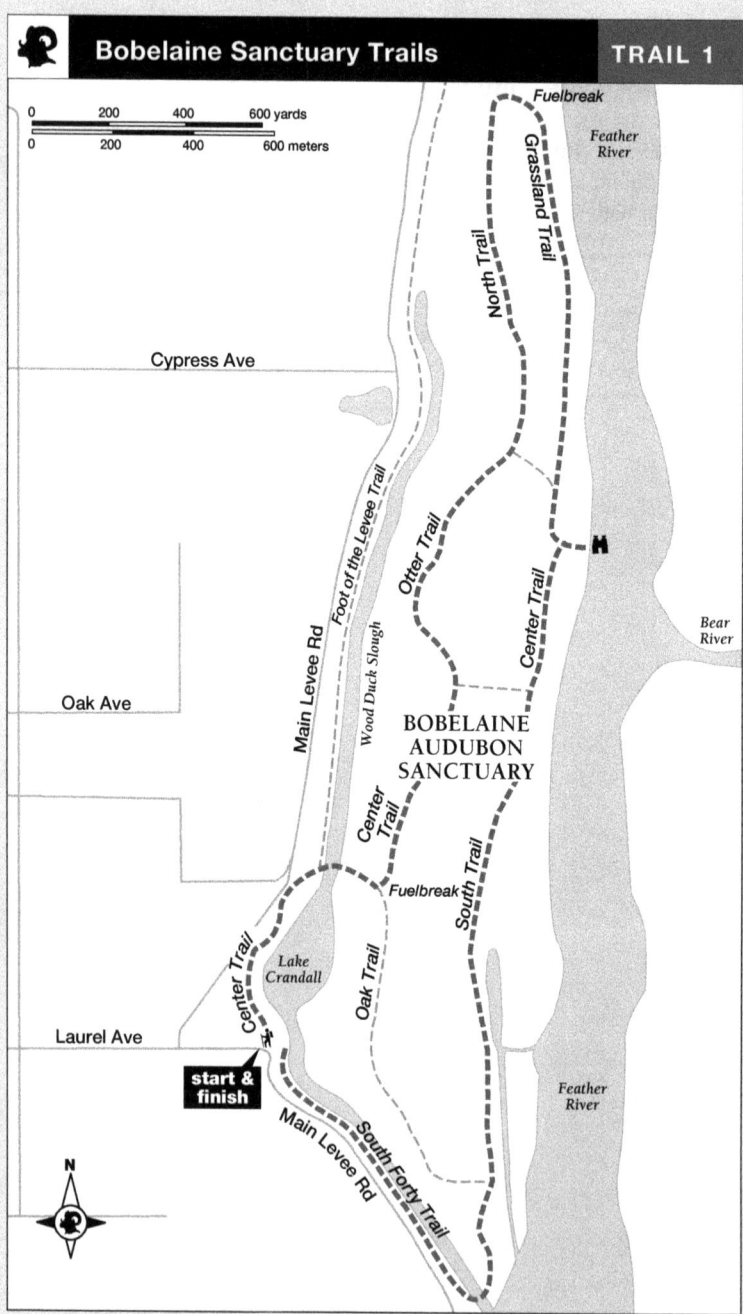

TRAIL 1 The Great Valley

Bobelaine Sanctuary Trails: Feather River

The Bobelaine Audubon Sanctuary on the Feather River provides a unique opportunity to explore the Central Valley's jungle-like riparian habitat. Maintained by the Sacramento Audubon Society, the 430–acre sanctuary has an extensive loop-trail system kept cleared by mowers so bird-watchers and hikers can make their way through the usually impenetrable forest to observe and appreciate the rich variety of wildlife that depends on this riverside habitat.

Best Time

Because the sanctuary is within the Feather River levee system, it may be flooded in the winter and spring. Summer days can be quite hot. Dawn, early morning hours, and dusk are the best times to observe birds and other wildlife.

Finding the Trail

From Sacramento, drive 8.3 miles north on Interstate 5 to the Hwy 70/99 exit. Drive north on highways 70/99 for 12.8 miles to the Hwy 99 interchange. Drive north 4.0 miles on Hwy 99, cross the Feather River, and continue north approximately 2.6 miles to Laurel Ave. Turn right onto Laurel Ave. and drive east about 0.8 mile to where it dead-ends at the Bobelaine Sanctuary parking lot.

TRAIL USE
Hike
LENGTH
5.3 miles, 2–3 hours
VERTICAL FEET
Minimal
DIFFICULTY
- 1 2 **3** 4 5 +
TRAIL TYPE
Loops (many options)
SURFACE TYPE
Dirt

FEATURES
Child Friendly
River
Meadow
Lake
Wetlands
Birds
Wildlife

FACILITIES
Porta-potty

Logistics

More than 144 species of birds, 39 mammals, and 126 plant species have been identified at the Bobelaine Sanctuary.

Be sure to bring binoculars and a bird book. Log onto the Bobelaine Sanctuary website at www.sacramentoaudubon.org/boblaine.htm for the latest visitor information. Also, consider sending a donation to the Sacramento Audubon Society for the management and protection of this important but privately maintained wildlife and habitat sanctuary.

Trail Description

From the Sanctuary parking lot, walk up the levee and proceed north. ▶1 On the river side of the levee, you will see **Lake Crandall**, an oxbow lake that was formerly the Feather River channel, until the river meandered eastward and left the lake unconnected with the river except during floods. River meander is an important ecological mechanism for the renewal of riparian habitat.

 Lake

Approximately 89 percent of the Great Valley's former riparian habitat has been lost to agricultural clearing, river channelization, and development. The remaining habitat provides homes to a wide variety of rare and endangered species, including the yellow-billed cuckoo, the valley elderberry longhorn beetle, and the bank swallow.

Follow the top of the levee northward until a road drops down off the levee on the right. ▶2 Drop down off the levee to the Center Trailhead, marked by a gate. Walk around the gate and proceed east through the riparian forest, past the unsigned junction with the Oak Trail on the right. At the beginning of a large fuel break in front of you, the Center Trail veers left (northward). Largely a mowed access road through riparian jungle, the trail makes its way past large cottonwood and sycamore trees, box elders, native grapevines, and blackberry brambles.

The Center Trail reaches the junction with the Otter Trail, which is heralded by a sign. ▶3 Turn left

Bobelaine Sanctuary Trails | TRAIL 1

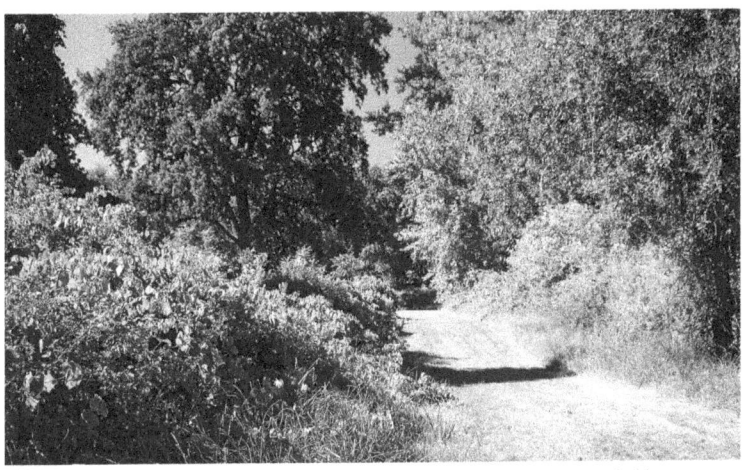

The cleared trails in the Bobelaine Sanctuary *provide access to the jungle-like riparian forest and excellent opportunities to view birds and other wildlife.*

and continue heading north on the much more trail-like Otter Trail, which follows a natural bench that is higher up from the river and supports less flood-resistant trees such as valley oaks, with a sprinkling of cottonwoods and sycamores. Occasionally, the trail breaks out into open areas ringed by cottonwood snags, possibly indicative of past fires. The habitat "edge" effect created by the transition from forest to open areas is one of the reasons that riparian habitat is so rich and supports so many species.

The Otter Trail ends at the unsigned junction with the North Trail, which connects from the right. Continue straight on the North Trail. ▶4 As the trail approaches the northern boundary of the sanctuary, the forest begins to thin out into patchy grassland.

At the northern boundary of the Sanctuary, the North Trail bends right and connects with the Grasslands Trail. ▶5 Go right on the Grasslands Trail and proceed southward through open meadows broken by occasional groves of cottonwoods and box elders. The **Feather River** soon comes into view on the left.

⸺ Meadow

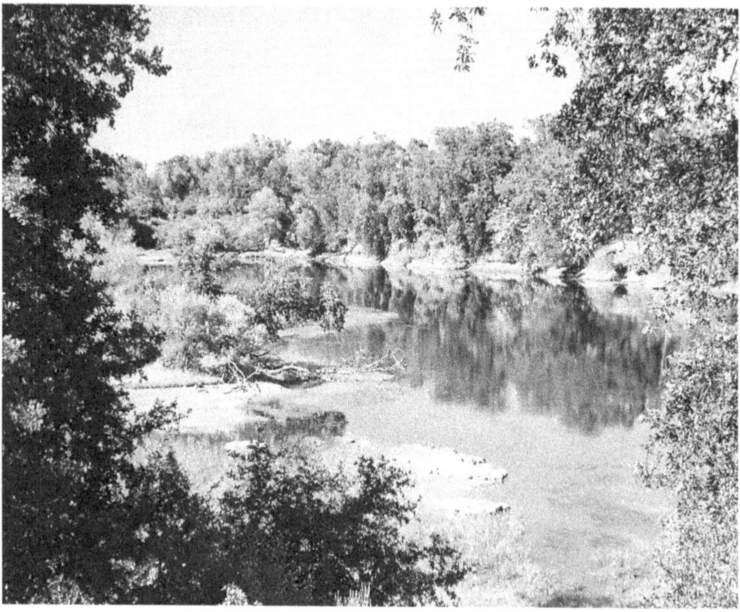

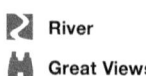

Lake Crandall in the Bobelaine Sanctuary is a former bend of the Feather River.

River

Great Views

The Grasslands Trail dead-ends at the North Trail. ▶6 Veer left at the sign and proceed a short distance to a clearing and the junction with the Center Trail. Turn left and walk a short way east to the **river overlook** on the bank of the Feather River. This is a good spot to stop for lunch and watch the river flow by. After enjoying the view, return to the North and Center trails junction and turn left. ▶7 The trail begins to leave the grasslands area behind, and reenters thick riparian forest.

The Center Trail reaches the junction with the South Trail. ▶8 For a shorter walk, simply continue straight ahead on the Center Trail back to the levee. For a longer walk, turn left on the South Trail and continue southward. The South Trail crosses a fuel break and continues south over a series of shallow drainages. ▶9 In this low part of the sanctuary, flooding occurs often, and the vegetation is quite

Bobelaine Sanctuary Trails | TRAIL 1

water tolerant. After dropping in and climbing out of the deep Sycamore Swale, the South Trail comes to its signed junction with the Oak Trail on the right. Continue on the South Trail, which soon crosses the even deeper Ringtail Bypass (which may retain water). This is the former Feather River bed extending downstream from Lake Crandall. If the channel is flooded, turn around and proceed back to the Center Trail.

If it isn't flooded, cross the channel and you will come to the junction with the South Forty Trail. ▶10 Turn right on this trail to proceed northwest along the slough draining Lake Crandall and along the foot of the Feather River levee on your left. ▶11 Follow the South Forty Trail to its junction with the Center Trail, at the foot of the levee from the Center Trailhead. Turn left, climb the levee and turn left again ▶12 to follow the levee back to the ▶13 Sanctuary parking area.

MILESTONES

- ▶1 0.00 From parking lot, walk up levee and proceed north
- ▶2 0.30 Drop down off levee to the Center Trailhead on the right
- ▶3 0.50 Otter Trail junction, turn left
- ▶4 1.10 North Trail junction, continue straight
- ▶5 1.85 Grassland Trail junction, turn right
- ▶6 2.60 North Trail Junction, turn left
- ▶7 2.80 River Overlook, retrace steps to North/Center junction, turn left
- ▶8 3.50 South Trail junction, turn left
- ▶9 3.75 Cross fuel break
- ▶10 4.25 Oak Trail junction, continue straight on South Trail
- ▶11 4.45 South Forty Trail junction, turn right
- ▶12 4.95 Return to Center Trail trailhead, climb levee, turn left, return to lot
- ▶13 5.30 Sanctuary parking lot

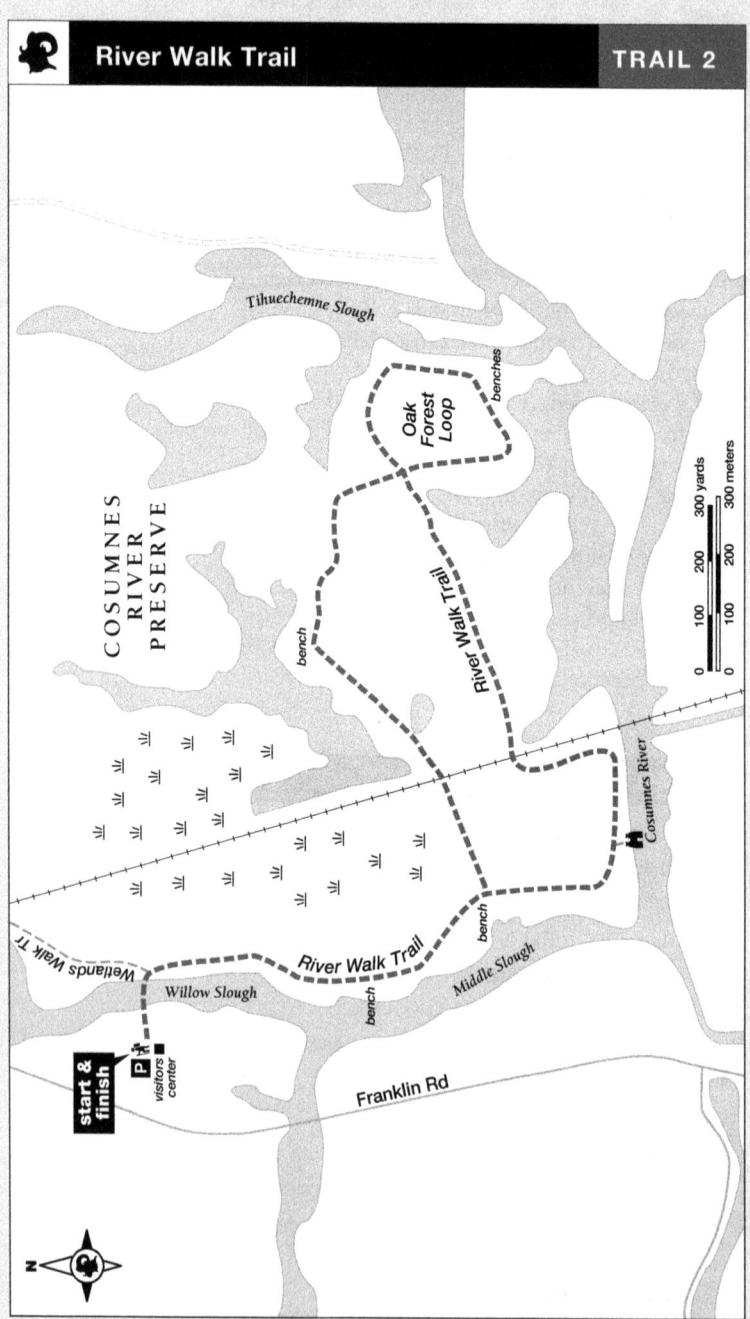

TRAIL 2 The Great Valley

River Walk Trail: Cosumnes River Preserve

The Cosumnes River is one of the few undammed rivers flowing from the Sierra Nevada into the Great Valley. Because its floodplain has been less developed than other valley rivers, the Cosumnes River Preserve provides an important opportunity for naturalists and scientists, as well as the general public, to study and enjoy the Great Valley as it once was. The River Walk Trail visits two rare Great Valley plant communities—riparian forest and freshwater marsh. These highly productive and rich habitats support more than 200 species of birds, including greater sandhill cranes and numerous other waterfowl. Birding and viewing wildlife are particular treats along the River Walk Trail. The preserve currently encompasses about 46,000 acres and is jointly owned and managed by The Nature Conservancy, Bureau of Land Management (BLM), Ducks Unlimited, California Department of Fish and Game, and other agencies.

Best Time

Much of the preserve may be flooded in the late winter and early spring. Summer afternoons can be quite hot. Dawn and dusk are the best times to observe birds and other wildlife. Later in the fall, from October on, is the best time to see and hear sandhill cranes and other waterfowl.

Finding the Trail

From Sacramento drive 19 miles south on Interstate 5 and take the Twin Cities Road exit. Turn left (east)

TRAIL USE
Hike
LENGTH
3.0 miles, 1–2 hours
VERTICAL FEET
±0
DIFFICULTY
- 1 **2** 3 4 5 +
TRAIL TYPE
Loop
SURFACE TYPE
Dirt

FEATURES
Child Friendly
Meadow
Wetlands
River
Birds
Wildlife
Photo Opportunity
Interpretive Signs

FACILITIES
Vault Toilets
No Water

Look for Swainson's hawks hunting for field mice and other small critters in the savanna.

over the I-5 overpass and drive 1.0 mile east to Franklin Road. Turn right on Franklin Road and drive 1.7 miles south to the Cosumnes Preserve visitors center. Park in the visitors center parking lot on the left.

Logistics

Much of the preserve may be flooded in the late winter and early spring. Call the preserve to check on flood conditions. This is an excellent birding area, so be sure to bring binoculars and a bird book. For more information about preserve access and scheduled activities, call the recorded information line at (916) 684-2816. For more detailed information about the preserve, visit www.cosumnes.org.

Trail Description

Park in the visitors center parking lot on Franklin road. ▶1 At dusk in the late fall, it is common to see and hear rare sandhill cranes in the wetlands directly west of the parking lot. Drop by the visitors center and pick up the River Walk brochure, which has interpretive notes corresponding to 14 numbered posts along the trail. Feel free to provide a donation to the preserve to support its restoration and education programs. The **River Walk Trail** begins just north of the visitors center. Go down a wheelchair accessible wood ramp and follow a boardwalk briefly north and then east. The trail crosses **Willow Slough** over a steel pedestrian bridge. An interpretive sign notes that the slough provides important habitat to juvenile salmon during high flows.

 Birds

After crossing the bridge, the trail comes to a **T** junction. The paved Wetlands Walk Trail heads off to the left. Turn right to follow the dirt River Walk Trail south. ▶2 The trail is on a low berm that parallels Willow Slough on the right and a freshwater

River Walk Trail | TRAIL 2

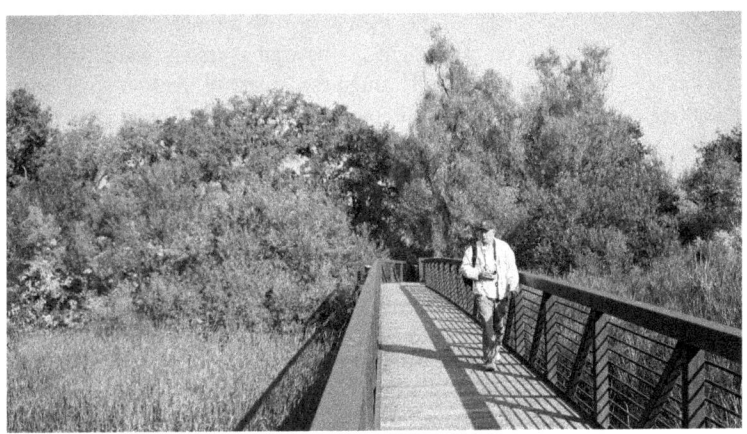

Bridge crossing slough *near the Cosumnes Preserve visitors center*

marsh filled with tules and cattails on the left. The route is well shaded by valley and scrub oaks, willows, buttonbush, and an occasional cottonwood.

The trail passes a maintenance road (closed to the public) on the left and a pump station on the right. Beyond this point, Willow Slough flows into the much wider **Middle Slough**, and the view opens up on the right to open water. This well-watered area is haunted by egrets and chittering kingfishers and surrounded by riparian forest. The trail continues along the berm, briefly losing its shading and then reentering the forest as it passes a bench and continues southward. As the riparian forest thickens, the trail turns east briefly and then south to cross a wood bridge over an unnamed slough.

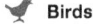 Birds

After crossing the bridge, the trail reaches another bench and a **Y** junction. The trail coming in from the left is your return route on the River Walk Loop. Continue straight ahead up a couple of wooden steps set in the earth ▶3 as the trail continues southward through a tunnel of overhanging oaks and cottonwoods. The trail soon breaks out to the edge of an open restoration area, where young oaks have been planted. Your route follows the

> **River**

edge of the open area, with a much older oak forest on your right as the trail veers eastward past two benches. Through the gallery of trees on your right, you will glimpse the **Cosumnes River**. ▶4 A short spur trail leads south a short distance through the forest to the river bank.

Now heading east, the River Walk Trail approaches a railroad track that crosses the Cosumnes River on a picturesque steel girder bridge. The trail reaches the railroad track and then turns left (north) to follow the track as it crosses the open area dotted with young oaks on a series of concrete trestles. The trail meets an access road running parallel to the track; a sign points the way east as the trail turns right ▶5 to go under the trestle.

> **Meadow**

On the east side of the trestle, the River Walk Trail enters a large, open grassland dotted with trees—a true oak savanna. The trail continues east along the edge of the savanna and the riparian forest just north of the river.

The trail comes to a four-way junction. ▶6 This is the Oak Forest Loop section of the River Walk Trail. Turn right as the trail reenters the oak and cottonwood forest, angles right to take you to the edge of the Cosumnes River, and then veers left (east) to parallel the river. The trail passes a ring of benches overlooking a placid section of the river and then bends left (north) where the river meets **Tihuechemne Slough**. As the trail veers north and then northwestward, it begins to follow the top of a low berm as it makes its way through the oak woodland. Soon you return to the four-way junction marking the end of the Oak Forest Loop, ▶7 turn right to continue on the River Walk Trail.

> **River**

The River Walk Trail leaves the oak woodland behind as it crosses the open savanna heading for a row of six large oaks in the middle of the grassland. The trail crosses a maintenance road closed to the public, crosses through the solitary line of oaks, and continues northwestward through the savanna. The trail crosses another maintenance road and continues straight to the edge of the savanna, marked by a willow-lined marsh. A large valley oak with spreading branches shades a bench at this spot, inviting hikers to sit a spell and listen for meadowlarks.

From the large valley oak, the trail turns sharply left and follows the savanna/riparian edge to the southwest. It approaches and then crosses under the concrete railroad trestle and then continues in a westerly direction. After crossing another maintenance road, the trail reenters the riparian forest as it approaches Middle Slough. Young cottonwoods along this section of the trail bear the characteristic gnaw marks of beaver.

 Wildlife

The trail returns to the River Walk Loop **T** junction, marked by a bench and the steps on the left. ▶8 Turn right to retrace your steps to the junction with the paved Wetlands Walk Trail. ▶9 Turn left and cross the bridge to return ▶10 to the visitors center parking lot.

MILESTONES

- ▶1   0.00   River Walk trailhead at the Preserve visitors center
- ▶2   0.15   Wetlands Walk Trail junction, turn right
- ▶3   0.53   River Walk Loop Trail junction, continue straight
- ▶4   0.66   Cosumnes River, continue on trail
- ▶5   0.90   Causeway road junction, turn right and go under trestle
- ▶6   1.20   Four-way junction, turn right to walk Oak Forest Loop
- ▶7   1.66   Back to four-way junction, turn right to continue River Walk Loop
- ▶8   2.40   Back to River Walk Loop junction, turn right
- ▶9   2.85   Back to Wetlands Walk Trail junction, turn left
- ▶10 3.00   Retrace steps to River Walk trailhead and visitors center

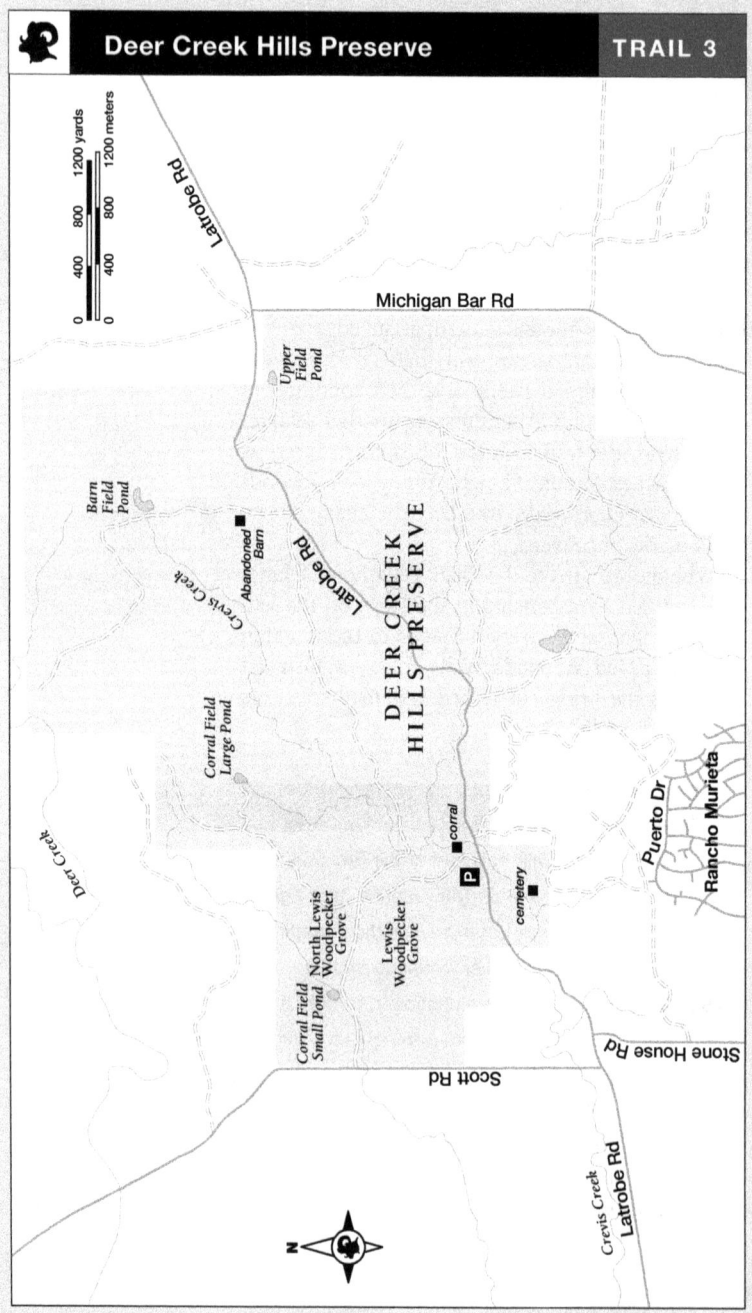

TRAIL 3 The Great Valley

Deer Creek Hills Preserve Trails

Without the vigilance and vision of the Sacramento Valley Conservancy and other conservationists, the Deer Creek Hills would have been just another exclusive enclave of McMansions that have leap-frogged over the eastern Sacramento suburbs into the lower Sierra Nevada foothills. But public concerns about leapfrog development, increased traffic on rural roads, and loss of open space in Sacramento County resulted in the establishment of the Deer Creek Hills Preserve. The Great Valley and the Sierra Nevada literally meet at this beautiful open space preserve. Its low rolling hills and shallow canyons are clothed in blue oak and live oak woodlands and open meadows and grasslands that put on fine spring wildflower displays. Public hikes ranging from 2–7 miles in length are led by Conservancy docents the fourth weekend of every month from January through May. Adoption of a management plan for the preserve in 2007 will eventually lead to the establishment of a permanent natural and cultural history trail that will be accessible to visitors on a daily basis. But for now, visitors need to make reservations for the monthly scheduled hike and pay a modest $10 fee to explore this beautiful area—not too high a price to pay to preserve and enjoy our region's rapidly disappearing open spaces.

Best Time

Spring is the ideal time to visit, with the hills clothed in green grass and wildflowers, and the blue oaks freshly leafed out.

TRAIL USE
Hike, Horse
(scheduled outings only)
LENGTH
2.0–7.0 miles,
up to 4 hours
VERTICAL FEET
±200
DIFFICULTY
- 1 **2 3** 4 5 +
(depending on specific hike taken)
TRAIL TYPE
Various
SURFACE TYPE
Dirt

FEATURES
Child Friendly
Streams
Meadows
Wetlands
Wildflowers
Birds
Wildlife
Historic values
Geologic Interest
Great Views
Photo Opportunity

FACILITIES
Porta-potties

Raptors floating on the thermals above the preserve are common, along with the song of the meadowlark in the open grasslands or the chatter of the acorn woodpecker in the oak woodlands.

Finding the Trail

The Deer Creek Hills Preserve is located off of Latrobe Road to the north of Rancho Murrieta and Hwy 16.

Logistics

The Sacramento Valley Conservancy organizes hikes on the fourth weekend of the month, from January–May. Visit www.sacramentovalleyconservancy.org to view the current schedule of hikes, or contact them via email at kelly_sacvalleyconservancy.com, or by phone at (530) 400-5922. Depending on the availability of docents, a couple of different hikes are typically available on the fourth Saturday, ranging from 2.0 to 7.0 miles and up to four hours in length. The outings usually focus on a natural value of the area, such as wildflowers, birds, geology, or natural history. Also, typically the fourth Sundays are reserved for equestrian rides (bring your own horse) of up to 10 miles. There are also opportunities to reserve special tours, group picnics and even overnight camping, as well as participate in service trips and docent training. Once you have made your hike reservation and paid your fee, the Conservancy will send you information about when and where to meet for the scheduled hike.

Trail Description

Since public use of the Deer Creek Hills Preserve is currently restricted to only scheduled docent-led outings, this more general narrative replaces the usual milestone-based hike description.

The Deer Creek Hills Preserve consists of 4000 acres of low-elevation Sierra Nevada foothills on the edge of the Sacramento Valley. **Deer Creek**, a large perennial stream, generally forms the preserve's northern boundary. The preserve is cut by

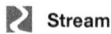 Stream

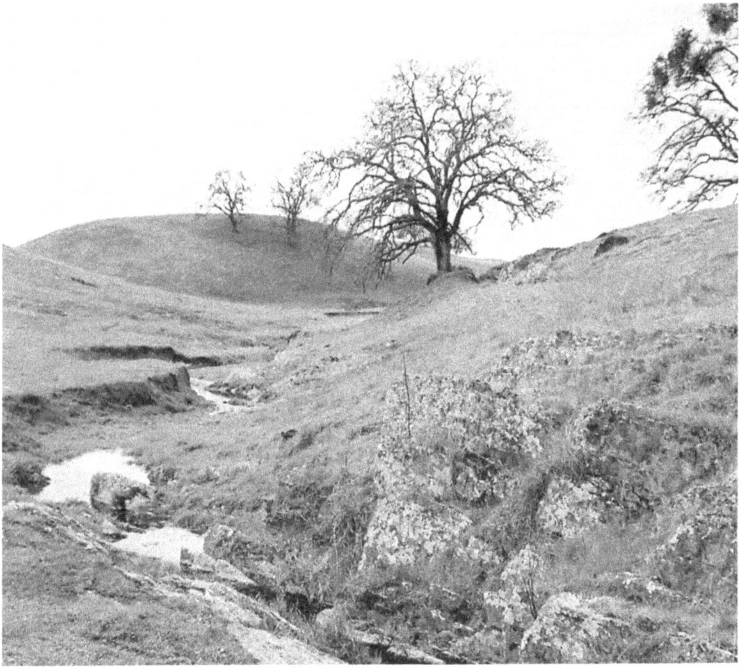

Deer Creek Hills Preserve Trails | TRAIL 3

The valley *meets the foothills in the Deer Creek Hills.*

numerous seasonally flowing shallow canyons and gullies, including **Crevis Creek**. A few artificial stock ponds provide important wetlands for waterfowl and a source of water for other wildlife and cattle that seasonally graze the area. The low rolling hills of the preserve are clothed in blue and live oak woodlands, separated by broad vistas of meadows and grasslands. Gray pines are found among the blue oaks, and an occasional large valley oak can be found in the rich alluvium of the canyon bottoms.

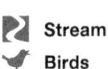 Stream
Birds

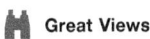 Great Views

Many of the docent-led hikes wander across country through the shallow canyons and to the top of the intervening ridges, although short segments of existing ranch roads and cow trails may also be followed for a short ways. Some of the hikes also require fording small streams, although

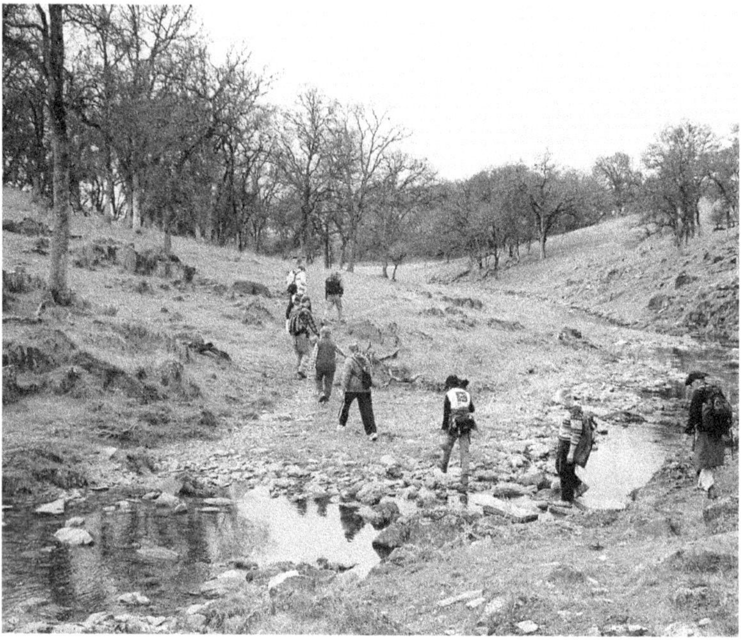

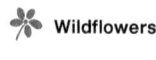

Seasonal stream crossing *in the Deer Creek Hills*

🌸 **Wildflowers**

🔨 **Geologic Interest**

Conservancy docents have established rock stepping stones at high-use stream crossings. Only the most onerous weather cancels a hike. In the rainy season, which runs November through April, hiking can be wet, muddy, and cold, but the hills are verdant with new grass and as the warmth of the sun increases, with a dazzling display of wildflowers.

The three major geological formations in the area—the Ione formation, Salt Springs slate, and Gopher Ridge volcanics—are marked by distinct vegetation changes as oak forests end abruptly at broad expanses of grasslands. Some parts of the preserve feature the upright and scenic "tombstone" rocks common to parts of the Sierra foothills. A 5.0–6.0-mile hike to the north boundary of the preserve features a dramatic view of perennially flowing Deer Creek from its scenic south canyon rim.

Deer Creek Hills Preserve Trails | TRAIL 3

More than 125 species of birds can be found migrating through or foraging and nesting in the preserve. The preserve also provides habitat for more than 40 wildlife species, including a few that are considered endangered or sensitive, such as the California red-legged frog, foothill yellow-legged frog, small-footed Myotis bat, and western pond turtle. The area is also rich in history and prehistory. Native American grinding holes are found in the bedrock outcrops along Crevis Creek and elsewhere. Ponds, ditches, and some hydraulic-mined areas were left behind by some of the less successful participants in the Gold Rush, and a few old homestead sites are remnants of the preserve's agrarian past.

The shorter docent-led hikes are suitable for families with children. Some of the longer hikes will please even the most die-hard trekkers.

 Birds

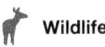 Wildlife

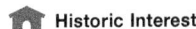 Historic Interest

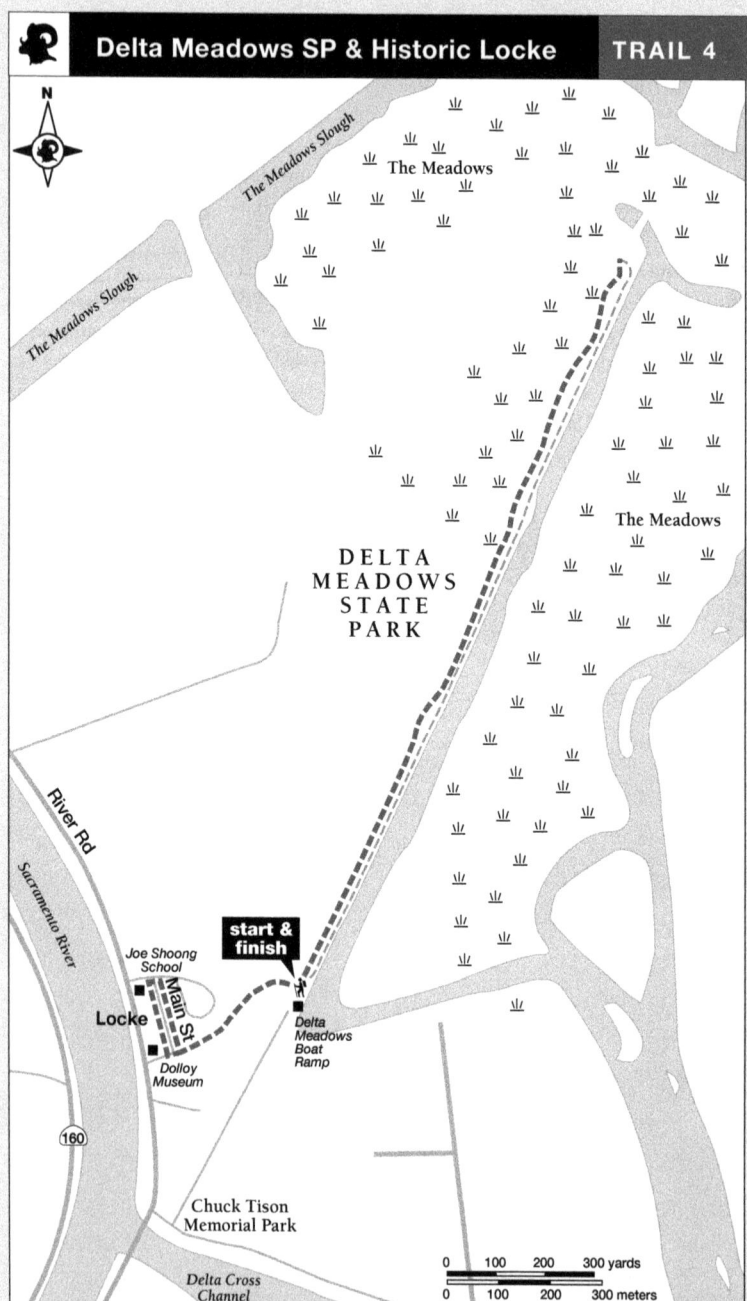

TRAIL 4 The Great Valley

Delta Meadows State Park and Historic Locke

Public areas and trails in the nearby Sacramento–San Joaquin Delta are few and far between. The undeveloped Delta Meadows State Park and the adjacent historic Chinese town of Locke offer a great opportunity to take a scenic drive through the west's largest estuary, enjoy some local history, and get a glimpse of the natural Delta as it existed before it was leveed and drained.

Best Time

This is a year-round walk. Summer afternoons can be hot.

Finding the Trail

From Sacramento, drive 20.4 miles south on Interstate 5 to the Twin Cities Road exit. Turn right on Twin Cities Road and proceed 6.3 miles east to River Road; turn left. Drive 2.0 miles south on River Road, which follows a levee parallel to the Sacramento River, to the historic town of Locke. Proceed 0.7 mile south on River Road past Locke, turn left before the bridge at the Chuck Tison Memorial Park. Make an immediate left on a gravel road with a DELTA MEADOWS RIVER PARK sign. Proceed 0.3 mile along the gravel road and park near the boat ramp.

Logistics

Bring money so you can shop for antiques and trinkets, and eat a meal in Locke. To learn more

---

TRAIL USE
Hike
LENGTH
2.44 miles, 1–2 hours
VERTICAL FEET
±0
DIFFICULTY
- **1** 2 3 4 5 +
TRAIL TYPE
Out & Back
SURFACE TYPE
Dirt
Wood Sidewalk
Pavement

FEATURES
Child Friendly
Dogs on Leash
River (Delta Slough)
Meadows
Wetlands
Birds
Wildlife
Historic
Photo Opportunity

FACILITIES
Porta-potty

Historically, more than a million salmon a year once migrated through the Delta on their way to the Sacramento and San Joaquin rivers and their tributaries.

about docent-led canoe trips at Delta Meadows State Park, call the Delta District Office of the California Department of Parks and Recreation at (916) 777-7701.

Trail Description

From the boat ramp, walk northeast on the levee that parallels the slough. ▶1 This levee was formerly the route of the Southern Pacific Railroad. The slough on the left was dredged to create the levee so that the tracks would be well above high tide and winter floodwaters. Almost immediately after leaving the boat ramp, you will pass a chain link fence enclosing a porta-potty. A trail leads to the left past the fenced enclosure and down off the levee. Keep this junction in mind for your return.

The trail follows the top of the levee, lined by shady oaks and cottonwoods. The levee parallels a slough on the right, which is easily viewable through the trees. The slough is one of the many waterways divided by leveed islands that make up the Delta.

River

The **Sacramento–San Joaquin Delta** is the largest estuary in the west. Through it flows all the water from rivers and streams that drain the west flank of the Sierra Nevada and the east slopes of the Coast Range. The estuary once abounded in native resident fish such as the tiny Delta smelt and Sacramento splittail. But major hydrological changes caused by upstream dams and by pumps that divert as much as 60 percent of the fresh water from the Delta for export south to feed San Joaquin Valley farms and southern California urban areas have decimated Delta fisheries. In addition, most of the Delta has been transformed from seasonally flooded tule marshes into farms protected by high levees. Water pollution from farms and cities has also contributed to the Delta's decline. Not surprisingly, the Delta is currently the focus of an intense effort by

Delta Meadows and Historic Locke — TRAIL 4

government agencies, agriculture, urban interests, and conservationists to restore its natural values and maintain its critical role as the hydrological heart of the Great Valley.

At **Delta Meadows State Park**, there is a rare opportunity to glimpse the Delta as it once was. Park rangers and docents lead weekend interpretive canoe trips on the slough that parallels the levee and on other waterways in the Park. The Park is one of the few relatively undeveloped natural areas in the Delta that is accessible to the public. As you continue northeast on the levee, the houses of Locke are replaced by open meadows and seasonally flooded wetlands punctuated by oak trees. Waterfowl and other wildlife abound on both sides of the levee.

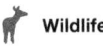
Wildlife

Approximately 1.0 mile from the boat ramp, the levee dead-ends at another slough. Here, a railroad trestle formerly crossed the water. At this point, you have the option of retracing your steps back along the levee or you can look for a use-trail leading down off the levee to the right, into the blackberry brambles and trees. ▶2 Follow this route to a rough trail that retraces your route back to the boat ramp along the edge of slough waters. Because this unofficial trail may not be maintained, watch for blackberry vines and poison oak, and keep in mind that this alternative return route may be flooded in the winter or spring. As the trail proceeds along the shoreline, it comes to a couple of open areas where anglers try their luck fishing in the slough. Just before reaching the boat ramp, the anglers trail climbs back to the top of the levee.

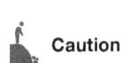
Caution

From the boat ramp, retrace your steps 100 yards northeast to the fenced enclosure with the porta-potty. Turn left on to the use-trail ▶3 and drop down off the levee and follow a well-defined path over an irrigation ditch and through vegetable gardens. The path soon connects with a street between two warehouses as you enter the historic town of

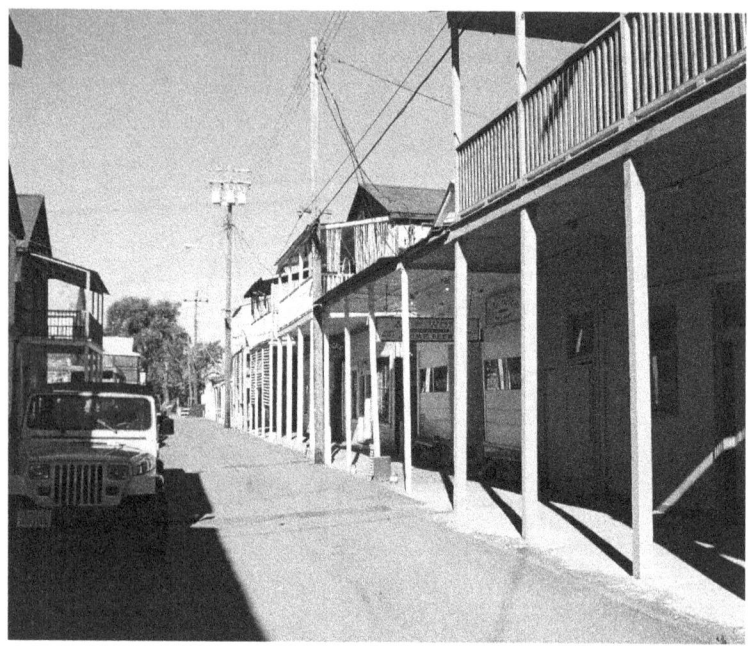

Explore *the nearby Chinese town of Locke.*

Locke. Please keep to the public streets and paths and respect the privacy and property rights of the residents. Continue straight on the apparently unnamed street past tidy bungalows and into the alley that leads you to Main St. in Locke. When you reach Main St., keep in mind the entrance of the alleyway next to the Dolloy Museum, on your left.

Turn right ▶4 and walk north on the east side of Main St. on the wooden boardwalk, window shopping as you go. Locke was founded in 1912 by Tin Sin Chan. It replaced Walnut Grove's former Chinatown, which was destroyed by fire. Approximately 1500 people lived in Locke in 1915, many of whom helped build the extensive levee systems along the Sacramento River and Delta waterways. Today, the town of Locke is on the National Register of Historic Places.

🏠 **Historic Interest**

Delta Meadows and Historic Locke | TRAIL 4

At the end and west side of Locke's short Main St. is the **Joe Shoong School**. Opened in 1926 and constructed with donated funds, the school inside looks much as it did 80 years ago, complete with wooden desks with inkwells. Historical news clippings and photos of graduates and community leaders hang on the wall. ▶5 Turn back at the school and walk south on the east side of Main St.

Cross Main St. to the **Dolloy Museum**, which is worth a visit if it is open. From the museum, proceed east into the alley next to the museum, ▶6 retracing your steps between the houses and warehouses, ▶7 to the garden path and then to the top of the levee to the parking area near the boat ramp.

MILESTONES

▶1	0.00	Start at Delta Meadows Boat Ramp, walk northeast on levee trail
▶2	1.00	Levee trail ends, turn right to follow anglers trail back to boat ramp
▶3	2.00	From boat ramp, walk 100 yards back to fenced enclosure, turn left
▶4	2.13	Walk east through Locke residential area to main street, turn right
▶5	2.22	Walk north on Main St. to Joe Schoong School, turn around
▶6	2.31	Walk south on Main St. to Dalloy Museum, turn left in alley
▶7	2.44	Retrace steps through residential area to boat ramp parking area

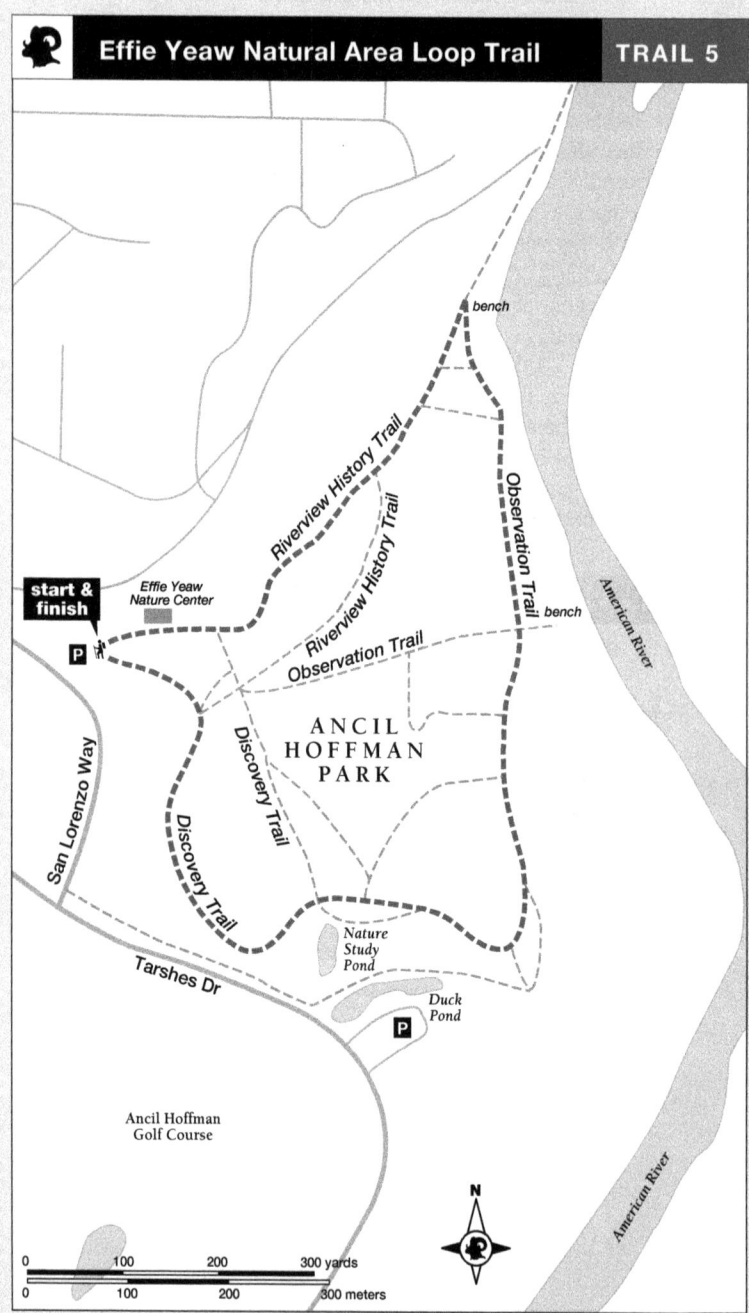

TRAIL 5 The Great Valley

Effie Yeaw Natural Area Loop Trail

The Effie Yeaw Nature Center and its adjacent Natural Area have a network of short interpretive trails perfect for families to explore and learn about the American River ecosystem, the life of the Nisenan Indians who formerly lived along the river, and the advent of gold mining that transformed the landscape and eventually led to the establishment of the American River Parkway. Although the trails are short and located in a relatively confined area, there is no better place to observe wildlife on a winter day. You may see deer and coyotes, and numerous avian species, including wild turkeys, great blue herons, kingfishers, acorn woodpeckers, and Cooper's hawks. By following different segments of the Observation, Riverview History, and Discovery interpretive trails, you can pretty much circumnavigate the entire natural area within about a mile, experience the many habitats of the Parkway, observe the river and a wetland, and start and end at the Nature Center itself so you can enjoy its exhibits and wildlife displays.

Best Time

The best time to observe wildlife is during the winter: check flood conditions on the American River before visiting. The cooler morning hours during the summer will also provide opportunities to observe wildlife.

TRAIL USE
Hike
LENGTH
1.0 mile, 30–60 minutes
VERTICAL FEET
±0
DIFFICULTY
- **1** 2 3 4 5 +
TRAIL TYPE
Loop (with Option)
SURFACE TYPE
Dirt

FEATURES
Child Friendly
Parking Fee
River
Wetlands
Meadow
Birds
Wildlife
Historic
Photo Opportunity

FACILITIES
Water
Toilets

Finding the Trail

> A large interpretive sign notes that much of this area was mined for gold by large dredges that operated well into the 1930s.

From Sacramento, drive 3.9 miles east on Business 80/Capital City Freeway to the Marconi Ave. exit. Turn right on Marconi Ave. and drive 5.1 miles. As Marconi crosses Fair Oaks Ave., it turns into Palm Ave. Continue east on Palm Ave. to the stop sign at California Ave. and turn right. Continue on California to Tarshes Dr., then turn left. Enter Ancil Hoffman Park (pay $5 at the entrance station). Continue a short distance on Tarshes Dr. to the stop sign, turn left at the stop sign on San Lorenzo Way, and proceed a short distance to the Effie Yeaw Nature Center parking lot on the right.

Logistics

The Effie Yeaw Nature Center and Natural Area are located in Ancil Hoffman County Park. There is a $5 vehicle fee to enter the park, which is open from dawn to dusk. There is no fee to visit the Nature Center or Natural Area. The Nature Center is open seven days a week (except Thanksgiving, Christmas, and New Year's Day), 9:00 a.m. to 5:00 p.m. February–October and 9:30 a.m. to 4:00 p.m. November–January. The Nature Center offers educational programs for school groups on weekdays and for families and other groups on weekends. For more information, you can contact the Effie Yeaw Nature Center at (916) 489-4918 or visit www.effieyeaw.org.

Trail Description

In addition to the three named interpretive trails, there are several connector trails. The various trail intersections are often unsigned and can be confusing, but every trail either leads back to the Nature Center or to another parking area south of the Nature Center Preserve on Tarshes Dr. If you reach

Effie Yeaw Natural Area Loop Trail | TRAIL 5

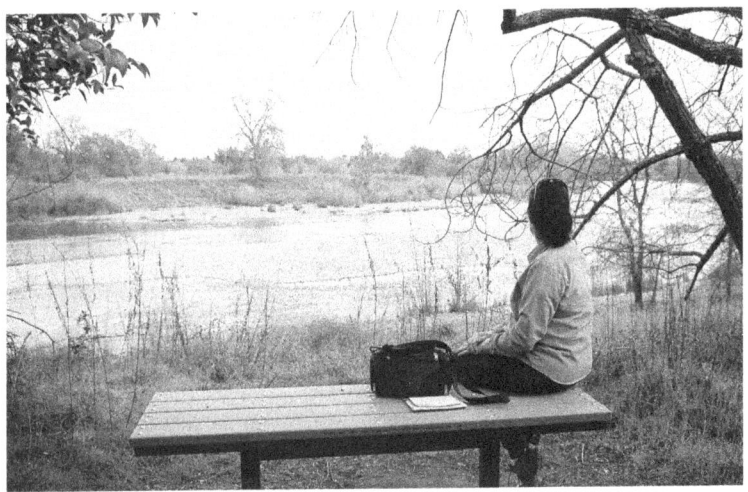

The Effie Yeaw Natural Area *offers some fine views of the American River.*

that point, simply turn around and head back to the Nature Center.

From the rear door of the Effie Yeaw Nature Center, proceed northeast on the combined routes that make up the **Riverview History** and **Observation trails**. ▶1 Within 100 feet, there is a **T** junction that marks the beginning of the Discovery Trail on the right. Continue straight on the Riverview History and Observation trails. Frequent interpretive signs offer insights into the ecology, habitats, and natural history of the area. The trail descends a slope and then drops in and out of a series of shallow swales that accommodate overflow from the American River during floods. Large valley oaks shade the trail as it makes it way through a typical riparian understory of blackberry brambles, box elder, and elderberry.

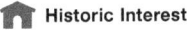 Historic Interest

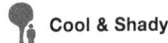 Cool & Shady

At the second **T** intersection, turn left to continue to follow the Riverview and Observation Trails to the northwest. ▶2 Go past a trail junction where the Observation Trail leads off to the right and another connector junction on the right farther

River

on. Continue a short way on the Riverview Trail to a small grassy opening in the woods with a large rock barbecue pit. A bench overlooks the **American River** to the east.

At this point, the Riverview Trail makes a sharp right turn and heads south. ▶3 Go past a connector junction on the right and then another right-hand junction where the Observation Trail reconnects with your route.

From this junction, the Riverview Trail turns right and heads back to the Nature Center. ▶4 Continue straight south on the Observation Trail as it makes its way through an open forest of blue oaks and coyote bush parallel to the cobbled bank of the American River on your left. The area was originally part of John Sutter's land grant. When gold mining ended, the river began restoring itself. Effie Yeaw was a teacher, conservationist, and environmental educator who began leading natural and cultural history walks in what was then known as the Deterding Woods, along the American River in Carmichael. She worked with William B. Pond, then Director of the Sacramento County Parks Department, to develop the concept of the **American River Parkway**. The Nature Center was completed in 1976 as the major interpretive facility of the Parkway and was named after the teacher whose dedication to nature and children still guides Nature Center activities today.

Continue south past a bench as your route ambles through oaks and brush. Go past a trail junction on the right, and continue south. At another right-hand trail junction, the Observation Trail heads back to the Nature Center. Continue south on your now unnamed trail, past another trail junction on the right. The trail crosses an old concrete pad with a large rusted iron trough on the left, equipment perhaps left from the gold dredging days. Your route continues south past a junction on the right.

Historic Interest

Effie Yeaw Natural Area Loop Trail | TRAIL 5

At the sixth trail junction on your southward journey, turn right and then proceed to a four-way junction at the end of a large pond edged by tules. ▶5 This pond is part of the natural overflow channels of the American River. It was lined with clay to enhance its ability to hold water year-round for waterfowl and other wildlife.

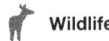 Birds

At the four-way junction at the end of the pond, ▶6 turn left and proceed along the edge of the pond past a trail junction on the right, which heralds the connection of the Discovery Trail. Continue straight as the Discovery Trail drifts away from the pond into a blue oak forest. The trail rambles through the forest until it comes to the edge of a large meadow just south of the Nature Center. This is a good spot to observe foraging deer late in the afternoon and early evening. The Observation Trail makes its way around the meadow and connects with the Riverview History Trail on its return leg to the Nature Center.

Wildlife

Turn left on the Riverview History Trail ▶7 and walk the short distance back to the ▶8 Nature Center.

MILESTONES

▶1	0.00	From the Nature Center, head northeast on the Observation Trail
▶2	0.30	Turn left on the Riverview History Trail
▶3	0.38	Riverview Trail reaches its northernmost point, bends south
▶4	0.42	Observation Trail junction, continue south on Observation Trail
▶5	0.48	Turn right at sixth trail junction
▶6	0.50	Turn left to connect with the Discovery Trail, go past pond
▶7	0.98	Turn left on Riverview History Trail
▶8	1.00	Return to Nature Center

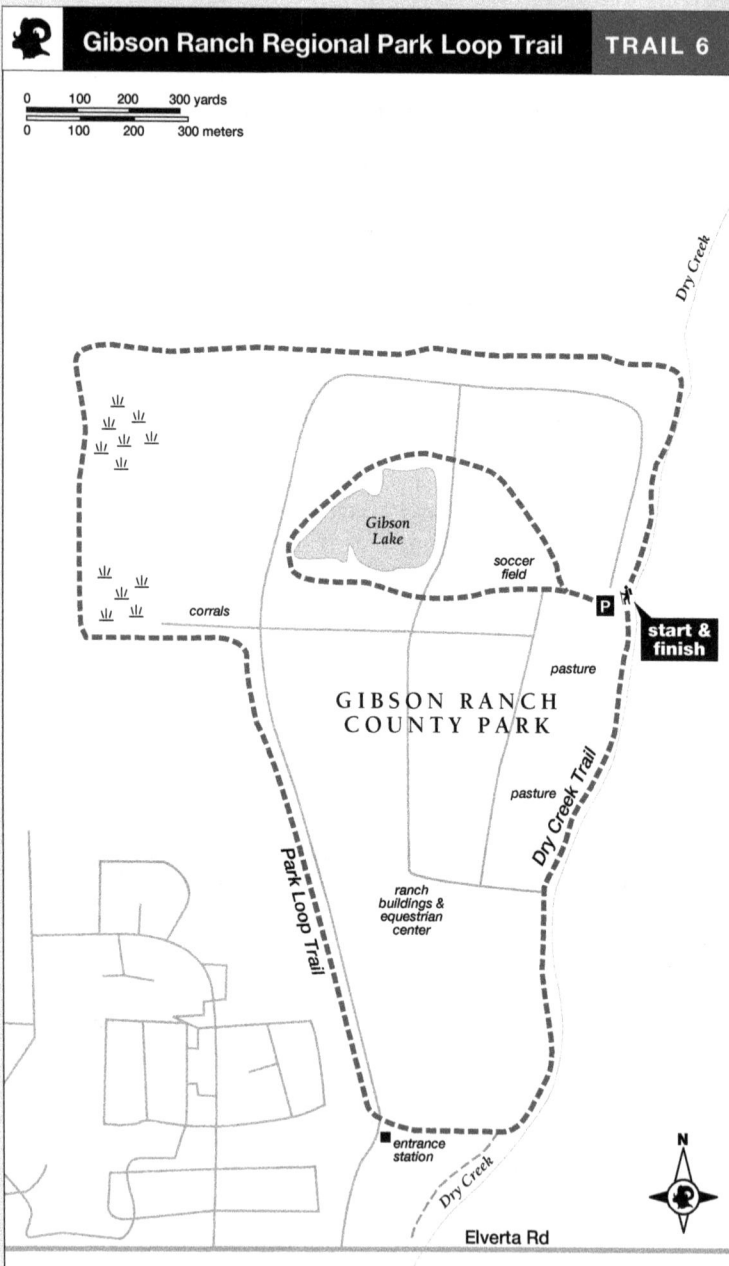

TRAIL 6 The Great Valley

Gibson Ranch Regional Park Loop Trail

Gibson Ranch provides a regional park experience for residents of the growing suburbs of northeastern Sacramento County and southeastern Placer County. The park was established to preserve a slice of the county's agrarian heritage, which is fast disappearing under suburban pavement. School children visit to learn about farm life, Civil War reenactors stage historic battles, and equestrians favor the park's extensive road and trail system. The 300-acre park also includes a large lake, an extensive wetland, and more than a mile of the Dry Creek Parkway. Hikers have several options, including the nearly 3.0-mile-long Park Loop, which circumnavigates the park's boundary; the 2.0 mile out-and-back stroll along Dry Creek; and a short stroll around scenic Gibson Lake. This description focuses on the Park Loop. The many short and level walking options, water attractions, and livestock make this a great destination for families with young children.

Best Time

Temperatures are best fall through spring. As is typical with most valley destinations, summer afternoons can be hot.

Finding the Trail

From Sacramento, drive east approximately 11 miles on Interstate 80. Take the Watt Ave. North exit. Drive 5.0 miles north on Watt Ave. to Elverta Road. A GIBSON RANCH PARK sign directs you to turn left on Elverta Road. Drive 2.2 miles west on Elverta

TRAIL USE
Hike, Run, Horse
LENGTH
2.86 miles, 1–2 hours
VERTICAL FEET
±0
DIFFICULTY
- 1 **2** 3 4 5 +
TRAIL TYPE
Loop
Out & Back Option
SURFACE TYPE
Dirt

FEATURES
Child Friendly
Dogs Allowed
Parking Fee
Entrance Fee
Stream
Meadow
Lake
Wetlands
Wildflowers
Birds

FACILITIES
Toilets
Water

> Some of the horses may wander over to their corral fence to say "hi" and to see if maybe you brought them a carrot or an apple.

Road. Just after crossing the Dry Creek Bridge, look for the Gibson Ranch Park sign, and turn right onto the park's entrance road. Pay the $4 fee at the entrance station and continue north on the road, past the Ranch and equestrian center on the right and Gibson Lake. The road curves right, around the lake, and then curves right at Dry Creek to dead-end at the Dry Creek parking lot. Park here. From the park entrance on Elverta Road to the parking lot is about 1.6 miles.

Logistics

For a short, scenic walk, the 2.14 mile out-and-back loop to the north and south ends of the Dry Creek Trail is your best bet. You can augment this hike by adding a .87-mile loop around scenic Gibson Lake. The 2.86-mile Park Loop includes the Dry Creek segment and can also be enhanced by adding the short Gibson Lake Loop.

Trail Description

From the Dry Creek parking lot, cross the access road to the **Dry Creek Trail**. ▶1 The trail follows a short berm that protects the rest of Gibson Ranch when Dry Creek floods. Proceed south along the trail as it parallels the creek's riparian forest, made up of some large valley oaks, smaller blue oaks, and cottonwoods. Dry Creek is the major drainage for much of northeastern Sacramento County. Steelhead formerly migrated up the stream, and efforts are underway to remove impediments to their migration and improve habitat. As you continue southward along the berm trail, use-trails to your left provide periodic access to the stream. At one of the larger streamside flats off the trail, you can see several cottonwoods that have been gnawed by beavers. On the right side of the trail are

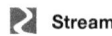 Stream

Gibson Ranch Regional Park Loop Trail | TRAIL 6

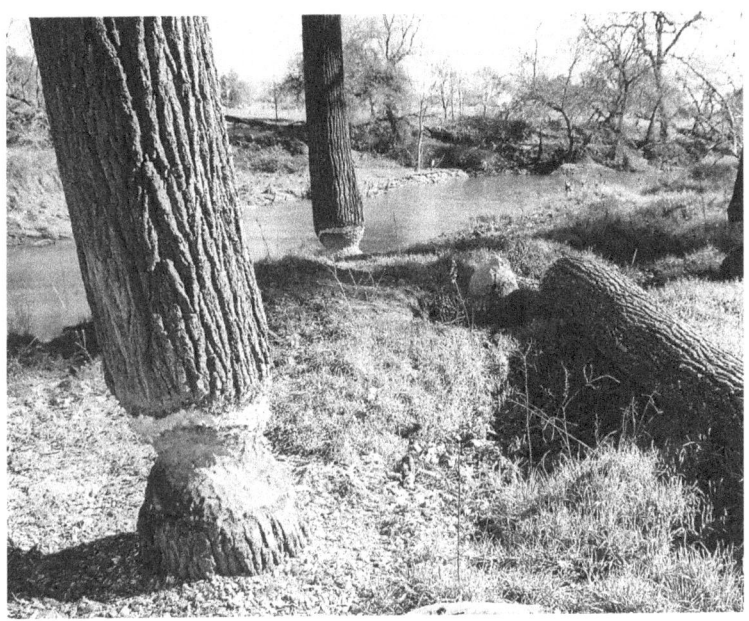

Dry Creek in the Gibson Ranch Regional Park provides exellent habitat for beaver.

pastures, where horses, cows, sheep, goats, llamas, and other livestock sometimes graze. Along the way, you cross two **T** intersections with service roads on your right. In both instances, continue straight and south along the Dry Creek Trail.

A bit over 0.5 mile from the parking lot, you will come to the third intersection with a service road, on your right. The sound and sight through the trees of traffic on Elverta Road will alert you to the imminent end of the Dry Creek Trail. If you are walking the there-and-back route along Dry Creek, you may continue another several hundred yards as the trail narrows considerably and ends at Elverta Road. Informal routes across the road suggest that the trail continues, but it does not, and crossing heavily trafficked Elverta Road can be quite dangerous. At this point, Dry Creek out-and-backers can turn around and head back to the northern end of the parkway. Hikers following the Park Loop should turn west at the third service road ▶2 and follow the road a short distance as it parallels a ditch and line of oak trees.

The **Park Loop Trail** crosses the park road at the entrance station. Then the trail turns right and parallels the road for slightly more than 0.5 mile, with the road on your right and a fenced residential area on your left. ▶3 This is the least interesting segment of the Park Loop.

The Park Loop Trail connects with a service road that leads westward from the main park road between several horse corrals and stalls. ▶4

The service road reaches the western boundary of the park. The Park Loop turns northward ▶5 along another service road as it parallels the park boundary. On your right, an extensive wetland of tules ringed by small trees marks the drainage that leads to **Gibson Lake**. Herons, ducks, and geese can be viewed in the shallow ponds.

🐦 Birds

Gibson Lake Loop

OPTIONS

To enjoy an 0.87-mile circuit of scenic Gibson Lake, proceed from the southwest corner of the parking lot along an unpaved service route. This route connects with a ditch spanned by a white bridge. Go past the bridge and continue west along the ditch, with a soccer field on your right. A second white bridge spans a 90-degree turn in the ditch. Cross here and climb up the berm in front of you, veering to the left to go around a small gray building that turns out to be restrooms. As you top the berm, you will see pretty Gibson Lake in front of you. The lake has several piers for fishing and is usually crowded with resident ducks and geese. Cross the paved service road on top of the berm, continue west around the end of the lake, and circle eastward back to the berm and the paved service road. Drop down off the berm and continue east, past the soccer field to the Dry Creek parking lot.

Gibson Ranch Regional Park Loop Trail | TRAIL 6

In slightly less than two miles from your starting point, you come to the northwest boundary of the park, which is marked by a large cell phone tower. ▶6 Turn right and proceed east along the park's northern boundary. As your route undulates in and out of a dry swale, a clear day will provide a good view of the Sierra Nevada beyond Dry Creek's forest line to the northeast. Swainson's hawks, northern harriers, and other raptors can be observed foraging for food in the open grasslands on both sides of the trail. About halfway along the northern boundary, the main park road begins to parallel the Loop Trail as it proceeds to the parking lot, which is your ultimate destination.

In a bit over 2.6 miles, the Loop Trail reaches the Dry Creek Trail. ▶7 Turn right and follow the Dry Creek Trail back ▶8 to the parking lot.

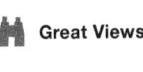

Great Views

Birds

MILESTONES

- ▶1 0.00 From the Dry Creek parking lot, head south on Dry Creek Trail
- ▶2 0.62 Turn right to follow service road
- ▶3 0.81 Cross road by entrance station, turn right on path parallel to road
- ▶4 1.36 Turn left on service road accessing horse corrals
- ▶5 1.60 Turn right on service road parallels to park's western boundary
- ▶6 1.92 Turn right at cell phone tower to parallel park's northern boundary
- ▶7 2.61 Turn right to follow the Dry Creek Trail
- ▶8 2.86 Return to Dry Creek parking lot

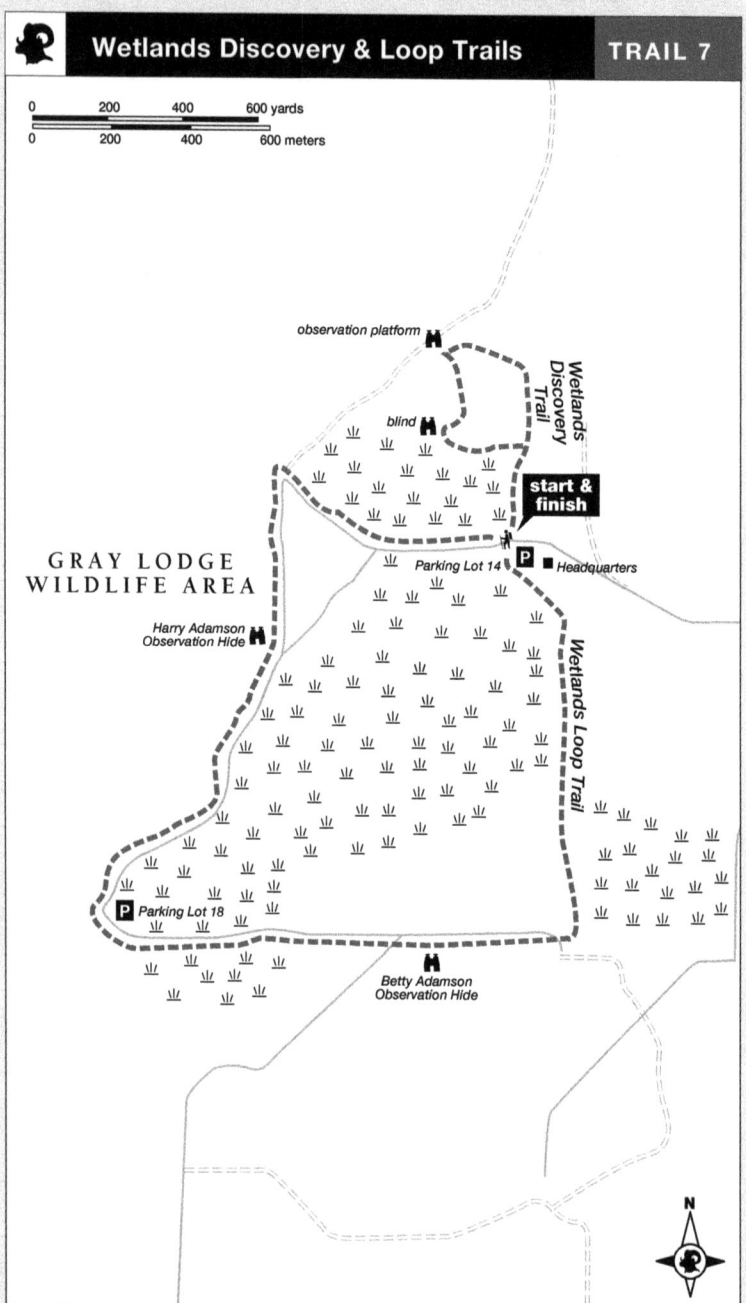

TRAIL 7 The Great Valley

Wetlands Discovery & Loop Trails: Gray Lodge Wildlife Area

More waterfowl visit the Great Valley than any other region along the Pacific Flyway. The Gray Lodge Wildlife Area, managed by the California Department of Fish and Game, is one of the best places to observe waterfowl and one of the state's oldest refuges. Established in the 1930s to provide habitat for migrating and seasonal waterfowl, Gray Lodge is 9100 acres and is one of the largest and most diverse refuges in the valley. It is also one of the most important stops for waterfowl along the Pacific Flyway, which has lost as much as 96 percent of its wetlands to development. Gray Lodge supports more than 300 species of wildlife, including more than 1 million ducks and 100,000 geese during the winter migration. Viewing the huge flocks of geese that rise to the sky every evening from Gray Lodge's wetlands is worth the short drive north from Sacramento. There are two trails for visitors to enjoy the wetlands and wildlife. They are short and easy, so plan on doing both during your visit.

Best Time

Mid-fall to early spring is the best time to view migrating waterfowl.

Finding the Trail

From Sacramento, drive north 8.4 miles to the Hwy 99/70 intersection. Proceed north 53.2 miles on Hwy 99 to the small town of Live Oak. In Live Oak, turn left on Pennington Rd. Drive west on Pennington Rd about 6.6 miles. Pennington does

---

TRAIL USE
Hike
LENGTH
Discovery Trail:
0.83 mile,
30–60 minutes.
Wetlands Loop:
2.64 miles, 1.5 hours
VERTICAL FEET
±0
DIFFICULTY
- **1 2** 3 4 5 +
TRAIL TYPE
Loops
SURFACE TYPE
Pavement
Dirt

FEATURES
Child Friendly
Dogs on Leash
Handicapped Accessible
Parking Fee
Wetlands
Birds
Wildlife
Great Views
Interpretive Signs

FACILITIES
Porta-potties

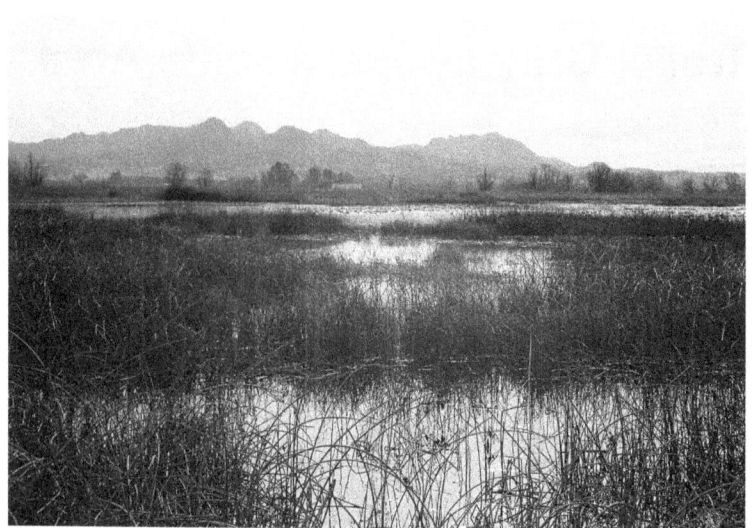

The Sutter Buttes *provide a scenic backdrop to the Gray Lodge Wildlife Area.*

a series of 90-degree turns and becomes North Butte Rd. Just past the intersection of North Butte Rd. and Powell, look for a brown sign on the right that says GRAY LODGE and has a binocular logo on it. Just past the sign, turn right on Almond Orchard Dr. Proceed north 1.7 miles (after crossing the Butte County line, Almond Orchard Dr. apparently becomes Pennington Rd. again) to Rutherford Rd., which is marked by another Gray Lodge sign. Turn left on Rutherford Rd. and proceed west 2.3 miles, past the wildlife area headquarters on your right and interpretive kiosk and small exhibit building on your left, to Parking Lot no.14. Both trails leave from this parking lot.

Logistics

From October through mid-February, visitors who aren't hunters are limited to these two trails and the 3.0-mile auto tour. Most of the refuge is open

Wetlands Discovery and Loop Trails — TRAIL 7

to the public (except for those areas signed CLOSED) the rest of the year. Gray Lodge is open from sunset to sundown. Free 1.5-hour-long naturalist-guided tours are available during the migration season on Saturdays at 9 a.m. and Sundays at 1 p.m. (cancelled if raining). Apparently, a $2.50 per adult visitors fee is charged. An iron ranger is located in Parking Lot no. 4, but at the time of writing, there were no envelopes available in which to place money.

For more information, visit www.dfg.ca.gov/lands/wa/region2/graylodge, or call the headquarters at (530) 846-7500 or the naturalist's office at (530) 846-7505.

> You may hear the extended chattering call of a belted kingfisher, and geese are likely to be found in the wetland.

Trail Description

Wetlands Discovery (Nature) Trail

The paved self-guided nature trail begins at the entrance to parking lot no. 14 and proceeds north. ▶1 Be sure to pick up the nature trail guide at the information kiosk in the parking lot, which is keyed to 14 numbered posts along the way. As you walk north, the pond on the left provides an immediate opportunity to view ducks, coots, egrets, and other waterfowl. A bench provides a good opportunity for visitors to sit and view the birds.

🐦 **Birds**

The paved trail branches left at the first trail junction (the dirt trail straight ahead is your return route). ▶2 Follow the paved trail to the left and proceed west, with wetlands on your left and dry upland habitat on your right.

At the second trail junction, leave the paved trail (which turns right) and go straight (west) on a dirt trail, which leads to an earth mound. ▶3 Climb the steps to the wildlife viewing blind on top of the mound, which provides a view to a larger wetland to the west. After observing the flocks in the wetland, turn around and drop down from the mound, turn

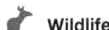 **Wildlife**

left and circle back to another junction with the paved nature trail. ▶4 Turn left here and continue north on the paved trail.

At another trail junction, continue straight (north) on the paved trail into a small grove of cottonwood, willow, and sycamore trees. ▶5 These were planted to increase habitat diversity in the refuge. The paved trail soon reaches a large raised wooden observation platform. ▶6 A spotting scope is provided to observe wildlife in the large wetland to the north. From here, you have an excellent view of the **Coast Range** to the northwest.

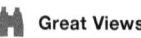
Great Views

After taking in the view on the observation platform, return to the Y intersection and veer left to follow the dirt path to the southeast. ▶7 This part of the trail meanders through small, open clearings defined by cottonwoods and blackberry brambles. This upland area provides important habitat and cover for rabbits, deer, quail, pheasants, and even great horned owls.

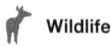
Wildlife

Eventually, the dirt path reaches the first trail junction and returns to the paved trail. ▶8 Follow the paved trail south ▶9 back to parking lot no.14.

Wetlands Loop Trail

From the southeast corner of parking lot no. 14, proceed south ▶1 on an unpaved road marked with a sign that says HIKING ROUTE and notes that wildlife blinds are 0.75 mile and 1.0 mile ahead. The trail heads straight for the **Sutter Buttes**, the remnants of an ancient volcano in the middle of the Great Valley. Your route parallels a canal on the left, and a large wetland on the right that should provide ample opportunity to view flocks of waterfowl.

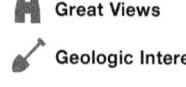
Great Views

Geologic Interest

Birds

In a bit over 0.5 mile, your route intersects with another road to your right. Turn right to follow the sign that says HIKING ROUTE. ▶2 This segment of the loop proceeds west along a row of cottonwood trees on your left. But soon the row of trees end and a large wetland comes into view to the left, typically hosting

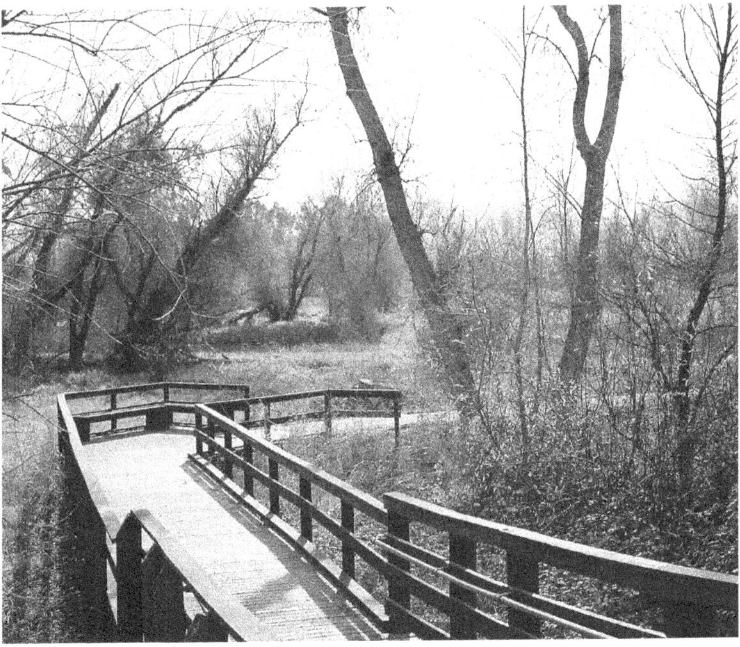

Wetlands Discovery and Loop Trails | TRAIL 7

Ramp leading down *from one of Gray Lodge's wildlife observation platforms*

large flocks of snow and Canada geese. Within about 0.75 mile, you reach the **Betty Adamson Observation Hide**, a cement brick building with south-facing windows for watching waterfowl in the adjacent wetland without disturbing them. The trail continues beyond the hide as it follows a road westward past wetlands, cottonwoods, and blackberry and wild rose brambles.

 Birds

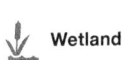 Wetland

A bit over a mile and a third into the loop, ▶3 you reach parking lot no. 18 on the auto tour route. Cross the parking lot and proceed due north on a trail marked by a sign that says HIKING TRAIL—FOOT TRAFFIC ONLY. ▶4 Nearly 2.0 miles into the loop, you will come to a four-way road intersection. Cross the road, and on your left is short trail that leads to the **Harry Adamson Observation Hide**, overlooking a pond to the west. After checking out the view from the hide, continue north on the trail as it parallels a canal on the left and a wetland on the right. Wild rose brambles line this route also.

Almost 2.25 miles into the loop, you will reach another four-way road intersection. Cross the road in front of you and make a sharp right turn ▶5 to follow the levee trail that parallels the road heading southeast back to parking lot no. 14. A large wetland to the north offers opportunities to observe more waterfowl. Make your way back ▶6 to parking lot no. 14 and your vehicle.

Wetlands Discovery and Loop Trails | TRAIL 7

MILESTONES

Wetlands Discovery (Nature) Trail

▶1 0.00 From Parking Lot no.14 entrance, proceed north on paved trail
▶2 0.15 Trail junction, turn left
▶3 0.26 Trail junction, continue straight on dirt trail to raised blind
▶4 0.36 From the blind, go left and circle back to the paved trail; turn left
▶5 0.46 Trail junction, continue straight on paved path to platform
▶6 0.51 Observation platform
▶7 0.56 Retrace steps to last trail junction, veer left
▶8 0.68 Return to first trail junction, continue straight on paved path
▶9 0.83 Return to parking lot no. 14

Wetlands Loop Trail

▶1 0.00 From parking lot no.14 head south on road marked "Hiking Route"
▶2 0.65 Road junction, turn right (west)
▶3 1.38 Reach parking lot no. 18, turn right (north)
▶4 1.94 four-way road intersection, continue north
▶5 2.24 Road junction, turn sharp right (southeast)
▶6 2.65 Return to parking lot no. 14

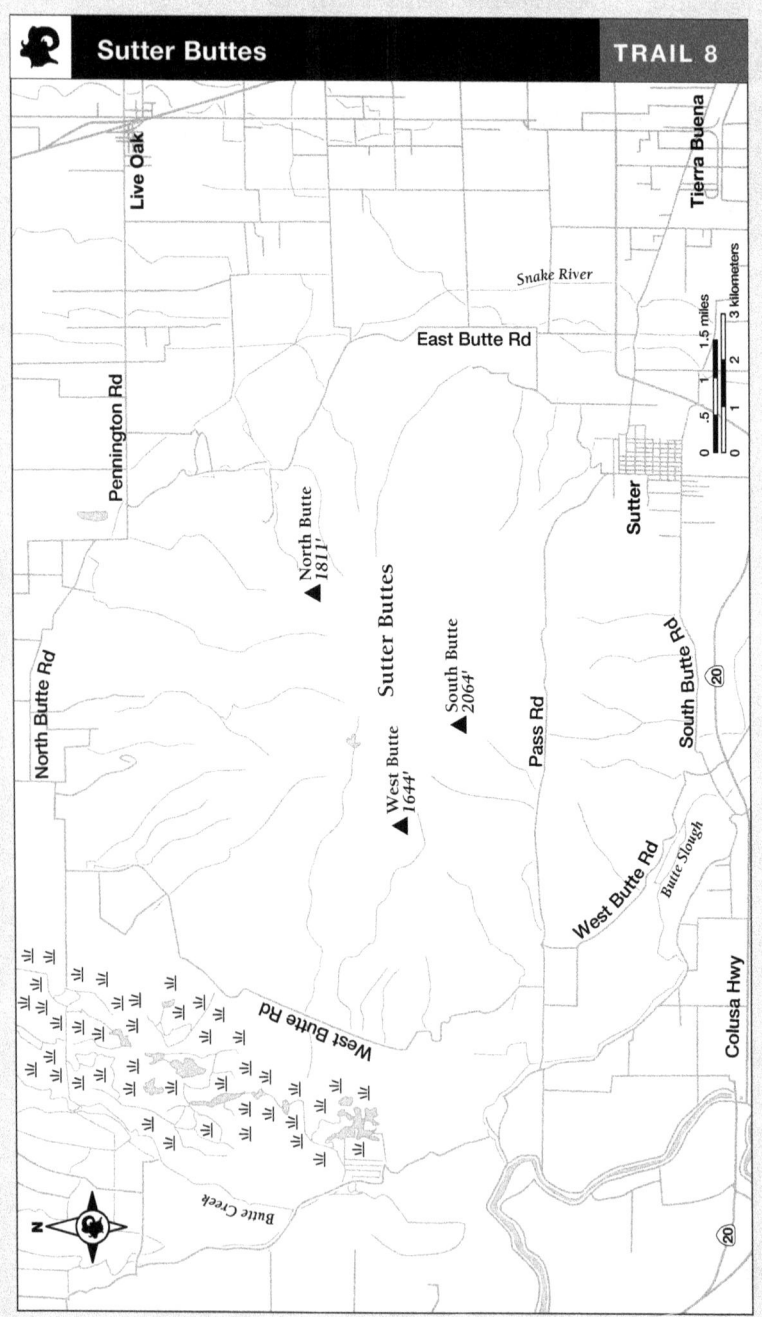

TRAIL 8 The Great Valley

Sutter Buttes Trails

Reputed to be the smallest free-standing mountain range in the United States, the Sutter Buttes rise more than 2000 feet from the Great Valley floor. The volcanic Buttes are literally an island of nearly pristine nature surrounded by the Valley's industrial farmlands. Most of the Buttes are privately owned, and public access is limited to hikes and outings led by the volunteer guides of the Middle Mountain Foundation. The Foundation works with local landowners to provide, for a reasonable fee, public access to the Buttes with an emphasis on education. The volcanic rock formations and dramatic topography of the Buttes, their rich oak woodlands and meadows, and their colorful tapestry of seasonal wildflowers are well worth the fee. The Foundation leads a wide variety of hikes and outings of varying difficulty, ranging in length from 2.0 to 8.0 miles. Many emphasize the natural history of the Buttes, including geology, wildflowers, birds, as well as Native American traditions and myths. Since visiting the Sutter Buttes is limited to the outings sponsored by the Middle Mountain Foundation, this is more a general description of the Buttes than a detailed trail description.

Best Time

Spring is the best time to visit the Sutter Buttes, if only to appreciate the magnificent wildflower display, newly leafed oak forests, and green meadows. The Middle Mountain Foundation schedules outings to the Sutter Buttes from October to May. June through September is generally too hot to visit the Buttes.

TRAIL USE
Hike
LENGTH
3.0–8.0 miles
VERTICAL FEET
±600–±1500 feet
DIFFICULTY
- 1 **2 3 4** 5 +
TRAIL TYPE
Variable
SURFACE TYPE
Dirt

FEATURES
Child Friendly
Hike Fee
Mountain
Canyon
Meadow
Wildflower
Birds
Wildlife
Historic
Great Views
Photo Opportunity
Interpretive
Geological interest
Steep

FACILITIES
Porta-potties

> One rare oracle oak (a hybrid between black and live oak) and a juniper can be found in the Buttes, indicative of the transitional nature of the Buttes' ecosystems.

Finding the Trail

Trailheads into the Sutter Buttes vary, depending on which hike you participate in. Middle Mountain Foundation hikes typically meet at the Sutter County Memorial Museum, 1333 Butte House Blvd., in Yuba City. To get to the museum from Sacramento, drive 7.0 miles north on Interstate 5 to the Hwy 70/99 exit. Drive north 12.8 miles on highways 70/99 to the Hwy 99/70 split. Take Hwy 99 and continue north 23 miles to the intersection with Hwy 20 in Yuba City. Turn left on Hwy 20 and drive approximately 0.2 mile west; turn right on Civic Center Dr. Go north on Civic Center Dr. approximately 0.3 mile and turn right on Butte House Road. The museum is on the left just before you drive under the freeway.

Logistics

Visit www.middlemountain.org to view the Middle Foundation's list of currently scheduled hikes and to reserve space on a hike. You can also call the Foundation at (530) 671-6116, or contact them via email at middlemountain@yahoo.com. Hikes are generally limited to 20 participants and fill up fast, so make reservations early. Most outings are on the weekend. The fee ranges from $35 to $55. You may also charter your own outing with the Foundation for a minimum of $300 for 10 people. Hikes range from easy to strenuous. Some of the less strenuous hikes are child- and senior-friendly, but many of the hikes require cross-country travel over rocky, uneven, and often wet ground. Some include seasonal stream crossings, as well as steep hill climbs and descents. Good hiking boots are required and poles or staffs are recommended. Poison oak and ticks are common. Seniors and families with children should check with the Foundation about a hike's difficulty before making reservations. Participants bring their own lunch and water. The

Sutter Buttes Trails | TRAIL 8

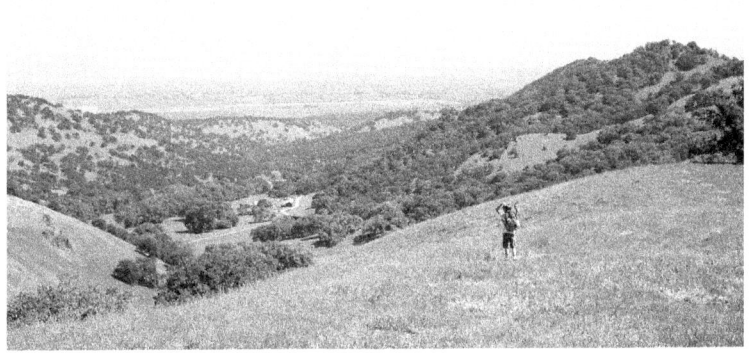

The Sutter Buttes *area is a volcanic island in the middle of the Great Valley.*

typical outing begins at the Sutter County Museum in Yuba City, where participants arrive as early as 8 a.m. to meet the hike leaders and form carpools. From there, carpools proceed via private roads and through locked gates to the trailhead. Hikes usually end around 3:30 p.m.

Trail Description

The **Sutter Buttes** are the remains of an extinct volcano that thrust itself up through the sedimentary layers of the Great Valley as it formed about 1.5 million years ago. The almost perfect circular perimeter of the Buttes implies that this was once one great volcanic cone, but in reality, the Buttes were formed by a series of eruptions in different places, each marked by a singular butte. The North Butte was the site of the last eruption.

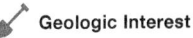 Geologic Interest

People have lived around the Sutter Buttes and appreciated their unique nature for more than 10,000 years. Prominent in the myths of the local Maidu Indians, the Buttes were called *Esto Yamani* ("The Middle Mountain"). The Maidu believed that the first man and woman were created in the Buttes, and that upon death, the souls of the Maidu

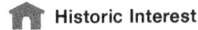 Historic Interest

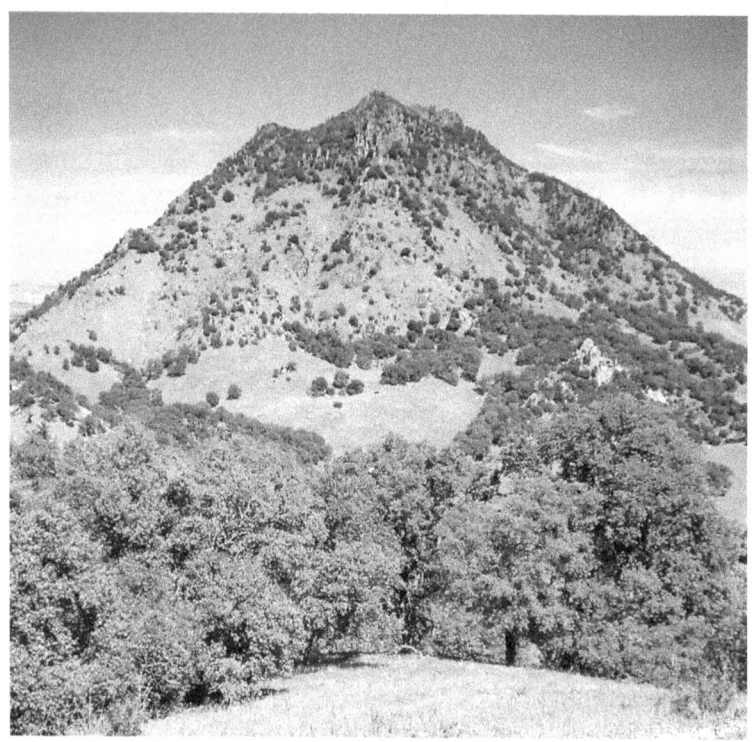

The North Butte *is the youngest of the Sutter Buttes' several volcanic cones.*

ascended to the highest peak. The Maidu did not live in these sacred mountains, but instead visited them for religious ceremonies and for hunting and the gathering of food.

🏠 **Historic Interest**

The Sutter Buttes were first sighted by a European in 1808, as Ensign Gabriel Moraga and his small party of Spanish soldiers explored the Great Valley for potential mission sites. Don Luis Arguello led another Spanish expedition into the area in 1817 and called the Buttes "Los Picachos" (the peaks). In 1828, the famous mountain man Jedediah Smith was the first American to see the Buttes as he explored the northern portion of the Great Valley on his way to Oregon. Hudson's Bay

Sutter Buttes Trails — TRAIL 8

Company trappers led by John Work first referred to them as "the buttes" in 1833, on a journey that unwittingly introduced smallpox, which ultimately devastated the local Indian tribes. Because of flooding in the valley, the Work party camped on the slopes of the Buttes for a month, which at the time teemed with elk, deer, antelope, and bears. John C. Fremont and his soldiers, along with scout Kit Carson, camped at the Buttes in 1846 while awaiting orders to participate in the Bear Flag Revolt, which ultimately led to the annexation of California by the United States. In 1849, gold was discovered on the American River, and California was changed forever. But the Sutter Buttes remain much as they have been for thousands of years.

A spring visit to the Sutter Buttes presents a dazzling array of wildflowers including poppies, popcorn flowers, lupine, blue dick, storks bill, soaproot, Dutch pipe vine (and its accompanying pipevine swallow-tail butterflies), cowbag udder, woodland star, lace pod, mule ears, creamcups, and some of the largest baby blue eyes you may ever see. Valley oaks dominate the lower elevations and meadow fringes of the Buttes, but these stately giants quickly give way to the smaller blue and live oaks on the slopes, upper canyons, and ridges. 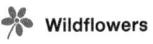 **Wildflowers**

Songbirds thrive in the oak woodlands and meadows, including phainopepla, meadowlarks, lark sparrows, yellow-rumped warblers, and Audubon warblers. Acorn woodpeckers and turkey vultures are common, and an occasional golden eagle can be seen enjoying thermals created by the Buttes. **Birds**

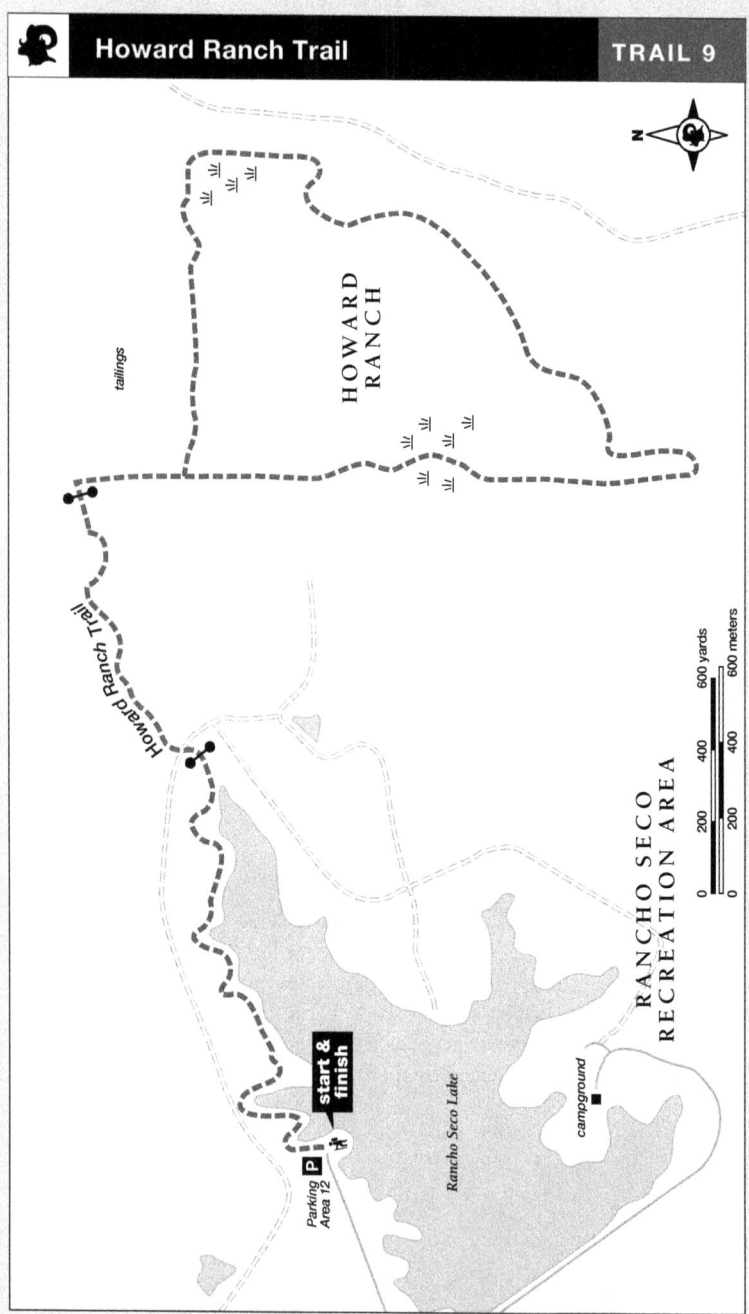

TRAIL 9 The Great Valley

Howard Ranch Trail

The Great Valley has lost 99 percent of its native grasslands. What hasn't been tilled for agriculture or paved for development has been overwhelmed by non-native grass species. Public opportunities to view the Valley's few remaining open grasslands are limited. The Howard Ranch Trail, which begins in Rancho Seco Park, provides perhaps one of the best opportunities to visit the Great Valley grassland (as transformed as it is by exotic grasses) and vernal pool ecosystem. The Nature Conservancy purchased the ranch in 1999 from the heirs of Charles Howard (of Seabiscuit fame) and then resold it to a local rancher while retaining conservation easements. The California Conservation Corps constructed the trail, which is maintained by the Sacramento Municipal Utility District (SMUD). SMUD also manages the adjacent Rancho Seco Park. The trail offers nice views of Rancho Seco Lake and provides access to the open, rolling grasslands at the base of the Sierra foothills. It circles a large area of vernal pools—shallow pools that provide important seasonal wetland habitat and a gorgeous display of spring wildflowers.

Best Time

Spring is absolutely the best time to view wildflowers and the green, rolling countryside. Spring comes early to this lowland (250–300 feet in elevation), so plan on a visit in March or early April.

TRAIL USE
Hike
LENGTH
6.83 miles, 2–3 hours
VERTICAL FEET
±50
DIFFICULTY
- 1 2 3 **4** 5 +
TRAIL TYPE
Loop
SURFACE TYPE
Dirt
Gravel

FEATURES
Child Friendly
Entrance Fee
Wildflowers
Wetlands
Lake
Meadows
Canyon
Birds
Great Views
Photo Opportunity

FACILITIES
Porta-potty

Typical vernal pool wildflowers include tidy tips, goldfields, and purple owl's clover.

Finding the Trail

From Sacramento, drive south 21 miles on Hwy 99. Take the Hwy 104 Jackson exit (also Twin Cities Rd. and Exit 277). Turn left on the frontage road and then left on Hwy 104 and drive over the Hwy 99 freeway. Drive east 12.3 miles on Hwy 104 and turn right on the road marked with the large sign saying RANCHO SECO PARK. Drive 0.3 mile, and turn left at a sign directing you to the Rancho Seco Recreation Area. Drive 0.5 mile to the park entry station; pay the $5 entrance fee. Continue 0.6 mile and turn left on the gravel road with a sign directing you to the Howard Ranch Trail. Drive 0.3 mile to parking area 12 and the Howard Ranch Trailhead.

Logistics

Water and a concession stand are available on the other side of Rancho Seco Lake, near the campground. No water is available at the trailhead or along the trail. The Howard Ranch is private land with public access allowed on the trail only. Please stick to the trail and do not harass or otherwise bother grazing cattle.

Trail Description

≋ **Lake**

From Parking Area 12, the trail follows the shoreline of **Rancho Seco Lake** eastward. ▶1 Built as an emergency water supply for the now defunct Rancho Seco nuclear power plant, the lake is a popular destination for local anglers, and the trail provides access to a couple of fishing piers. The lakeshore is lined with willows, cottonwoods, bulrushes, and blackberry brambles, and hosts a variety of waterfowl, including ducks, geese, and swans. Along this first leg of the trail, hikers will be treated to the colorful displays of blue dicks and other flowers in the brodiaea family. As it parallels the meandering lakeshore, the

Howard Ranch Trail | TRAIL 9

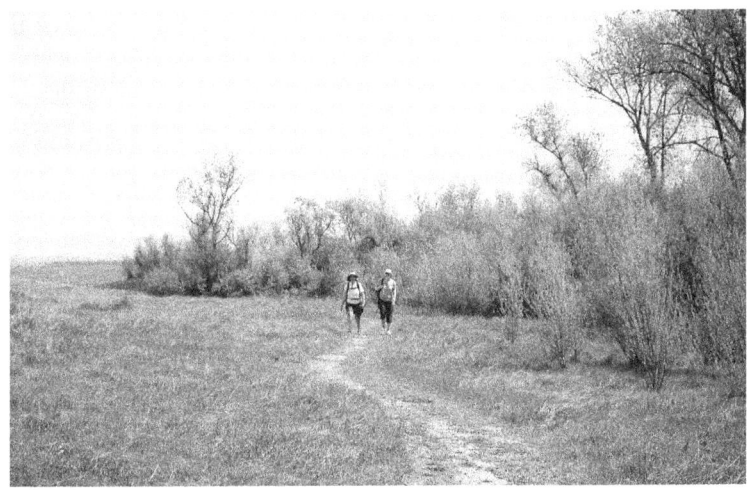

Hikers *on the Howard Ranch Trail*

trail crosses shallow tributary drainages on sturdy boardwalks. Eventually, the trail comes to the end of the lake and reaches a fence line.

A bit over 1.0 mile from the trailhead, the trail passes through a green pedestrian gate in the fence, leaving Rancho Seco Park behind and entering the privately owned **Howard Ranch**. ▶2 Be sure to close the gate after you. From the gate, the trail climbs easily up a grassy drainage in a northwest direction. A broad expanse of rolling, green grasslands surrounds you as the trail climbs toward some low mounds of dredge tailings. On the distant horizon, you may see the snowy peaks of the Sierra Nevada. Small frying pan poppies and buttercups sprinkle the trailside. Singing meadowlarks and horned larks are common in this area. Red-tailed hawks circle overhead. Fiberglass wands occasionally mark the trail.

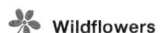 **Wildflowers**

The trail reaches another fence line and second green gate a bit over 0.5 mile from the last gate. ▶3 Go through the second gate (again making sure that it closes behind you) and turn right to follow the firebreak that parallels the fence line southward. On your left are small mounds of dredge tailings, either from an unsuccessful gold mining attempt or perhaps left over from the construction of Rancho Seco Lake. Behind the tailings, cottonwoods are revegetating shallow ponds. These provide the only shade found along the trail. The trail continues south along the fence and crosses an ephemeral drainage.

Just past the crossing, you will come to a trail junction—this is the beginning and the end of the vernal pools loop of the Howard Ranch Trail. A wand lying on the ground notes that this junction is either mile 2.0 or mile 5.0 of your walk, depending on which direction you're going. My mapping program says it is 1.85 miles—close enough. ▶4 Turn left at the junction and proceed east on a slightly raised trail bed of gravel that parallels the shallow drainage you crossed just before the junction. The trail crosses two wooden walkways and skirts the edge of the tailings and some ponds with a lone stand of cottonwoods on the left.

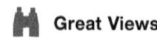
Great Views

The trail reaches the brink of a wide drainage running from north to south and delineated by a fence line. At this point, the trail bends, turning south-southwest and follows the rim of the shallow canyon. From here, you will have an even better view of the Sierra Nevada and its oak-studded foothills, which appear tantalizingly close but remain out of reach. The broad expanse to the right is dimpled by vernal pools. Here you will have an excellent opportunity to explore the pools and their bright rings of wildflowers, which advance inward as the shallow pools dry up during the spring.

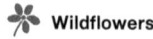
Wildflowers

As the trail follows the rim of the shallow canyon, there is a fine view of the beginning of the Sierra foothills just to the east, as well as a bucolic swath of pasture and wildflowers, grazing cattle, and a large stock pond just to the south. The trail zigzags

Howard Ranch Trail — TRAIL 9

southwest as it follows the peninsulas and drainages that carve the rim of the mini-canyon.

Nearly 3.66 miles into your hike, the trail reconnects with the fence line and firebreak that you left at Milestone 4. Turn right and follow the fence line northward. ▶5 To the northwest are the brooding cooling towers of the Rancho Seco nuclear plant and the shoreline vegetation hiding Rancho Seco Lake. To the right is the largest complex of vernal pools on the hike. At one point, the trail/firebreak moves away from the fence line to avoid a particularly deep set of pools, but it soon returns to its parallel course. You may find large clumps of lupine along this trail segment.

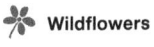 **Wildflowers**

Return to the **T** junction at Milestone 4. ▶6 Retrace your steps through the second and first gates to Rancho Seco Lake and return ▶7 to the trailhead parking area.

MILESTONES

- ▶1   0.00   Trailhead parking area next to Rancho Seco Lake, proceed east
- ▶2   1.05   First gate at end of lake, continue straight (east)
- ▶3   1.64   Second gate, turn right (south) and follow firebreak along fence
- ▶4   1.85   Trail junction, turn left to follow vernal pool loop
- ▶5   3.63   Trail junction, turn right and follow firebreak north along fence
- ▶6   4.53   Return to first trail junction, go straight to retrace steps to trailhead
- ▶7   6.83   Return to trailhead parking area

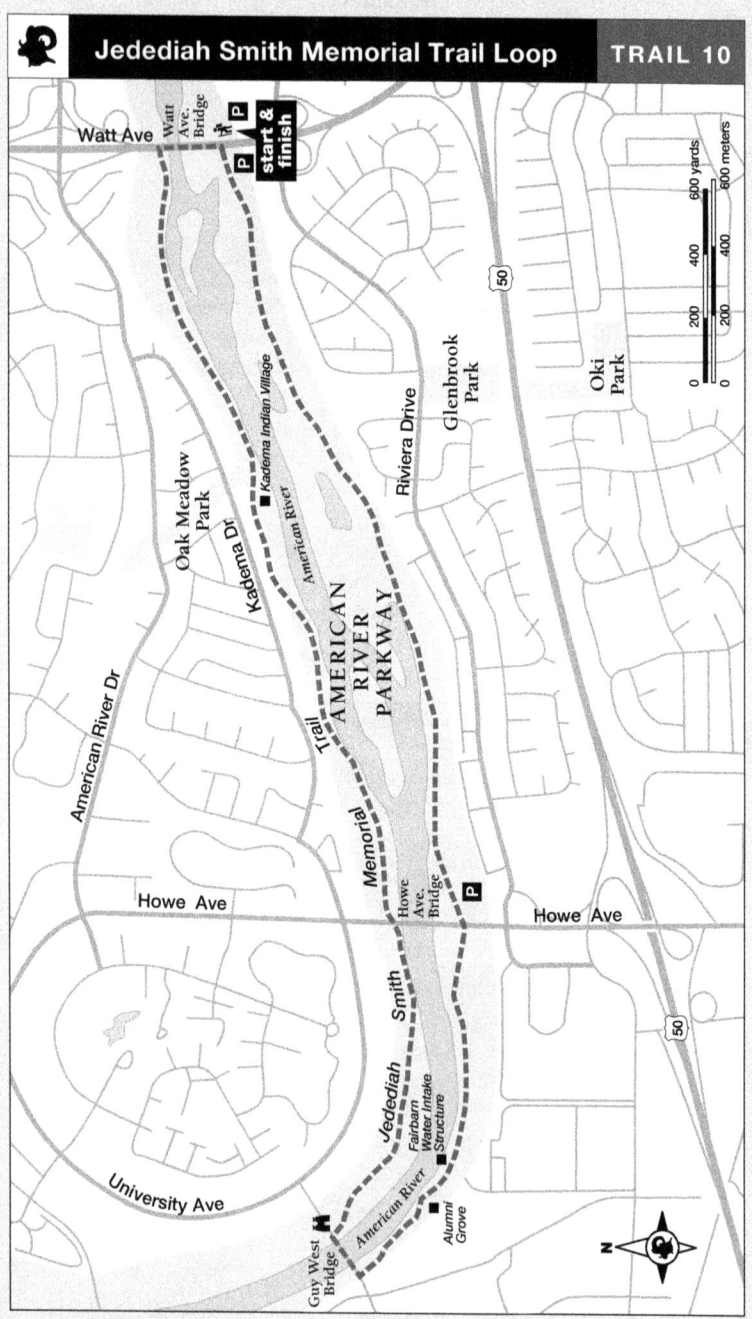

TRAIL 10 The Great Valley

Jedediah Smith Memorial Trail Loop: American River Parkway

The Jedediah Smith Memorial Trail is a popular 31-mile paved bicycle and pedestrian route that begins at Beals Point in the Folsom Lake State Recreation Area and follows the American River Parkway eastward to Discovery Park, at the confluence of the American and Sacramento rivers. For those who prefer a more intimate introduction to the trail and the parkway, this is one of several sections of the trail suitable for exploring on foot. This section of the Parkway has reciprocal trails on the north and south sides of the river, which allows for a 4.2 mile loop along the river and through its wildlife-rich riparian forest.

Best Time

Pretty much anytime is a good time to walk this loop. You can avoid hot summer afternoons and see more wildlife by walking in the morning. Because this loop trail is entirely located on the river side of the levee system, it would be a good idea to check on flood conditions in the American River Parkway before walking this loop in the winter or spring.

Finding the Trail

From Sacramento, drive east on Hwy 50 to the Watt Ave. exit. Go north on Watt Ave. and just before the American River bridge, turn right on La Riviera Dr. Make a U-turn at the first left turn lane and backtrack to Parkway entrance just before the bridge, turn right. Pay your $4 parking fee at the kiosk and then drop down over the levee to the parking areas east and west of the bridge.

TRAIL USE
Hike, Run, Bike
LENGTH
4.2 miles, 1.5–3 hours
VERTICAL FEET
±0
DIFFICULTY
- 1 2 **3** 4 5 +
TRAIL TYPE
Loop
SURFACE TYPE
Paved

FEATURES
Child Friendly
Handicapped Accessible
Dogs on Leash
Parking
River
Birds
Wildlife
Historic
Interpretive Signs
Great Views
Photo Opportunity

FACILITIES
Toilets
Water

After becoming the first European explorer to cross the Sierra Nevada, mountain man Jedediah Smith camped along the American River in 1827, which he named the "Wild River."

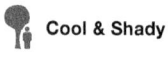
Cool & Shady

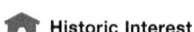
Historic Interest

Logistics

A $4 fee is charged for parking. Call the Sacramento County Parks Department at (916) 875-6672 to check on potential flood conditions in the American River Parkway during winter and spring. The parking area can fill up fast on high-use summer weekends. Despite its wild appearance, this is an urban park and trail. It's always a good idea to walk with a friend, be done well before dusk, and do not leave valuables in your car.

Trail Description

Proceed to the west end of the Watt Ave. parking area. The paved southside trail begins there by heading into the riverside forest consisting of cottonwoods, sycamores, and willows. ▶1 The trail is frequented by bicycles, so be sure to walk along the dirt shoulder to give bicycles plenty of room to pass. As you head west through the forest, with the river levee on your left, you will notice several opportunities to follow use-trails down to the river's edge. Shortly after leaving the Watt Ave. parking area, the trail rises out of the forest, and follows a bench midway along the levee.

Much of what is now the **American River Parkway** consisted of piles of cobbles left over from the gold mining era, some 150 years ago. After the mining era, the riparian forest began reestablishing itself, and Sacramento began to recognize the natural and recreational values of the river. The first trail was built along the river in 1896 by early bicyclists. As Sacramento grew in the 1960s, community visionaries established a parkway between the river levees. The American River Parkway would soon grow to attract millions of visitors annually, who picnic, swim, boat, fish, hike, and bicycle its length through the heart of the state's capital.

Jedediah Smith Memorial Trail Loop — TRAIL 10

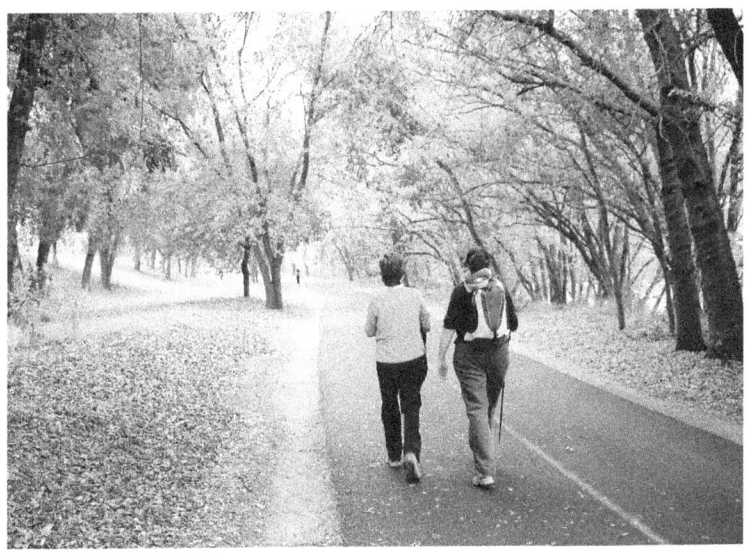

The Jedediah Smith Trail *is suitable for walking, running, and bicycling.*

About 1.5 miles west of your starting point, the trail reaches the Howe Ave. parking area and it proceeds under the Howe Ave. bridge. Vault toilets and water are available here. Continue west on the trail. ▶2 Wildlife is common along the trail, including geese, ducks, raptors, and even deer. As you proceed west down the trail, you will see a large structure in the river. This is the City of Sacramento's Fairbarn Water Intake Structure. Shortly after passing the structure, the trail reaches an open area with grass and picnic tables shaded by oaks. This is the **Alumni Grove** of the California State University, Sacramento. The busy campus is just over the levee on the left.

 Wildlife

Just past the Alumni Grove, the trail reaches the **Guy West Bridge**, which provides pedestrian and bicycle access across the river. Turn right to cross the bridge ▶3 and enjoy the scenic views up and down the river.

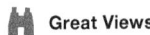 Great Views

River

After crossing the bridge, turn right again to connect with the **Jedediah Smith Memorial Trail**, ▶4 which extends from Beals Point in the Folsom Lake State Recreation Area 31 miles west, along the American River to Discovery Park, at the confluence of the American and Sacramento Rivers. The Jedediah Smith Memorial Trail became a recognized national trail in 1974.

The Jedediah Smith Trail is heavily used by bicycles. Be sure to walk along the shoulder to avoid collisions with speeding bicyclists. As you proceed east on the paved Jedediah Smith Trail, you will notice that a dirt equestrian trail parallels your paved path. If you want to enjoy a more natural walk that leads you into the trees along the river and away from the bicycle traffic, feel free to meander along the equestrian trail. As you walk along the north bank, you can't help but notice that the character of the vegetation is much more open and dry. Oaks and coyote bush tend to dominate the landscape, as compared to the more water-loving cottonwoods and sycamores on the south bank. Whether this is because the north bank vegetation represents a more mature vegetative succession or because the south bank faces north and captures more rain and therefore is more conducive to moisture-loving vegetation is for the ecologists to debate.

About 0.5 mile after crossing the Guy West Bridge, the trail reaches and passes under the Howe Ave. bridge, ▶5 where you'll find benches, a portapotty and a water fountain. Continue east on the Jedediah Smith Trail or its parallel equestrian trail. About 0.5 mile east of the Howe Ave. bridge, the trail reaches a interpretive sign informing trail users

Historic Interest

that this is the site of the **Kadema Indian Village**. Nisenan Maidu Indians lived here for more than 1500 years, fishing for salmon, hunting for deer, and gathering acorns. It supported as many as 500 Maidu and was one of the largest and most

Jediah Smith Memorial Trail Loop | TRAIL 10

permanent villages along the river. Urban development and the north levee now cover most of the village site, but the sign at least reminds us that Jedediah Smith or some other European did not "discover" the American River at all. It in fact had been the home of local people for hundreds of years. Benches and a water fountain are available at the Kadema site.

About 0.5 mile east of Kadema, the Jedediah Smith Trail reaches the north side of the Watt Ave. bridge, where you'll find a vault toilet and drinking water. Follow the connector path to the left that climbs the levee and connects with the sidewalk along the west edge of the bridge. ▶6 Turn right and follow the sidewalk over the bridge to the north bank of the river. As you cross the bridge, look for anglers fishing from drift boats anchored downstream of the bridge. The American River provides important spawning habitat for Chinook salmon and steelhead trout.

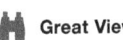 **Great Views**

After crossing the bridge, turn right to drop down to the Watt Ave. bridge parking area ▶7 and return to your car.

MILESTONES

▶1	0.00	From the Watt Ave. parking area, head west on southside trail
▶2	1.50	Continue west on trail under Howe Ave. bridge
▶3	2.00	Turn right, cross river on the Guy West pedestrian/bicycle bridge
▶4	2.10	After crossing bridge, turn right on Jedediah Smith Trail
▶5	2.60	Continue east on Jedediah Smith Trail under Howe Ave. bridge
▶6	4.10	Turn right, cross river on Watt Ave. bridge
▶7	4.20	Turn right and drop down from the levee to return to parking area

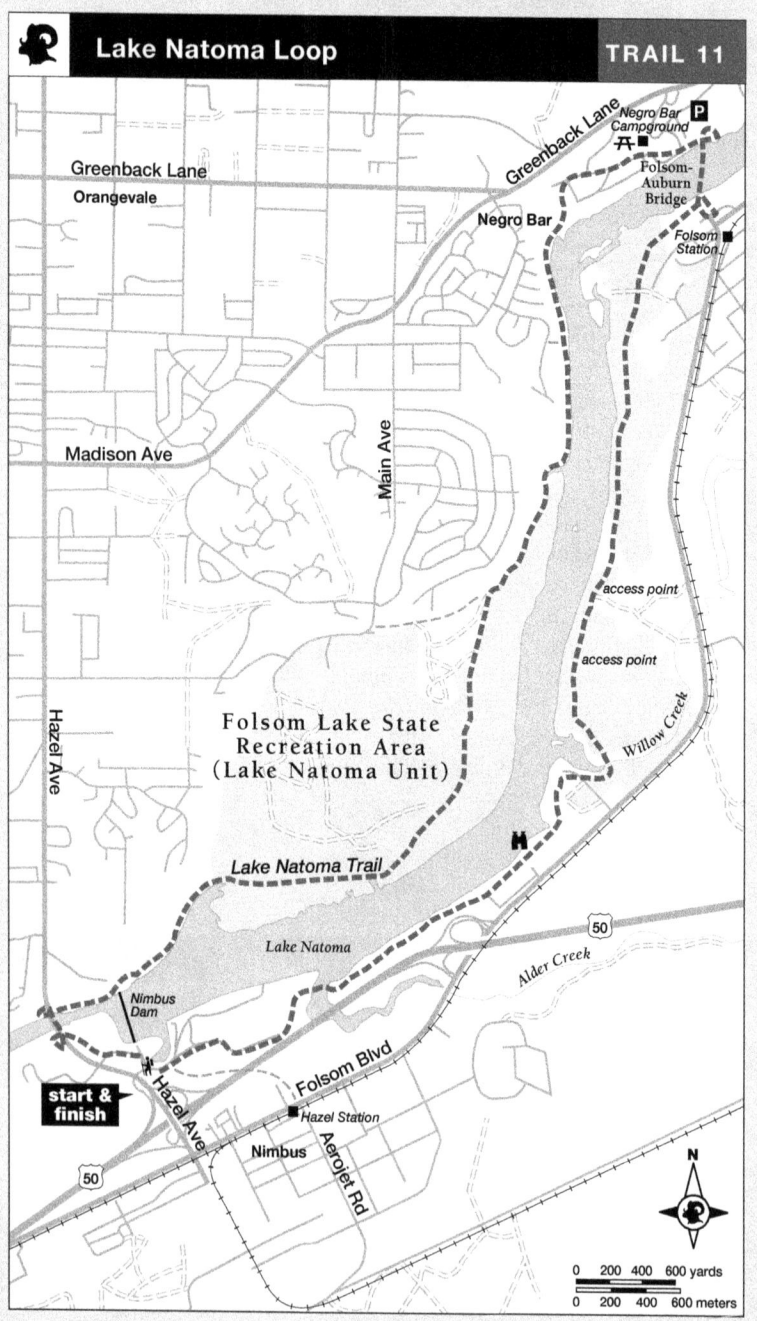

TRAIL 11 The Great Valley

Lake Natoma Loop: Folsom Lake State Recreation Area

Scenic Lake Natoma is the focus of this paved loop trail, and it offers a number of options for exploration by foot, bike, or even kayak. The end points of the loop have easy access to light rail public transportation, which means you can leave your car at home. It also means that you can do half the loop and make your way back to your starting point via light rail. Wildlife abounds in the marshes and oak woodlands along the loop, which also provides glimpses of Gold Rush history.

Best Time

Fall and spring are the best times to use this loop trail. Early morning treks are advisable in the summer to avoid the heat. Clear winter days can also be quite pleasant.

Finding the Trail

Drive east on Hwy 50 to the Hazel Ave. exit. Turn left (north) on Hazel Ave. and cross over the freeway. Just before the Hazel Ave. bridge, turn right into the Lake Natoma Unit of the Folsom State Recreation Area. If you come to the light with the CSUS Aquatic Center on your right and the Nimbus Fish Hatchery on your left, you have driven about 100 feet too far. Avoid the temptation of free parking in the park-and-ride lot, and continue to the entrance of the State Recreation Area, pay the $5 entrance fee, and park in the lot just beyond the entrance station. The bike path/loop trail starts at the eastern end of the lot.

TRAIL USE
Bike, Hike, Run, Horse

LENGTH
10.3 miles, 4–5 hours

VERTICAL FEET
±50 feet

DIFFICULTY
- 1 2 3 **4** 5 +

TRAIL TYPE
Loop

SURFACE TYPE
Dirt
Paved for Bikes

FEATURES
Child Friendly
Handicapped Accessible
Dogs on Leash
Parking Fee
Lake
River
Wetlands
Birds
Wildlife
Historic
Interpretive Signs
Great Views
Photo Opportunity

FACILITIES
Water
Toilets

Lake Natoma is a popular recreation destination for bicyclists, canoers, kayakers, and birders.

Bike riders and hikers can access this trail by light rail and avoid parking hassles and reduce air pollution as well. To get to the trailhead by light rail, take the Folsom line east to the Hazel Station on Folsom Ave. From the Hazel Station, walk east on Folsom Ave. 0.2 mile to the intersection with Aerojet Road. Cross Aerojet Road and then turn left at the light and cross Folsom. A bike path leads north between the freeway off ramp on the left and the car lot on the right. This bike path goes over Hwy 50 and connects with the Lake Natoma Loop Trail just east of the trailhead parking lot.

People who want to do just the first 4.5 miles of this hike (from the trailhead to the Auburn–Folsom Road Bridge in Folsom) may turn left at Auburn–Folsom Road (instead of right to cross the bridge) and proceed 100 feet south to Folsom light rail station. From there, they can take a westbound light rail train to the Hazel Station.

Logistics

The entire loop is paved and provides one of the most enjoyable bike rides in the region. A dirt path for hikers and equestrians roughly parallels the south side of the loop, so the route also provides an enjoyable walk. If you don't want to walk the entire 10.3-mile loop, you can walk from Hazel Ave. to Folsom and take light rail back to Hazel Ave., or vice versa. The north side of the loop also has a dirt path along its shoulder.

Trail Description

Pick up the bike path along the edge of the Lake Natoma Unit parking area ▶1. As you head east on the path, it leaves the parking area behind and follows a service road (a sign says CLOSED AREA, but that means closed to motor vehicles) through an

Lake Natoma Loop | TRAIL 11

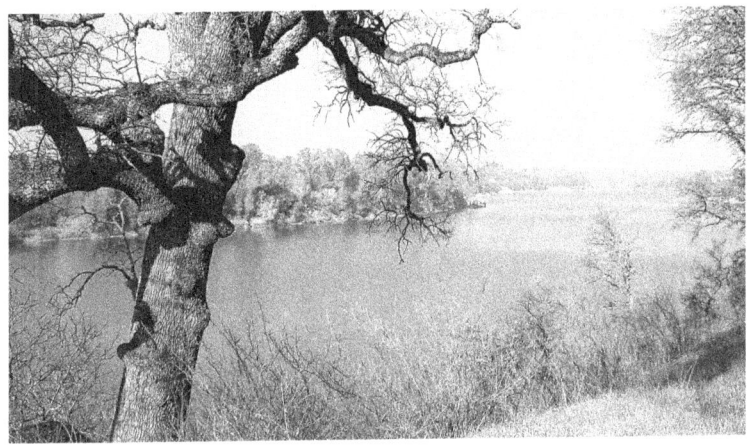

Scenic Lake Natoma *is the heart of this loop trail.*

oak forest. Within 0.5 mile, a path breaks off to the right—this is the path to the bike/pedestrian bridge crossing Hwy 50 and leading to the Hazel light rail station. Continue straight on the service road, past another bike path junction on the left. Just beyond, you come to a Y junction; veer right off the service road, and continue east on the bike path.

The path crosses the mouth of **Alder Creek** on a foot/bike bridge and continues eastward ▶2 through pleasant oak woodlands with views of **Lake Natoma** on your left and occasional glimpses of the Hwy 50 freeway on your right. Soon the path moves away from the freeway and, after passing another bike path junction on your right leading to Folsom Blvd., it climbs slightly and comes to a bluff overlook with a beautiful vista of Lake Natoma. The path parallels the bluff as it passes occasional picnic tables. An interpretive sign notes that the gray pines visible on the north side of the lake provide a rookery for nesting herons.

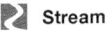 Stream

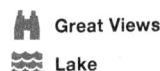 Great Views
Lake

Lake Natoma is a steady-state reservoir created by Nimbus Dam on the American River. Nimbus Dam was intended to divert water into the

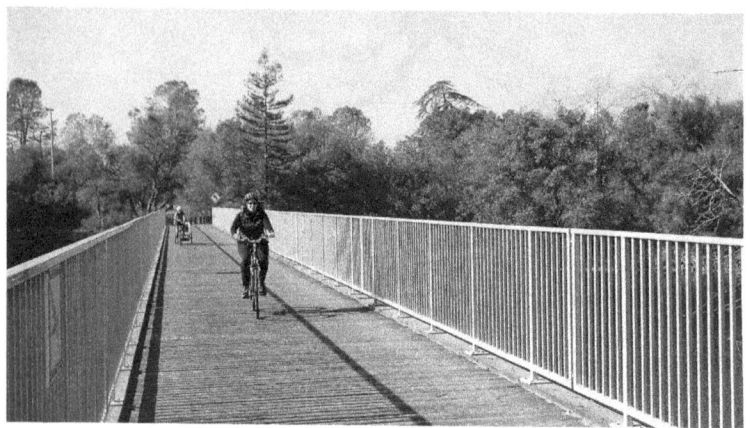

One of several bridges *crossing various inlets to Lake Natoma*

Folsom-South Canal, but a lawsuit by conservationists ultimately prevented much of the diversion, which threatened to dewater the American River. Today, it is managed by the California Department of Parks and Recreation as part of the Folsom State Recreation Area. The American River Parkway begins just downstream of Nimbus Dam.

🏠 **Historic Interest**

The bike path drops down into a grove of gray pines punctuated by mounds of rounded river rock—debris left over from the Gold Rush mining days. Go past two more bike path junctions on your right (both leading to Folsom Boulevard) and continue east to the Willow Creek parking area. Water and restrooms are available here.

Stream

Continue east on the path as it crosses ▶3 **Willow Creek** on a foot/pedestrian bridge and then makes its way through more gray pines, live oaks, and rock mounds. More picnic tables on the left offer places to stop and view the lake. This portion of the trail is somewhat urbanized, as it parallels a power line overhead, and occasional buildings are visible over the trees on the right. Despite the urban intrusions, you may hear geese honking on the lake.

Lake Natoma Loop | TRAIL 11

As you continue east on the south side of the lake, enjoy the view of the high, clay bluffs that rim the north shore. You may glimpse bicycle riders or walkers making their way along the foot of the bluffs as they follow the western leg of the loop. Your current path continues east past a bike path junction on the right leading to Parkshore St. It climbs out of the river bottom, past another bike path junction on the right leading to Folsom Ave., and then proceeds under the relatively new **Folsom–Auburn Bridge**.

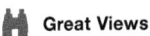 Great Views

Just after crossing under the bridge, ▶4 turn right into the Lake Natoma Inn parking area. Continue in a 180-degree loop to the right as your path climbs the southeast abutment of the bridge to the bike/pedestrian walkway along the bridge's east side. If you are doing this segment as a point-to-point hike, turn left here to go to the Folsom Light Rail Station. If you are doing the full loop, turn right to cross the bridge. As you cross the Folsom–Auburn Bridge, stop at one of several benches to admire the view of the architecturally interesting and old Rainbow Bridge, upstream.

After leaving the bridge, you come to the intersection of Folsom–Auburn Road and Greenback. ▶5 Turn right to follow the sidewalk along the Greenback for about 20 feet until you come to a green BIKE PATH sign and another sign that says NEGRO BAR PARK ACCESS. Turn right at this sign to follow a narrow bike path as it switchbacks steeply downward. The final switchback leads you westward, past a bike path junction on the left leading to a parking lot; then your path connects with an access road.

Continue west on the access road, past the Negro Bar Group Campground and then past another parking lot. Veer left off the access road and back onto the paved bike path. Continue west to a large flat, which is used by equestrians. An interpretive sign notes that this area was once the bustling

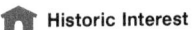 Historic Interest

mining town of Negro Bar. William Leidesdorff acquired it as part of a 35,521-acre land grant in 1848. It was purchased by J. L. Folsom in 1849, when the Gold Rush was in full swing. The area was mined by African Americans, and the town had a population of 700 people. It was supplanted in 1855 by the town of Folsom on the other side of the river.

Just past the equestrian area, the high, clay bluffs close in from the right. The path follows the foot of the bluff along the north side of the lake. Just past a gully that breaks the façade of the bluffs, the path reaches the junction with the Snowberry Trail on the right. Continue straight as the path begins the longest (but still modest) climb of the loop to the Mississippi Bar area. At the top, the path makes it way through a largely open area punctuated by rock mounds and groves of live oaks.

The path reaches another junction on the right, leading to Main Ave. A sign says HAZEL AVE.—3.5 MILES, pointing the way west. Continue straight across Mississippi Bar and past several equestrian trail junctions on the right. Soon the bluffs close in again from the north. Across the lake, you can see the California State University Sacramento Aquatic Center and the top of Nimbus Dam. The path curves around a fenced-in transformer area and passes the north end of Nimbus Dam. For the first time, you can see the American River beginning at the foot of the dam and large gravel bar favored by anglers for salmon and steelhead. The path continues downstream, past a bike path junction leading up the northeastern side of Hazel Ave., and then proceeds ▶6 west under the Hazel Ave. Bridge.

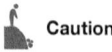
River

Just after crossing under the bridge, the path climbs steeply up to the right along the northwest bridge abutment and then turns right to connect with the narrow walkway on the west side of the bridge. Cross carefully, as the walkway is heavily

Caution

Lake Natoma Loop | TRAIL 11

used by pedestrians and bike riders. As you cross the bridge to the south side, you get a good view of the Nimbus Fish Hatchery just downstream.

▶7 After crossing the bridge, the path drops down to the right along the southwestern bridge abutment and comes to a **T** junction. Turn sharply right and proceed north to the river. Turn right again and cross under the Hazel Ave. Bridge, and then turn right once again to climb the bridge's southeastern abutment. ▶8 After you climb the abutment, the path's ascent flattens as it reaches the Hazel Ave./Nimbus Road/Gold River Road intersection. Follow the path to the left as it crosses the entrance to the Aquatic Center parking lot, and then circles the lot as it proceeds southeastward to the Natoma Unit parking area. ▶9 The path goes past the Aquatic Center buildings on the left, across the gate structure spanning the Folsom–South Canal, and to the Natoma Unit entrance. ▶10 Proceed to the parking area.

MILESTONES

▶1	0.00	Start at the Lake Natoma Unit parking area
▶2	0.77	Cross the Alder Creek bridge, continue straight
▶3	2.24	Cross the Willow Creek bridge, continue straight
▶4	4.45	Cross under Folsom–Auburn Bridge, circle right to cross bridge
▶5	4.55	Turn right at Greenback, follow Negro Bar bike path to the right
▶6	9.70	Go under Hazel Ave. Bridge, circle to the right to cross
▶7	9.90	After crossing the bridge, follow the bike path to the right
▶8	10.00	Circle under Hazel Ave. Bridge and follow bike path to the right
▶9	10.10	Go left and circle the Aquatic Center parking lot, cross canal
▶10	10.30	Return to Lake Natoma Unit parking area

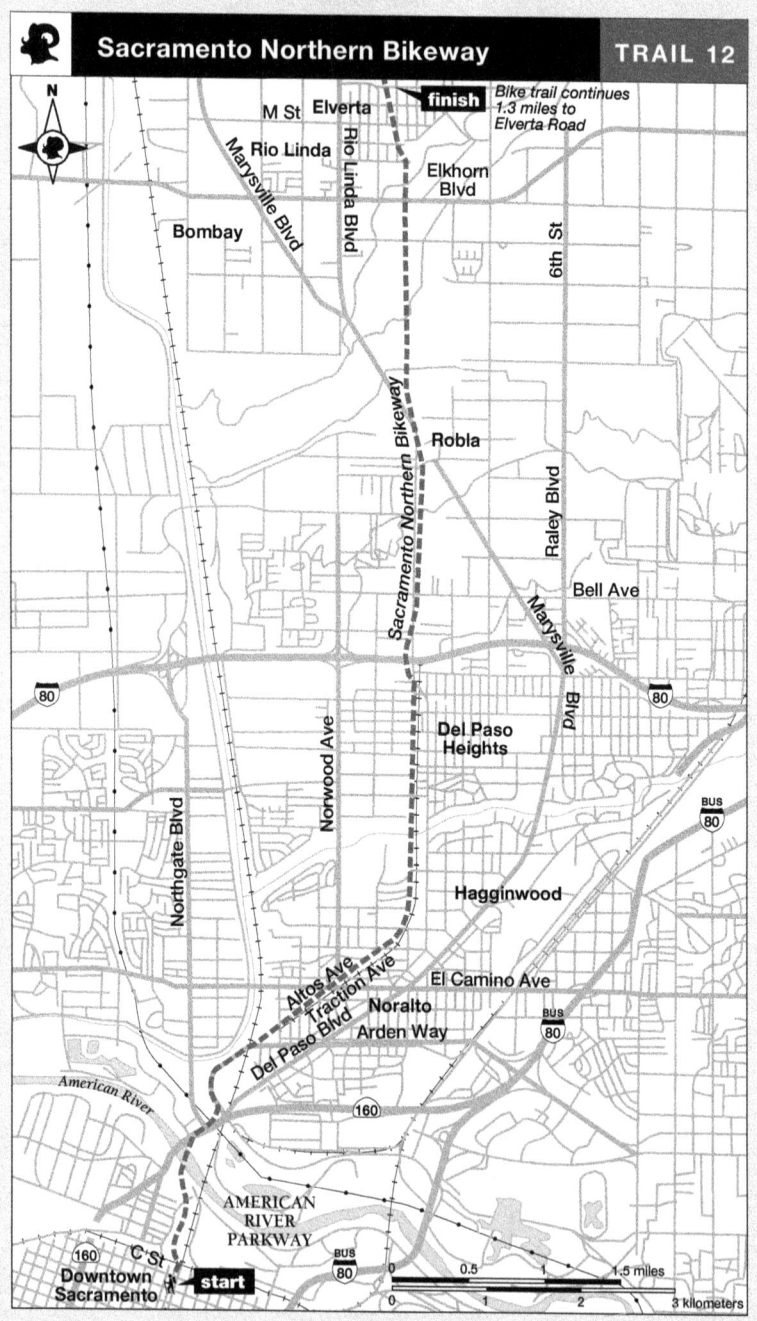

TRAIL 12 The Great Valley

Sacramento Northern Bikeway

This scenic bikeway runs from downtown Sacramento to the semirural community of Elverta in northern Sacramento County. It follows the route of the historic Sacramento Northern Railroad. Along the way, it crosses the American River and its scenic Parkway, several small neighborhood creeks, and the wooded floodplain of Dry Creek (a parkway in the making). It also connects downtown Sacramento with the northern neighborhoods and communities of Noralto, Del Paso Heights, Robla, Rio Linda, and Elverta. This is an excellent excursion for those who would like to explore this region of Sacramento by bike.

Best Time

This is a year-round bikeway. To avoid summer heat, it's best to ride in the morning or early evening. The more rural portions of the bikeway are quite scenic in the spring, with green pastures, poppies and other wildflowers, and newly-leafed oak trees lining the route.

Finding the Trail

The bikeway begins on C St. between 19th and 20th streets in downtown Sacramento, and out-and-back trips would also end here. Another option is to bike one way, to Elverta, and return by car shuttle. To drop off a vehicle for a car shuttle, drive north approximately 3.0 miles on Interstate 5 from downtown Sacramento to the junction with Interstate 80. Turn east on Interstate 80 and drive approximately

TRAIL USE
Hike, Run, Bike
LENGTH
10 miles one way, 4–5 hours
VERTICAL FEET
±0
DIFFICULTY
- 1 2 3 **4** 5 +
TRAIL TYPE
Point to Point
Out & Back
SURFACE TYPE
Paved

FEATURES
Child Friendly
Handicapped Accessible
Dogs on Leash
River
Streams
Wetlands
Meadows
Wildflowers
Birds
Wildlife
Historic

FACILITIES
Pavilions

Scattered stands of blue oak close in on both sides of the bikeway.

6.0 miles to the Raley/Marysville Blvd. exit. Take this exit, turn left, and go over the freeway, driving 0.2 mile north to Bell Ave. Turn left and drive 0.3 mile on Bell Ave. Turn right and drive 1.3 miles north on Marysville Blvd. Turn right on Rio Linda Blvd. and drive 3.7 miles north on Rio Linda to Elverta Road. Just before reaching the Elverta Road intersection, turn right into the small parking area that serves a pavilion at the end of the bikeway.

Logistics

See above for the one-way trip with car shuttle option. The lower portion of the bikeway goes through some of Sacramento's more economically depressed neighborhoods. For safety purposes, ride this bikeway with a friend and don't ride it after dark. Bring water on your bike ride, as trailside water fountains are largely not working. The bikeway north of the American River is for the most part handicapped accessible—the section that crosses the American River climbs and drops steeply over levees, which may be problematic for wheelchairs.

Trail Description

An archway on C St. announces that this is the entrance to the **Sacramento Northern Bikeway**, which follows the former right-of-way of the Sacramento Northern Railroad. Pass under the arch and proceed north ▶1 on the bikeway, which passes under the Union Pacific Railroad (UPRR) main east/west line and parallels the UPRR main north/south line on the right. On the left is the Diamond Nuts industrial plant, from which emanates the pleasant smell of roasting nuts.

At its peak, the Sacramento Northern Railroad was one of the largest electric interurban railways in the nation. It ultimately covered 185 miles,

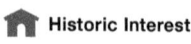 Historic Interest

Sacramento Northern Bikeway | TRAIL **12**

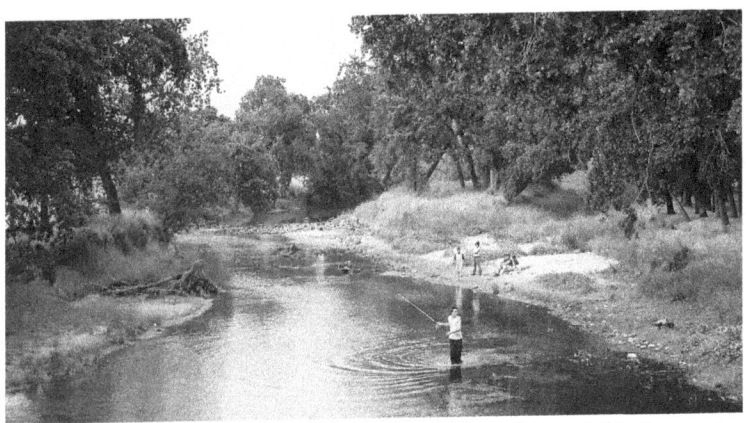

The Dry Creek Parkway is one of the scenic features of the northern end of the Sacramento Northern Bikeway.

connecting San Francisco with Sacramento and Chico. The Sacramento–Chico section began as the Northern Electric Railroad in 1904, and became a subsidiary of the Western Pacific Railroad in 1921. The northern link was merged with the San Francisco–Sacramento Railroad in 1928. SNRR trains crossed Suisun Bay by ferry, negotiated the Oakland hills, and stopped at the Oakland waterfront. Direct service to San Francisco began when the Oakland Bay Bridge was completed in 1938. The electric system switched to diesel locomotives in 1941. Passenger use declined after World Way II, and passenger service to the Bay Area was discontinued in 1951. The SNRR continued to run freight trains between Sacramento and Chico for several years, often astounding college students as they left downtown Chico bars at 2 a.m. only to find a SNRR train slowly proceeding up tracks on Main St. The entire line was discontinued when the SNRR was acquired by Union Pacific Railroad in 1983.

The bikeway turns left and follows the northern fence line of the Diamond plant. It reaches a Y junction with a bike path connector to 16th St.

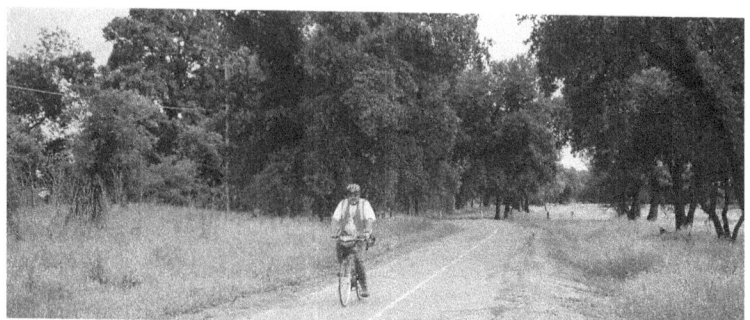

The Sacramento Northern Bikeway crosses the blue oaks and meadows of the Dry Creek floodplain.

River

Turn right and continue north on the Sacramento Northern Bikeway, which crosses the American River over a steel-girder bridge. As you cross the river, you can see the UPRR bridge upstream and the Hwy 160 bridge downstream. After crossing the river, the bikeway drops down into the Woodlake Area of the **American River Parkway**, noted by a trailside sign. The bikeway passes the end of Northgate Blvd. on the left, and then curves left to go under the Hwy 160 overpass, and then curves right to reach the junction with the **Jedediah Smith Memorial Trail** (JSMT).

Turn left on the JSMT ▶2 and then cross Del Paso Blvd. (after first carefully checking for traffic). Almost immediately, this short segment of the combined JSMT and Sacramento Northern Bikeway reaches a Y junction. Veer right to leave the JSMT ▶3 and to follow the Sacramento Northern Bikeway up a levee. The bikeway follows the top of the levee as it curves right and to the north to parallel for a short distance the Natomas East Main Drain Canal (more positively known as Steelhead Creek by the locals).

Stream

The bikeway crosses the UPRR north/south tracks and then drops down off the levee and goes under the Arden St. overpass. Bike path connectors lead off to the right on each side of the overpass to link with local streets. From here, the bikeway continues in a northeast direction under an arch announcing that you are entering the northern Sacramento neighborhood of Noralto. After crossing Colfax St., the bikeway follows the broad and nicely landscaped former right-of-way of the SNRR. Altos and Traction avenues parallel both sides of the linear bikeway park as it enters a residential area. Occasional connector paths lead off to the right and left. Bicyclists, dog walkers, families, and other local residents clearly enjoy and use this section of the bikeway.

The first of several pavilions providing shade and benches where you can rest and enjoy the bikeway park is located at the bikeway's crossing of El Camino Ave. Although each of these pavilions is equipped with drinking fountains, most have either been vandalized or disconnected. It is advisable to use the pedestrian crossing button and wait for the walk signal before crossing heavily trafficked El Camino.

Continuing in a northeast direction, the bikeway crosses Eleanor Ave. and curves to the north. After crossing a small drainage channel, the bikeway spans the much larger Arcade Creek flood control channel and then passes under an arch marking the **Del Paso Heights** neighborhood.

Continuing true north, the bikeway crosses Ford St. and goes past another pavilion. It then crosses South and Grand avenues before reaching Rio Linda Blvd. Unfortunately, there is no pedestrian signal crossing for busy Rio Linda Blvd., so bike riders should use extra caution before crossing. After crossing Rio Linda, the bikeway turns left, crosses the Rose St. cul-de-sac, and then goes right to cross North Ave. next to its intersection with Rio Linda. The bikeway then proceeds under Interstate 80.

Another arch announces the **Robla** neighborhood. The surrounding countryside is more rural in

Robla, with larger lots and some open pastures ripe for new urban development.

The bikeway crosses Jessie Ave. and then busy Bell Ave., a bit over 5.0 miles from its start on C St. in Sacramento. ▶4 Another pavilion is located near the Bell St. crossing. The bikeway continues due north, climbs a short levee, and crosses **Robla Creek** (also known as Magpie Creek). The bikeway then crosses Marysville Blvd. at its intersection with Rio Linda Blvd. You will definitely need to follow the traffic signal at this busy intersection.

After crossing Marysville Blvd., the bikeway enters a relatively undeveloped area. It makes its way across open meadows and pastures and then crosses the south branch of Dry Creek, which flows year-round. The more natural landscape of the Dry Creek floodplain is slated for protection in the Sacramento County General Plan as part of the 6.0-mile-long Dry Creek Parkway (which begins in Gibson Ranch Regional Park). Ultimately, bike paths will follow the levees to the north and south of the creek, but today, the primary access to this section of the Dry Creek Parkway is via the Sacramento Northern Bikeway. Wildlife depends on this bit of linear open space. Meadowlarks sing, pheasants run across the bike path, and you may have to dodge some suicidal squirrels.

After crossing the south branch of Dry Creek, the bikeway parallels the creek for several hundred yards. It soon begins to follow the western boundary of Rio Linda's **Central Park**. A connector path to the park leads off to the right, crossing Dry Creek on a bridge. Just north of Central Park, the bikeway crosses Elkhorn Blvd., another busy street where use of the pedestrian crossing signals is advisable. The bikeway continues north, crosses the barely flowing north branch of Dry Creek, and parallels the western boundary of the **Rio Linda–Elverta**

Sacramento Northern Bikeway | TRAIL **12**

Community Center Park on the right, which includes a small rodeo arena.

In case you missed the large water tower on the left, which says RIO LINDA in large letters, another arch lets you know that you have reached this rural Sacramento County community. The bikeway passes the former Rio Linda train station (now the headquarters of the local Chamber of Commerce), which has a small adjacent parking lot right across from a fire station.

Just past the old Rio Linda railroad station and about 8.2 miles from your start on C St. in Sacramento, the bikeway crosses M St. in Rio Linda. ▶5 It continues north through a combination industrial and residential area. The bikeway designers used a bit more creativity in this stretch, curving the path back and forth along the right-of-way. This relatively new part of the bikeway was recently landscaped, and the scenery will definitely improve in the coming years as the newly planted trees and other vegetation mature.

The bikeway continues northward through a residential area, with newer homes on the right and older homes to the left. After crossing Q St., the bikeway begins to parallel Rio Linda Blvd. on the left. Over the next mile or so, the bikeway crosses U St. and Delano St., and then ends ▶6 at a pavilion and small parking area just before reaching Elverta Blvd. near its intersection with Rio Linda Boulevard.

MILESTONES

- ▶1 0.00 Bikeway begins on C St., head north.
- ▶2 1.14 Junction with Jedediah Smith Memorial Trail, turn left.
- ▶3 1.15 Trail junction, veer right and up the levee
- ▶4 5.18 Bell St. pavilion, continue north
- ▶5 8.21 M St. in Rio Linda, continue north
- ▶6 10.02 Bikeway ends at Elverta Road pavilion and parking area

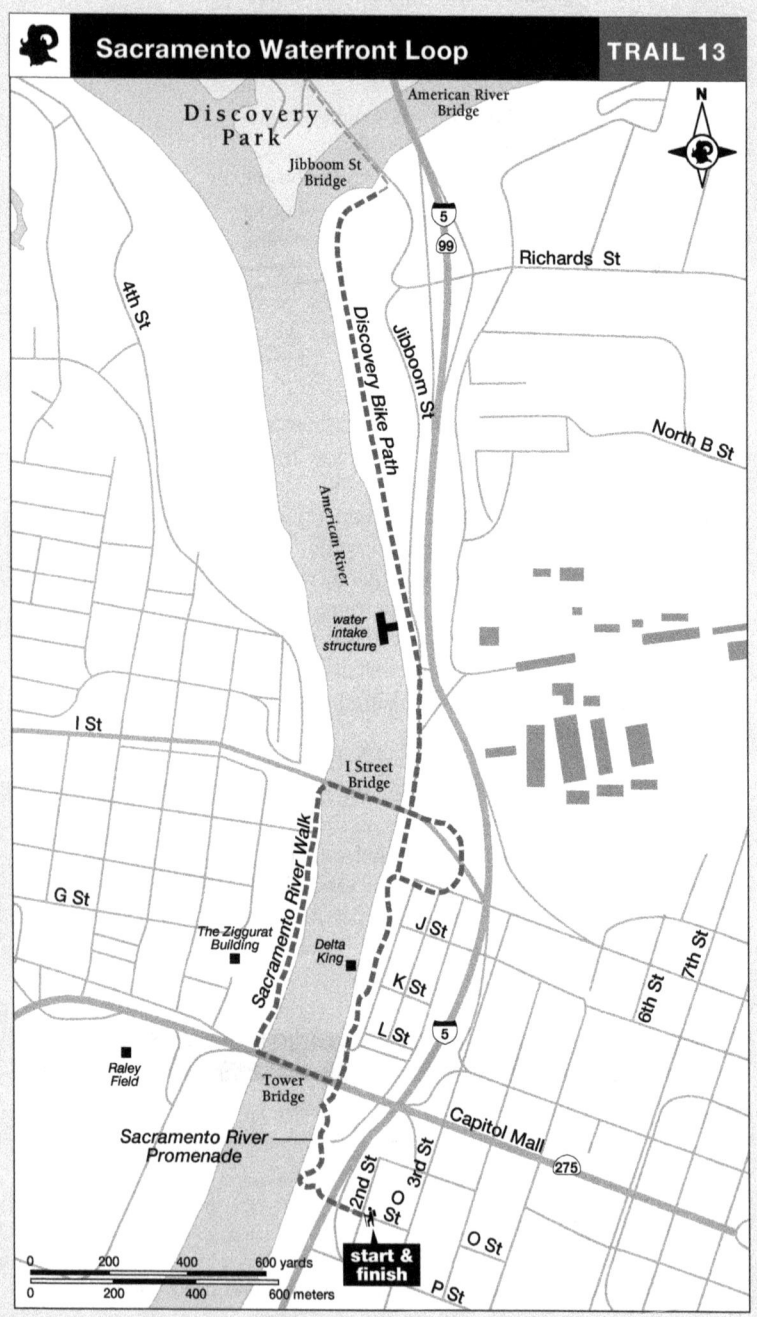

TRAIL 13 The Great Valley

Sacramento Waterfront Loop

This urban walk showcases the history of the Old Sacramento waterfront and the recreational amenities of the Sacramento River Promenade on the east bank and the River Walk on the west bank. The route crosses two historical but quite different bridges, and provides great views of the Sacramento River and the increasingly distinct urban skyline surrounding the river. It also features a short out-and-back side trip along the bike path to Discovery Park, past the City's unique water intake structure to the confluence of the American and Sacramento rivers. Plan on doing this hike in conjunction with visiting the various nearby museums and tourist establishments in Old Sacramento.

Best Time

This is a fine year-round walk. Mornings and evenings are best in the summer to avoid the heat.

Finding the Trail

From downtown Sacramento, drive west on Capitol Mall or L St. and turn left on 3rd St. Turn right on O St. and park in the vicinity of O and 2nd streets. The walk proceeds west on O St., across the I-5 overpass and Front St. to the Sacramento River Promenade.

Logistics

The Old Sacramento Historic District and its surroundings can be quite crowded, and parking is at a premium in the summer and on most sunny

---

TRAIL USE
Hike, Run, Bike
LENGTH
3.4 miles, 2–3 hours
VERTICAL FEET
±20
DIFFICULTY
- 1 **2** 3 4 5 +
TRAIL TYPE
Loop
Out & Back
SURFACE TYPE
Paved

FEATURES
Child Friendly
Dogs on Leash
Handicapped Accessible
River
Birds
Great views
Photo Opportunity
Historic
Interpretive Kiosks

FACILITIES
Picnic Tables
Restrooms
Water

Paddle-wheel boats moored here provide an idea of what the waterfront must have looked like in the 1800s.

weekends. Bring quarters to feed the meters (except Sundays and evenings) for on-street parking at O and 2nd streets or use the adjacent surface fee lot. You can also park in the parking structure (for a fee) at Front and Capitol Mall, at the east end of the Tower Bridge.

Some portions of the Promenade, River Walk, Old Sacramento waterfront boardwalk, and the Discovery Park bike path are wheelchair accessible. Unfortunately, the I St. Bridge is not.

Trail Description

From the corner of O and 2nd streets, ▶1 proceed west on O St. across the I-5 overpass and Front St. O St. dead-ends at the **Sacramento River Promenade**, which parallels the east bank of the Sacramento River.

Turn right and proceed north along the Promenade, ▶2 stopping occasionally to read the educational kiosks recounting local river history. Pass the Embassy Suites Hotel on the right, along with a small memorial plaza to the maritime industry, and cross Capitol Mall at the crosswalk.

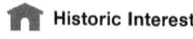 Historic Interest

▶3 Turn left and cross the historic **Tower Bridge**. Built in 1936, it is the only historically significant vertical lift bridge in California. This means that the center span of the bridge between its two towers rises straight up to allow for the passage of tall boats. Pedestrians should take care when sharing the bridge's narrow walkway with bicyclists, who definitely should walk their bikes across the bridge (widening of the bridge's walkway is scheduled for completion in 2008).

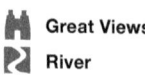 Great Views
River

Take the opportunity to look upstream from the center of the bridge. The bridge provides a good opportunity to view the Sacramento River and the historic **Old Sacramento** waterfront.

Sacramento Waterfront Loop | TRAIL 13

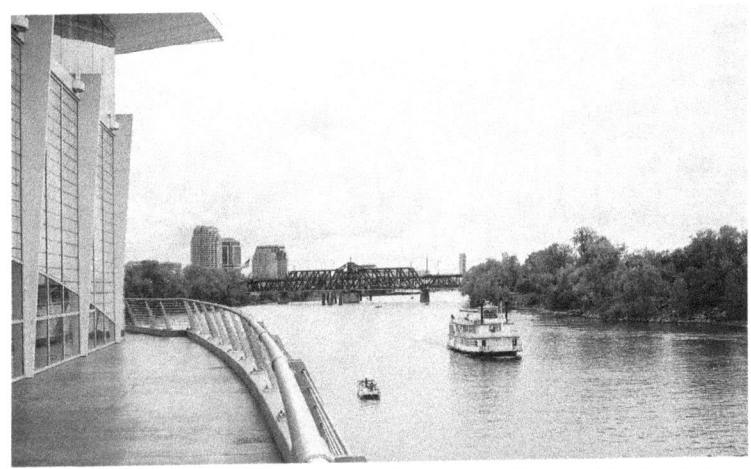

View of the Sacramento River waterfront *from the City of Sacramento's unique water intake structure*

The larger of the two boats moored here is the *Delta King*. Built in 1927, the *Delta King* plied the Delta between San Francisco and Sacramento until 1940 and is now a permanent floating (but stationary) hotel and restaurant. The smaller boat, the *Spirit of Sacramento*, actually cruises up and down the river. It was constructed in 1877 and was formerly the ferryboat *Newark*. Another more modern boat, the faux paddle-wheeler named the *Matthew McKinley*, is also often moored in Old Sacramento.

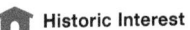 **Historic Interest**

After crossing the Tower Bridge, ▶4 turn right (north) to enter West Sacramento's **River Walk**. This pleasant river parkway was established in 1998. It provides a scenic walk along the river with access to the river's edge, adorned by large cottonwood trees. The River Walk offers benches, picnic areas, and swaths of lawn as well. The nearly 0.33-mile walkway also boasts a number of interpretive signs highlighting the human and natural history of the Sacramento River. The City of West Sacramento plans to eventually extend the River Walk north of the I St. Bridge and south of the Tower Bridge.

The Great Valley

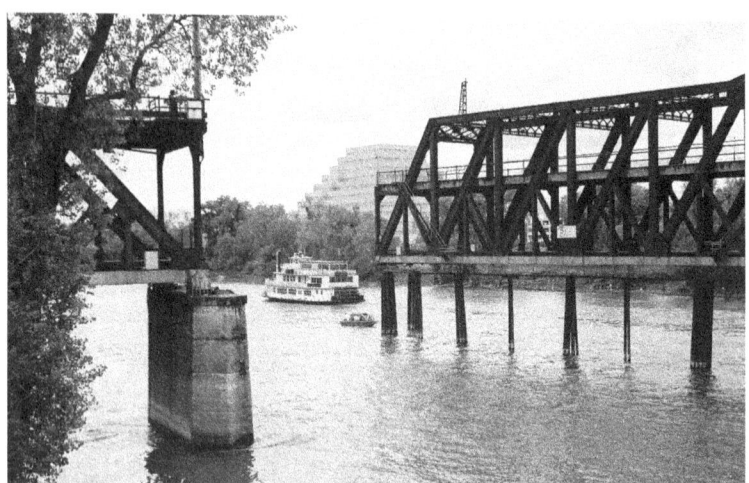

The I Street Bridge *rotates 90 degrees to allow for boat passage along the Sacramento waterfront.*

Visitors on the River Walk quickly discover from the many interpretive signs that this section of the Sacramento River was the location of the first salmon cannery built on the Pacific Coast. Also in this area was the first bridge to cross the Sacramento River. It was completed in 1858 and was used by the Pony Express. Visitors may also discover that this very urbanized river still supports salmon, egrets, and other wildlife.

Looming over the middle of the River Walk is one of the more curious and recent architectural achievements in the area. The Ziggurat Building in West Sacramento was constructed in 1998 as a private office building, but now provides offices for a state agency. The golden-colored terraced pyramid certainly offers a unique silhouette in the rapidly developing urban skyline along the river.

Continue north past the Ziggurat on the River Walk, which ends just short of the **I St. Bridge**. Keep walking south along the gravel levee road to the steep stairs that climb up to the rusty, double-decker bridge. Bicyclists will have to carry their bikes up these stairs, which unfortunately completely impede wheelchairs. Built in 1911, the historic but decidedly utilitarian I St. Bridge is the main east/west route of the Union Pacific Railroad and Amtrak passenger trains. The center span of the bridge rotates to allow for the passage of tall boats.

After climbing the stairs, turn right again ▶5 and proceed east over the bridge. From the center of the span, there are good views downstream to the Tower Bridge and upstream to the unique water intake structure in the river, which provides a good destination for a side trip.

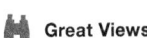 Great Views

After crossing the I St. Bridge, proceed 20 feet west through the intersection of I and Jibboom streets. Just past the intersection, a crosswalk crosses the eastbound lane of I St. ▶6 Cross here and follow the ramp that switchbacks down below the I St. and I-5 overpasses. Ironically, the maze of concrete overpasses in this area provides nesting sites for one of the few populations of purple martins in California, which attracts birders from all over the state.

The switchback ramps lead to the corner of "old" I St. (the street as it was before it was routed over the I St. Bridge) and 2nd St. At this point, you will be facing the popular **California State Railroad Museum** in Old Sacramento. Cross 2nd St., ▶7 jog left, and then turn right on old I St. past the Railroad Museum, proceeding westward about 0.1 mile, past the Discovery Museum and History Center, to the street's dead-end at the railroad tracks. Cross the tracks to ▶8 the **Sacramento River Overlook**. Here, an interpretive sign allows you to contemplate the watery grave of the sailing vessel *LaGrange*, which served as the city's floating jail from 1849 to 1859, until it sank in a week-long storm.

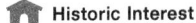 Historic Interest

As you stand at the overlook, below you is one of the few points where the massive concrete flood wall that defends Sacramento from inundation has been removed, allowing people access to the river's edge. You can reach the river by taking the sloping pathways to the north and south of the overlook. Take the time to stop and watch the river flow by and perhaps see salmon jump and roll during their seasonal migrations.

From the Sacramento River overlook, turn right and proceed north on the **Discovery Park Bike Path**. The path drops under the I St. Bridge and continues north past an old abandoned concrete warehouse building and stately cottonwood trees that line the east bank of the Sacramento River. About 0.5 mile from the overlook, the path reaches a park plaza and fountain that herald the entry on the left to the City of Sacramento's unique Water Intake Structure. Built in 2004, this futuristic structure in the middle of the river can be explored during daylight hours ▶9 by walking out to it. There you'll have fine views up and down the river, and see an interpretive kiosk that recounts more of the river's natural history.

Great Views

After checking out the structure, return to the bike path, ▶10 turn left, and continue north about 0.4 mile on the bike path to **Discovery Park**. Here, a sandy beach at the confluence of the American and Sacramento rivers beckons seasonal waders and swimmers (who should be mindful of the river's cold water, uneven bottom, and strong currents). The park also offers cottonwood-shaded picnic tables, BBQs, and restrooms.

River

After enjoying Discovery Park, ▶11 retrace your steps south on the bike path about 0.8 mile to the Sacramento River Overlook in Old Sacramento. Continue south ▶12 on the wooden boardwalk parallel to the railroad track on the left, to the gang-plank structure that provides access to the *Delta King*. Turn left at this point ▶13 and cross the track to the corner of K and Front streets, turn right on Front St., and proceed past the historic school house

Sacramento Waterfront Loop | TRAIL 13

and not-so-historic parking structure to the crosswalk at Capitol Mall. ▶14

Cross Capitol Mall and retrace your steps along the Promenade to O St., turn left at O St., and cross over the I-5 overpass to your starting point ▶15 at the corner of O and 2nd streets.

MILESTONES

▶1 0.00 Start at the corner of O and 2nd streets, go west over I-5
▶2 0.08 Cross Front St. and turn right on the Sacramento River Promenade
▶3 0.16 Cross Capitol Mall, turn left to cross the Tower Bridge
▶4 0.30 West end of Tower Bridge, turn right to enter the Sacramento River Walk
▶5 0.68 Climb I St. Bridge stairs, turn right to cross I St. Bridge
▶6 0.90 Cross eastbound lane of I St., follow ramp down to Old Sacramento
▶7 0.98 Cross 2nd St. and proceed east on old I St. to Sacramento River
▶8 1.17 Sacramento River overlook, turn right on the Discovery Park bike path
▶9 1.67 Turn left to check out the water intake structure
▶10 1.72 Return to Discovery Park bike path, turn left
▶11 2.13 Reach Discovery Park, turn around and retrace steps to Old Sacramento
▶12 3.09 Sacramento River overlook, continue south along Old Sacramento waterfront
▶13 3.17 Turn left at *Delta King* and then right on Front St. proceed south
▶14 3.24 Cross Capitol Mall and retrace steps to O and 2nd streets
▶15 3.40 End walk at the corner of O and 2nd streets

The Great Valley

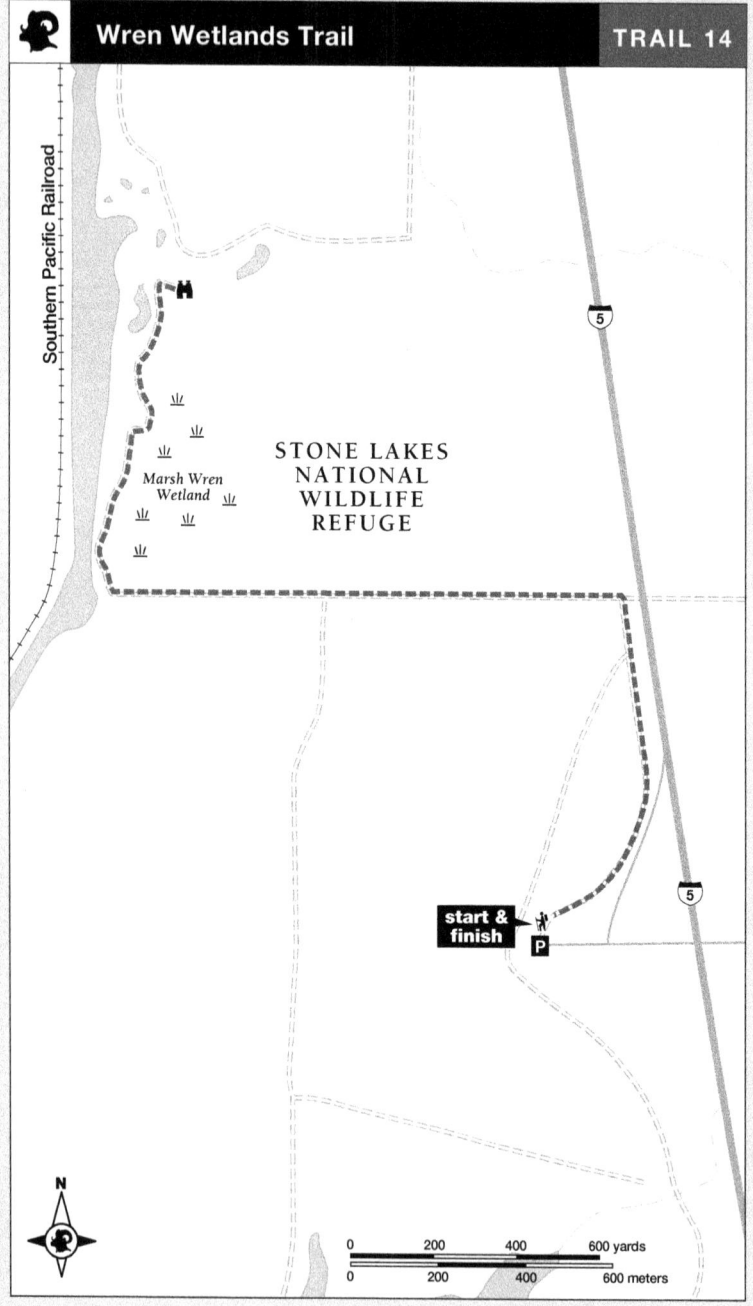

TRAIL 14 The Great Valley

Wren Wetlands Trail: Stone Lakes National Wildlife Refuge

The Stone Lakes National Wildlife Refuge is a promising and relatively recent addition to the Sacramento area's diverse array of outdoor experiences. The refuge offers a rich mosaic of perennial and seasonal wetlands, grasslands, woodlands, and riparian habitat, attracting hundreds of species of waterfowl and other wildlife. Some local landowners and developers vociferously opposed the establishment of Stone Lakes in 1995 as the nation's 505th refuge in the National Wildlife Refuge System. As a result, land acquisition to fill out the proposed 18,000-acre refuge has been sporadic, and the refuge has been slow to develop visitor services. A new visitors center, additional trails, and boat access to South Stone Lake are planned for 2009. In the meantime, public access is limited the Wren Wetlands Trail on two weekends a month. Despite this restricted access, you can enjoy sandhill cranes, white pelicans, Canada geese, and many other species of waterfowl and wildlife. This is a nice walk for families with children.

TRAIL USE
Hike
LENGTH
3.68 miles, 1–2 hours
VERTICAL FEET
±0
DIFFICULTY
- 1 **2** 3 4 5 +
TRAIL TYPE
Out & Back.
SURFACE TYPE
Gravel

FEATURES
Child Friendly
Wetlands
Slough
Meadow
Birds
Wildlife
Interpretive (Docents)

FACILITIES
Porta-potty

Best Time

November–March is the best time to view migrating sandhill cranes, geese, and other waterfowl. Because of the diversity of habitats, the refuge offers good wildlife viewing year-round. Early morning is usually the best time to view wildlife. Summer afternoons can be quite warm.

Just a few of the waterfowl species that may be observed in these wetlands are egrets, black-necked stilts, coots, white pelicans, and on the far side of the wetlands, sandhill cranes.

Finding the Trail

From Sacramento, drive approximately 12 miles south on Interstate 5 to the Elk Grove exit. Once off the freeway, turn right and proceed to the parking area. On visitor days, you will usually find a table staffed by volunteers to provide maps and other information.

Logistics

The trail is open to the public every second and fourth Saturday of the month except in July and August. The gate opens at 7:30 a.m. and closes at 3 p.m. A free docent-guided hike starts from the parking area at 9 a.m. Docents are often stationed along the way with powerful spotting scopes, providing the visitor an opportunity to use the scopes to view wildlife. Be sure, however, to bring your own binoculars and a bird book, so you can identify the many waterfowl and other bird species found along the entire trail. To find out when the Refuge is open for visitors and to get the latest update on visitor improvements, visit www.fws.gov/stonelakes, or call (916) 775-4420.

Trail Description

From the parking area, proceed north on the gravel road ▶1 that (unfortunately) parallels the freeway for about 0.5 mile. There usually isn't much to see along this stretch, with I-5 on your right and grazed grasslands owned by Sacramento County on your left. But ahead and to your right, you can see flooded wetlands and woodlands promising some good wildlife viewing.

You come to a road intersection. The road ahead is marked CLOSED. ▶2 Turn left and continue west on the gravel road. On your right are seasonally flooded wetlands.

Wren Wetlands Trail — TRAIL 14

After about 0.75 mile heading west, the gravel road reaches a line of woodlands and riparian habitat that parallel a slough created when the old railroad bed on the other side was raised above the floodplain. If you are quiet and it is early in the morning, you may see river otters and beavers in the slough, as well as the ubiquitous great blue heron. Northern harriers and Swainson's hawks use the trees to spot prey and forage in the nearby grasslands. At this point, turn right and follow the considerably narrower road north ▶3 as it skirts around a smaller area of open water on the right named the **Marsh Wren Wetland**. A side trail curves farther right, providing access to the east side of the wetland, but the main route continues north on the road and slightly to the left, with open grassland and wetlands on the right and a line of trees on your left.

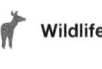 Wildlife

 Wetland

The trail enters a grove of cottonwoods ▶4 and reaches a raised viewing platform. Proceed up the ramp to the platform, which provides a view of the slough to the west through the screen of cottonwoods and a view of the large seasonal wetland to the east. Some benches provide a nice opportunity to stop, listen to bird sounds, and maybe munch on a snack.

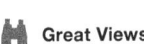 Great Views

 Birds

Retrace your steps ▶5 to the parking area.

MILESTONES

- ▶1 0.00 Elk Grove Exit parking area, head north on gravel road
- ▶2 0.57 T intersection, turn left (west)
- ▶3 1.35 Big bend at the slough, follow road to the right (north)
- ▶4 1.84 Viewing platform
- ▶5 3.68 Return to parking area

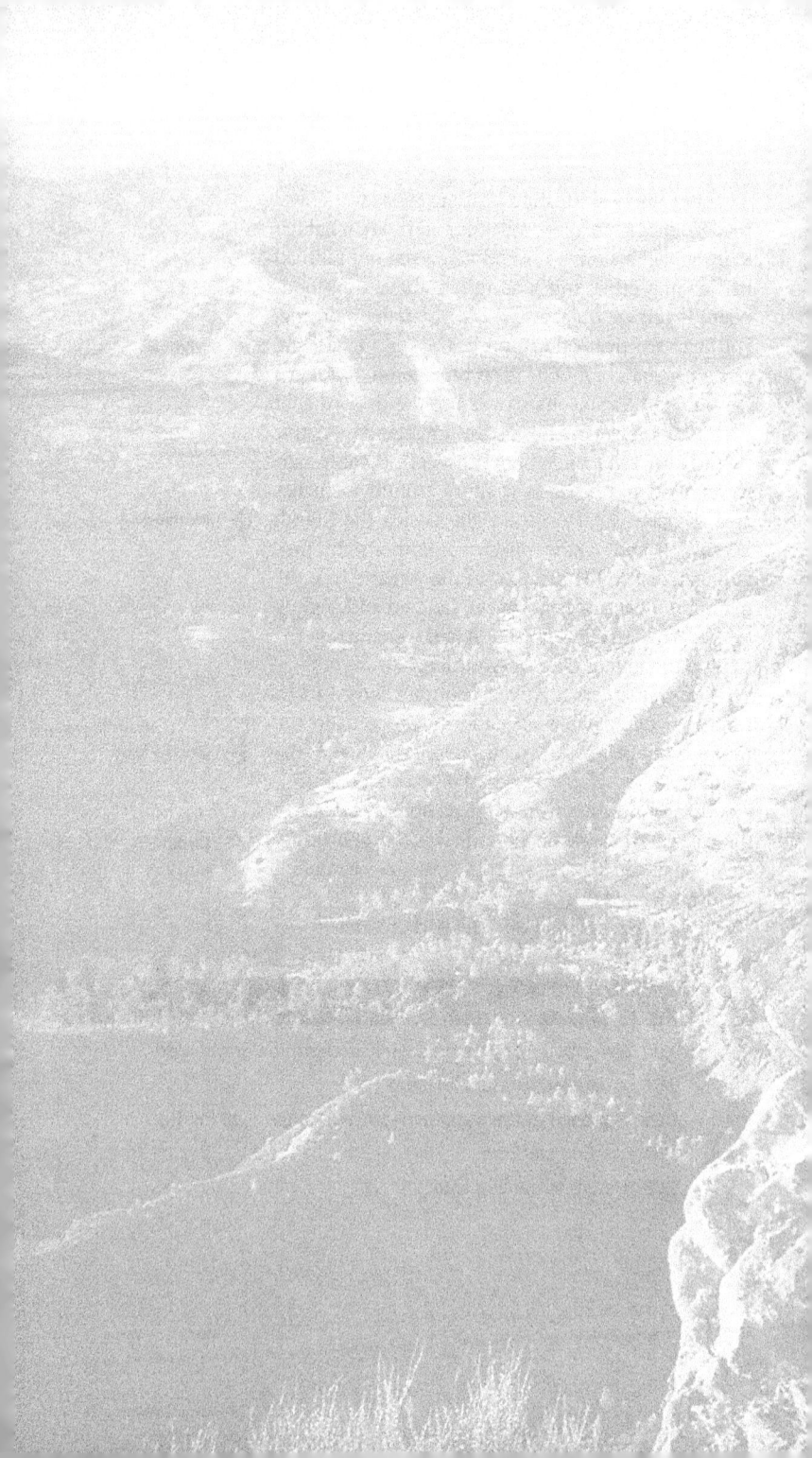

CHAPTER 2

The Coast Range

15. Blue Ridge Trail: Cache Creek Natural Area
16. Cache Creek Ridge Trail: Cache Creek Natural Area
17. Redbud Trail: Cache Creek Wilderness
18. Cold Canyon–Blue Ridge Loop Trail: Stebbins UC Reserve

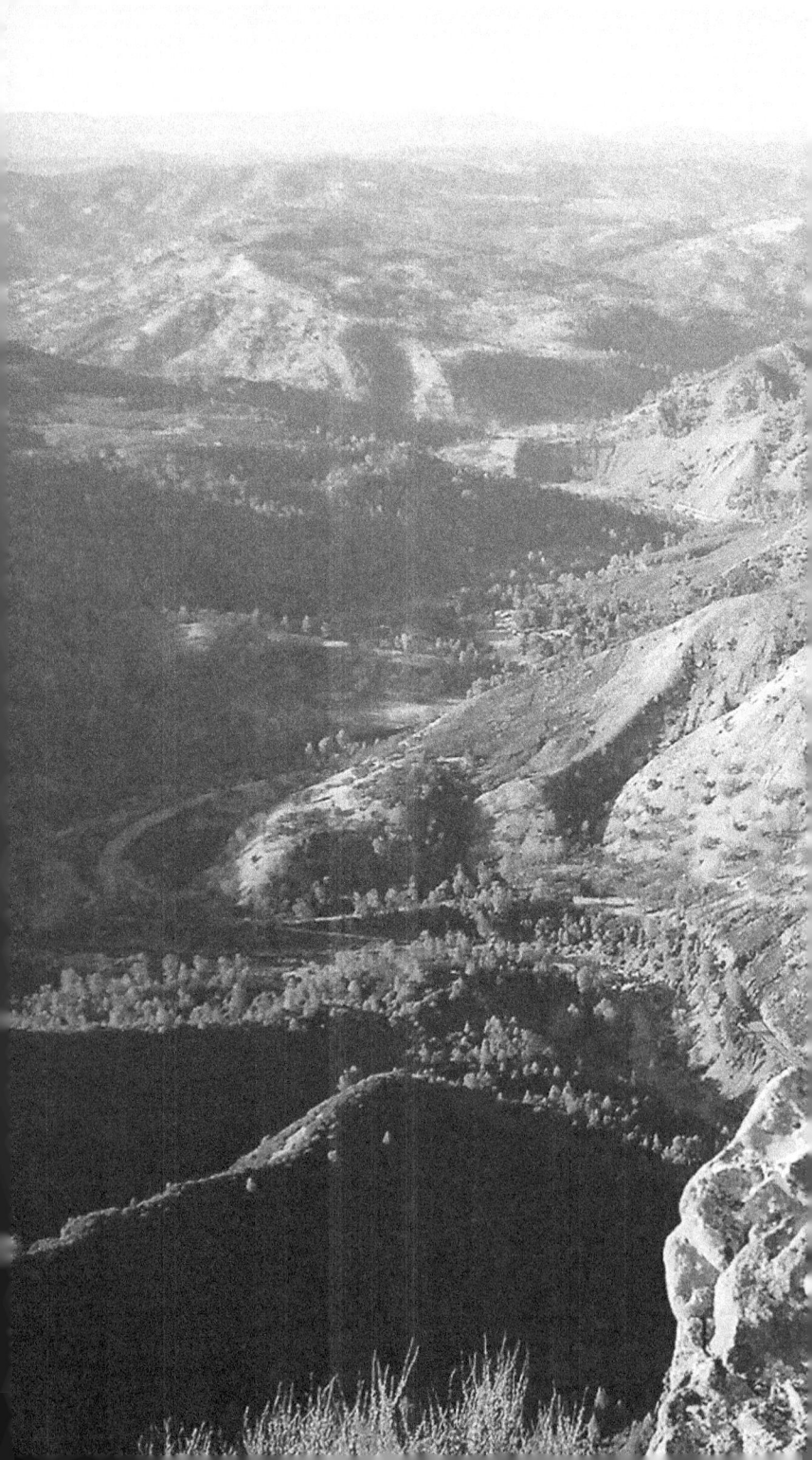

AREA OVERVIEW

The Coast Range

Until a few decades ago, the Cache and Putah Creek watersheds in the Coast Range seemed almost a forgotten part of the mountains that define the western boundary of the Great Valley. To the north are the higher and more well known peaks of the Snow Mountain and Yolla Bolly wildernesses. To the south lies an extensive network of public parks and open space areas well known to many Bay Area residents. But these Coast Range watersheds were largely privately owned until recent public land acquisitions by the BLM and other agencies introduced the area to public exploration and enjoyment. This region of the Coast Range shares many similarities with the Sierra Foothills. Both ranges were created by uplift and faulting, and the California Woodlands and Interior Chaparral Ecoregion occupies the same 500–4000-foot elevations in both ranges. But the little sister range to the east lacks the higher-elevation uplands that the Sierra Foothills enjoy, making the Coast Range drier and hotter in the summer, but still a spectacular place to visit in the fall, winter, and spring.

Maps and Permits

USGS 7.5-minute quad maps best identify topography and physical features. Many of the trails opened relatively recently to the public for hiking, biking, and equestrian use follow old road and jeep trails systems that are still accurately depicted on the USGS maps. Some new foot trails have been built and more are under construction. Check out the appropriate managing agency website for the latest information. As of press time, no permits are needed to visit these areas.

Overleaf and opposite: *Cache Creek and Glasscock Mountain seen from the top of Blue Ridge (Trail 15)*

AREA MAP

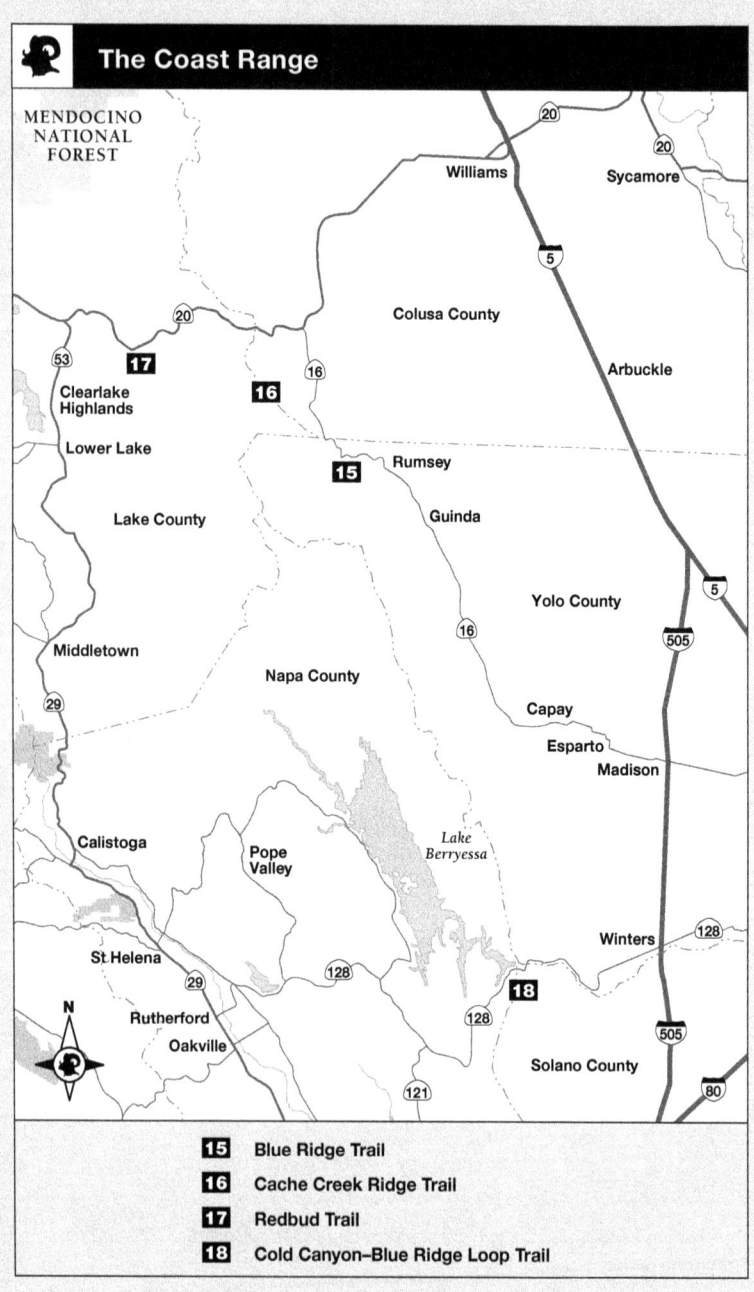

- 15 Blue Ridge Trail
- 16 Cache Creek Ridge Trail
- 17 Redbud Trail
- 18 Cold Canyon–Blue Ridge Loop Trail

TRAIL FEATURE TABLE

The Coast Range

TRAIL	Difficulty	Length	Type	USES & ACCESS	TERRAIN	FLORA & FAUNA	OTHER
15	5	5.56	↗	Hiking, Dogs Allowed	River/Stream, Wetland, Mountain	Wildflowers, Birds	Great Views, Historic Interest, Steep, Secluded
16	4	9.9	V	Hiking, Horses, Running, Biking, Dogs Allowed	River/Stream, Meadow, Wetland, Mountain	Wildflowers, Birds, Wildlife	Historic Interest, Steep, Camping
17	3	4.02	↗	Hiking, Horses	River/Stream, Meadow, Mountain	Wildflowers, Birds, Wildlife	Historic Interest, Steep, Camping, Photo Opportunity
18	5	4.9	V	Running, Child Friendly, Handicap Access	River/Stream, Meadow, Wetland, Mountain	Wildflowers, Birds, Wildlife	Historic Interest, Great Views, Secluded, Photo Opportunity

USES & ACCESS
- Hiking
- Horses
- Running
- Biking
- Child Friendly
- Handicap Access
- $ Fee
- Permit Required
- Dogs Allowed

TYPE
- Loop
- Out & Back
- Point-to-Point
- V Variable

DIFFICULTY
- 1 2 3 4 5 +
less   more

TERRAIN
- River or Stream
- Waterfall
- Lake
- Wetland
- Meadow
- Canyon
- Mountain

FLORA & FAUNA
- Wildflowers
- Fall Colors
- Birds
- Wildlife

FEATURES
- Historic Interest
- Geologic Interest
- Great Views
- Steep
- Secluded
- Camping
- Photo Opportunity

TRAIL SUMMARIES

The Coast Range

TRAIL 15
Hike
5.56 miles, Out & Back
Difficulty: 1 2 3 4 **5**

Blue Ridge Trail:
Cache Creek Natural Area 127
If you want to burn off some energy and get some great views as a reward, there is no better way than making the steep climb to the top of Blue Ridge. From this 2600-foot-high spot, you can enjoy some great vistas of this portion of the Coast Range, including a dramatic view of Cache Creek and all the way across the Great Valley to the Sierra Nevada.

TRAIL 16
Hike, Bike, Horse
9.9 miles, Point to Point
Difficulty: 1 2 3 **4** 5

Cache Creek Ridge Trail:
Cache Creek Natural Area 133
As it meanders through oak woodlands, meadows, and chaparral, this ridgetop trail parallels the boundary of the newly designated Cache Creek Wilderness. Each little bump in the ridge provides different views of Snow Mountain to the north, Mt. Konocti to the west, Blue Ridge to the east, and Cache Creek to the north. Quiet and persistent hikers may catch a glimpse of one of the many bald eagles that cruise Cache Creek Canyon or tule elk that graze the ridgetop meadows.

Redbud Trail:
Cache Creek Wilderness 141

The Redbud Trail provides access to the scenic Cache Creek Wilderness and the Wild River. Look for bald eagles and tule elk as the trail winds its way through wildflower-studded meadows and oak woodlands to the top of a ridge overlooking the rugged canyon of Cache Creek. Although this trail description ends at Baton Flat, hikers and overnighters may want to cross the creek to explore Wilson Valley in the heart of the Wilderness.

TRAIL 17

Hike, Backpack, Horse
4.0 miles, Out & Back
Difficulty: 1 2 **3** 4 5

Cold Canyon–Blue Ridge Loop Trail:
Stebbins UC Reserve 147

Families who just want to take a stroll can walk 1.6 miles round-trip to the old homestead site in the Stebbins UC Reserve. The trail is relatively easy, if rocky in some places. Those looking for more of a challenge may want to continue past the homestead site and climb 1200 feet to the top of this section of Blue Ridge for dramatic views of Berryessa Reservoir and the surrounding ridges of the Coast Range.

TRAIL 18

Hike, Run
4.9 miles, Loop
Difficulty: 1 2 3 4 **5**

Blue Ridge Trail

TRAIL 15

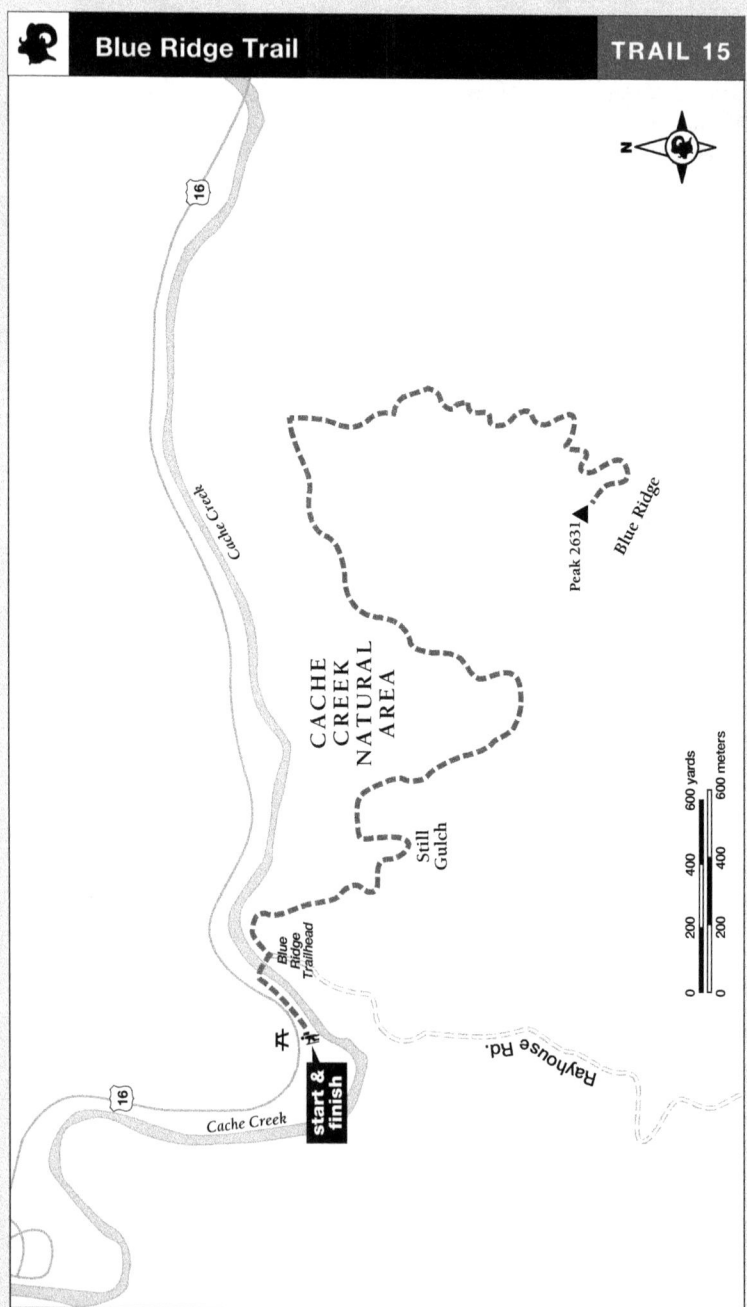

TRAIL 15 The Coast Range

Blue Ridge Trail: Cache Creek Natural Area

When the cold days of winter have closed in and the holiday excesses have you feeling slothful, there is no better cure than climbing to the top of Blue Ridge to take in the outstanding views of the Coast Range and California's latest Wild & Scenic River—Cache Creek. Cache Creek was designated a California Wild & Scenic River by the state legislature in 2005, and is one of 12 Wild & Scenic Rivers, which are protected by law from new dam development.

Built by volunteers, this challenging trail provides access to public lands that stretch along Blue Ridge south to Berryessa Peak. Tuleyome, a Yolo County-based conservation group, has recently acquired land in order to increase public access to this little-visited area, with the ultimate goal of designating much of the ridge as a federally protected wilderness.

Best Time

This is definitely a fall-winter-spring trail. The relatively low elevation, exposure, and uphill nature of the hike all make summer hiking challenging.

Finding the Trail

Drive north 24 miles on Interstate 5 to the City of Woodland. Take the Hwy 16–Esparto exit. Turn left, drive over I-5, and continue southeast for 3.1 miles on Hwy 16 to its intersection with Main St. Turn right and continue west on Hwy 16 through the small towns of Esparto and Capay, past the incongruous sprawl of the Cache Creek Casino in

---

TRAIL USE
Hike
LENGTH
5.56 miles, 3–5 hours
VERTICAL FEET
±2500
DIFFICULTY
- 1 2 3 4 **5** +
TRAIL TYPE
Out & Back
SURFACE TYPE
Dirt

FEATURES
Dogs on Leash
Streams
Canyon
Mountain
River
Wildflowers
Birds
Great Views
Geological Interest
Secluded
Steep

FACILITIES
Vault Toilets

> Blue Ridge's rocky summit towers on the left, hinting at the climb ahead.

the middle of the otherwise bucolic Capay Valley, and through the even smaller towns of Guinda and Rumsey. Hwy 16 enters Cache Creek Canyon and follows the creek. Approximately 65.6 miles from Sacramento, turn left at the sign that says CACHE CREEK CANYON REGIONAL PARK—LOWER SITE. Park here and walk down Rayhouse Road and across the Cache Creek low-water bridge to the trailhead.

Logistics

The gate on the Rayhouse Road is closed and locked during the rainy season, so this trail description begins at the Cache Creek Regional Park Lower Site parking area. If you are foolish enough to hike this trail in the summer, you can drive down Rayhouse Road, cross the low-water bridge, and park just on the other side of the bridge. The trailhead is inaccessible when Cache Creek swells above 1000 cubic feet per second from winter and spring rains and flows over the low-water bridge. To check Cache Creek flows, visit www.dreamflows.com.

Trail Description

From the Cache Creek Canyon Regional Park Lower Site parking area, ▶1 proceed down **Rayhouse Road** on your left to **Cache Creek**. The gate across this road is typically closed and locked during the rainy months. Cross the low-water bridge over the creek (avoid during high flows).

Just after crossing the bridge, another gated road heads off to your left and a sign says BLUE RIDGE TRAIL. ▶2 Follow this road a short distance until you reach a large flat next to Cache Creek. In the summer, the flat provides camping for white-water rafters.

As you enter the flat, you will see the Blue Ridge trailhead on your right marked by another BLUE RIDGE TRAIL sign. ▶3 The sign also says BLUE

Stream

Blue Ridge Trail | TRAIL **15**

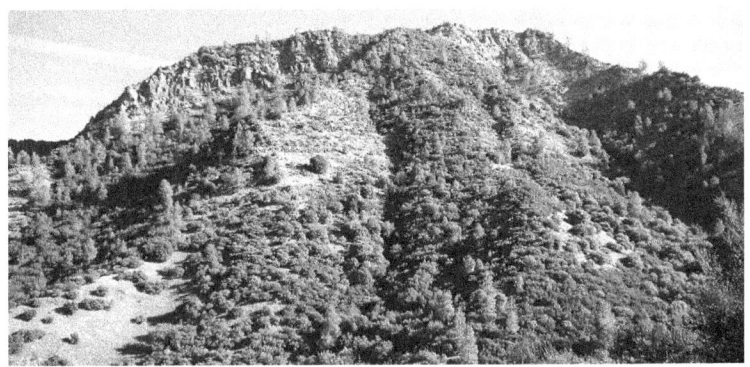

The hike to the summit of Blue Ridge is steep, *but well worth the spectacular views.*

RIDGE—3.0 MILES, FISKE PEAK—4.0 MILES, FISKE CREEK ROAD—8.5 MILES. A stone monument to the right of the trailhead commemorates Ada Merhoff, a Sierra Club volunteer instrumental in mobilizing the volunteers who helped build the Blue Ridge Trail.

The trail proceeds uphill in a southerly direction through gray pines, live oaks, and manzanita. This initial section of trail is well built, and climbs at a moderate pace up a side ridge that branches off from Blue Ridge to the northwest. Soon, you pass a fiberglass wand noting that you have climbed to an altitude of 1000 feet.

The trail drops down briefly from the side ridge ▶4 and crosses seasonally flowing **Still Gulch**. It then traverses the slope on the other side of the gulch through toyon (Christmasberry) and chamise. It soon bends east with views of the Cache Creek Wild & Scenic River and Hwy 16 below. In short order, the trail crosses the end-point of another side ridge and then begins climbing to the south, to the top of a ridge with nice views to the west through the thick chaparral. The trail follows the ridge upward and then crosses ▶5 a second gully with seasonal flows.

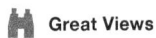 **Great Views**

After crossing the second gully, the trail begins ascending **Blue Ridge** proper, traversing its north

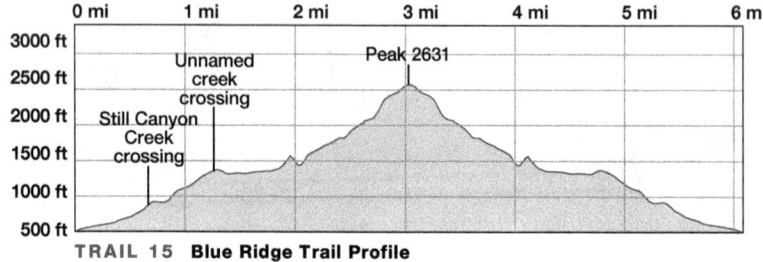
TRAIL 15 Blue Ridge Trail Profile

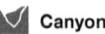 Canyon

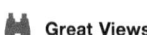 Great Views

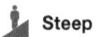 Steep

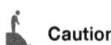 Caution

slope, with Cache Creek Canyon below. The tread narrows and becomes more uneven, frequently broken by rocks and mossy boulders. Take care as you negotiate some awkward drops and upward steps. More nice views of Cache Creek are found along this section.

About 0.66 mile from the second gully, the trail rounds the steep north end of Blue Ridge. ▶6 Stop to catch your breath and appreciate the views west of the Capay Valley and the Sacramento Valley. From here, the trail traverses south as it climbs the east face of Blue Ridge through thick chaparral, laurel, and scrub oak. As you pass the 2000 foot marker, you can see the brushy summit of Blue Ridge, still high above you.

The trail ascends via several switchbacks, its tread in places quite narrow and rough. At one point, the trail comes to the brink of a landslide and climbs steeply up and around the landside's headcut on narrow and crumbling tread (use particular care here), and then drops down to its original route. Beyond the landslide, the trail continues up several more switchbacks, past the 2500-foot marker. The trail traverses southward a couple of hundred feet below the ridgetop a short ways and enters a recently burned area that is regenerating nicely. Another set of switchbacks, this one thankfully short, brings you to the brushy top of Blue Ridge between two knolls.

Blue Ridge Trail | TRAIL 15

▶7 The trail to 2868-foot-high Fiske Peak (visible about a mile to the south) branches to the left. To get an immediate "view" fix, follow a use-trail through the brush on the right as it climbs to the top of the 2631-foot-high knoll on Blue Ridge. ▶8 Some well-placed rocks provide an excellent lunch spot. Some of the whitewashed rocks confirm that golden eagles and other local birds of prey also love this perch and use it to survey the surrounding landscape for prey.

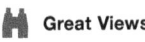 Great Views

From here, you enjoy spectacular views in all directions, but particularly of the geologically tortured canyon of Cache Creek and of Glasscock Mountain just across the canyon to the north. To the west, you can see much of the newly designated Cache Creek Wilderness, with Mt. Konocti near Clear Lake and Mt. St. Helena near Napa Valley looming on the horizon. To the east are even more expansive views of the Capay and Sacramento valleys, and on a clear day, the Sierra Nevada establishes the eastern horizon line.

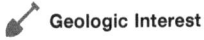 Geologic Interest

Eat, rest, drink in the view, and when you are satiated, retrace your steps carefully ▶9 back to the trailhead and parking area.

MILESTONES

- ▶1 0.00 Cache Creek Regional Park Lower Site parking area
- ▶2 0.20 Rayhouse Road to Cache Creek Flat Road
- ▶3 0.30 Blue Ridge Trailhead
- ▶4 0.58 Still Gulch crossing
- ▶5 1.11 Second gulch crossing
- ▶6 1.76 North ridgepoint
- ▶7 2.69 Blue Ridge–Fiske Peak Trail junction
- ▶8 2.78 Peak 2631
- ▶9 5.56 Return to Lower Site parking area

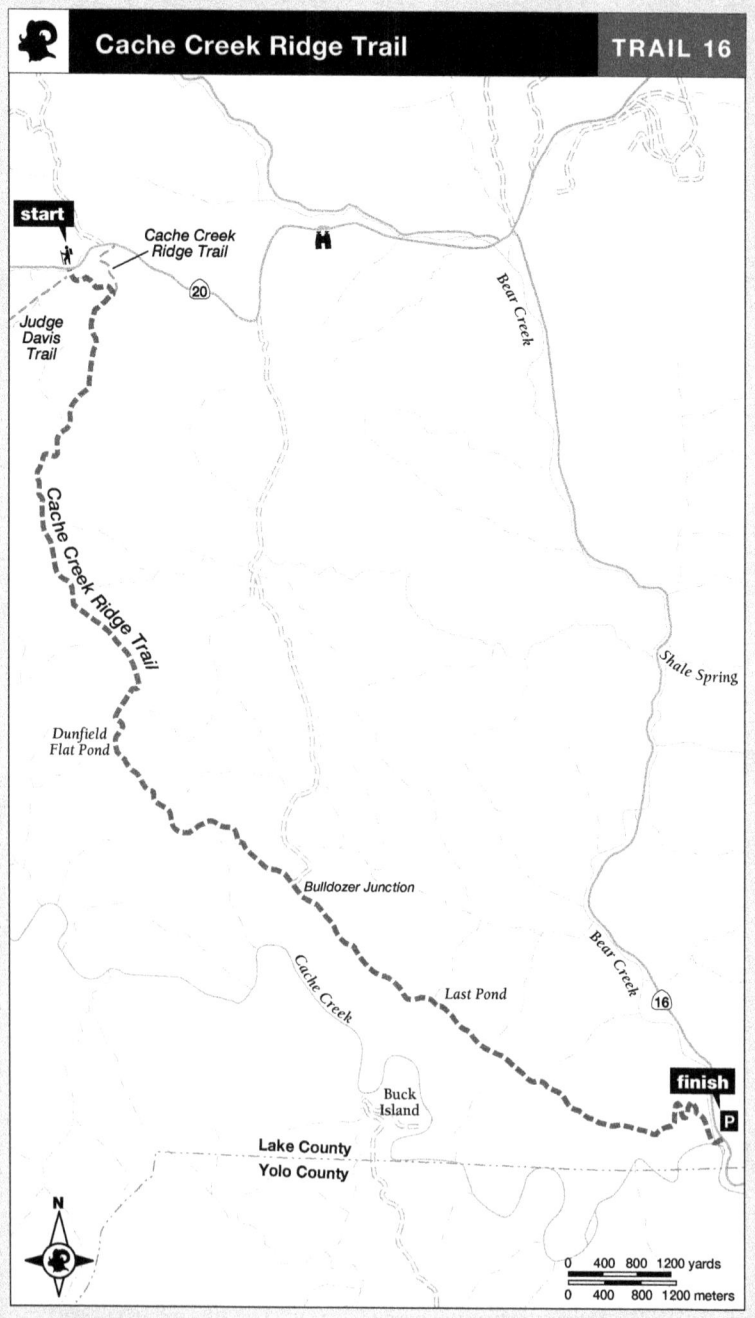

TRAIL 16 The Coast Range

Cache Creek Ridge Trail: Cache Creek Natural Area

Just a few years ago, this trail was located on the privately owned Payne Ranch, which blocked public access to much of the existing public land to the south and east encompassing the wild canyon of Cache Creek. But a determined effort by the BLM to acquire the 12,769-acre ranch resulted in expansion of the Cache Creek Natural Area to more than 70,000 acres. The trail follows the ridgetop that creates the boundary between the former Payne Ranch and the Cache Creek Wilderness, which was designated in 2006. From the ridge, hikers enjoy frequent views of sinuous Cache Creek, which was added to the California Wild & Scenic Rivers System in 2005. The trail makes its way through classic low-elevation Coast Range habitat, including blue oak woodlands, grasslands, and chaparral on serpentine-based soils. The possibility of viewing wildlife is high, since this area is home to one of the largest free-roaming tule elk herds in California, as well as one of the largest wintering populations of bald eagles. Except for some seasonal stock ponds, this ridgetop trail is dry for most of its length, so be sure to bring plenty of water.

Best Time

The ridgetop is verdant with fresh grass, newly leafed oaks, and wildflowers in the spring. Spring rains also fill the stock ponds along the ridge, which provide a handy source of water if you have a filter. This can be a pleasant hike on sunny late-fall or winter days. Hot summer days can turn this hike into a waterless survival march.

TRAIL USE
Hike, Run, Bike, Horse
LENGTH
9.9 miles, 4–7 hours
VERTICAL FEET
±1500
DIFFICULTY
- 1 2 3 **4** 5 +
TRAIL TYPE
Point to Point
Out & Back
SURFACE TYPE
Dirt

FEATURES
Dogs on Leash
River
Canyon
Meadow
Wetlands
Wildflowers
Birds
Wildlife
Great Views
Camping
Secluded

FACILITIES
Vault Toilet

> The trail continues south along the ridgetop for about a mile, dropping in and out of mixed oak woodland and chaparral.

Finding the Trail

From Sacramento, drive north 24 miles on Interstate 5 to the city of Woodland. Take the Hwy 16–Esparto exit. Turn left, drive over I-5, and continue southeast for 3.1 miles on Hwy 16 to its intersection with Main St. Turn right and continue west approximately 10 miles on Hwy 16 to its intersection with Interstate 505. Cross over I-505 and continue west on Hwy 16 approximately 31 miles (driving through the small towns of Esparto and Capay, past the incongruous sprawl of the Cache Creek Casino in the middle of the otherwise bucolic Capay Valley, and through the even smaller towns of Guinda and Rumsey). Hwy 16 enters the Cache Creek Canyon and parallels the creek. Drive past the Lower, Middle, and Upper Cache Creek Canyon parks managed by Yolo County. Approximately 31 miles after crossing I-505, Hwy 36 enters Colusa County. There is a small pull-out on the left at the 7.08-mile marker on Hwy 16, just above the confluence of Cache and Bear Creeks. Leave one car here and then proceed north approximately 7.0 miles on Hwy 16 to where it dead-ends at Hwy 20. Turn left and drive west on Hwy 20 for approximately 3.7 miles. Just past a large grassy flat to the left and a sign on the right noting that you are entering Lake County, begin to slow down. The highway curves to the left and the Judge Davis Trailhead is on the left. It is marked by its parking lot and vault toilet (but no sign on the highway). Carefully turn left into the parking area and park. The trail begins from the parking lot.

Logistics

This trail works best as a long one-way hike or overnight backpack with a car shuttle. If you have a filter, water is generally available in the spring from stock ponds. There is no available water in the summer and early fall.

Cache Creek Ridge Trail | TRAIL **16**

Trail Description

From the Judge Davis Trailhead parking lot, ▶1 proceed southeast up the old jeep trail (closed to public motorized use) that climbs 350 feet up the ridge, which is covered in blue oaks, gray pines, and tree-sized manzanita. In about 0.5 mile, the trail reaches a saddle, and then your ascent moderates as you traverse the slope of the 2153-foot-high hill on your left. Soon, you reach the top of the ridge as it heads in a southerly direction and you get your first but not last view of Cortina Ridge to the east and the broad grassy flat where headwater streams gather to form **Thompson Canyon**. You are reminded that this is a former cattle ranch and is still actively grazed under a permit from the BLM as your trail passes a couple of stock ponds and a saucer-like guzzler installed for tule elk by the Department of Fish and Game.

 Great Views

 Canyon

In about 1.3 miles, you come to a junction with a spur trail on the right that connects with the Judge Davis Trail, which eventually drops down into Wilson Valley, in the middle of the Cache Creek Wilderness. ▶2 But your route veers left to follow the now-single-track Cache Creek Ridge Trail, which begins to climb gently up a wooded draw. In a little bit over 1.6 miles from the trailhead, the trail climbs out of the draw to a broad grassy saddle, with an even better view eastward of Cortina Ridge and Thompson Canyon Flat.

 Great Views

The trail reaches a **T** junction on the saddle. A barely discernable trail heads off to the left, but your route follows an overgrown jeep trail that climbs the hill on your right. ▶3 As you crest the hill, you get your first view of volcanic Mt. Konocti near Clear Lake to the west. The ridge route levels off as you continue south past a junction with a trace of a trail leading off to the right that also connects with the Judge Davis Trail. Continue south on the Ridge Trail as it begins another moderate climb. All the land sloping away to your right is part of the newly designated **Cache Creek Wilderness**. As the trail nears a 2200-foot-high point on the ridge, serpentine soils abruptly change the vegetation to chaparral consisting of chamise, buckbrush, and manzanita, topped by an occasional gray pine. If it has been raining recently and cattle have been using the trail, be prepared to deal with some rough tread, because the cattle hooves churn the clay soil, making walking difficult.

The trail continues south along the ridgetop for about a mile. If you turn around and look north, you may glimpse the white flanks of the Snow Mountain Wilderness on the horizon. In a shallow saddle between two high points on the ridge, you'll come to a trail on the right heading down toward a stock pond. Another barely discernable track leads off to the left toward Thompson Canyon. Continue straight south over another high point, then drop down through open oak woodland to another saddle with some overgrown use-trails heading off to the left.

The Cache Creek Trail continues straight, climbing gently upward through mixed oaks, chaparral, and gray pines. The trail reaches an electric fence used to control cattle. The gate through the fence consists of a single wire with a plastic handle hooked to the fence post. Simply grasp the plastic handle (avoiding the bare wire), unhook it from the post, step through, and be sure to rehook the wire to the post to keep cattle from drifting into sensitive areas.

Eventually, the trail climbs gently upward to a trail **T** junction at the edge of **Dunfield Flat**, nearly 2.5 miles from the trailhead. A trail to the left leads to Dunfield Spring and Thompson Canyon. ▶4 Veer right to Dunfield Flat, a pleasant grassy meadow studded by large blue oaks and featuring a large stock pond. From this high flat, you can see Cache

⏤ **Meadow**

Cache Creek Ridge Trail | TRAIL 16

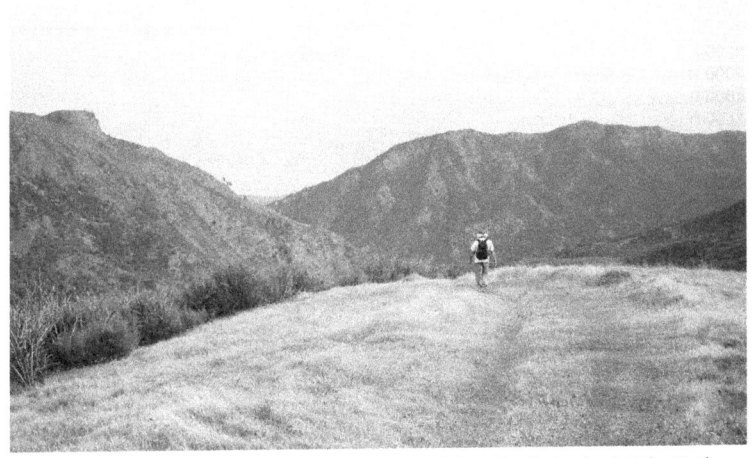

Blue Ridge (right) and Glasscock Mountain (left) *from the Cache Creek Ridge Trail*

Creek Ridge sloping down to the foot of Cortina and Blue Ridges, at the confluence of **Cache Creek** and **Bear Creek**—your eventual destination. Also to the east, you can see a large stock pond (really a small lake) at the headwaters of Brophy Canyon.

From Dunfield Flat, the trail continues climbing and following the ridgetop in a southerly direction, and in less than 0.5 mile from the flat, reaches a 2192-foot-high point. This high part of the ridge continues southeast for nearly a mile through blue oaks before reaching a 2127-foot-high knob. From here, you have even better views of Snow Mountain to the north, Mt. Konocti to the west, and for the first time, Cache Creek to the south as it flows through Kennedy Flats. The vistas make this a great place to have lunch under an oak tree.

 Great Views

From this high point on the ridge, the trail turns east and drops somewhat steeply downward 500 feet through open oaks woodlands and thick fields of chamise. Wet serpentine soils churned by cow hooves can make walking difficult along this segment. The trail intersects with another electric fence

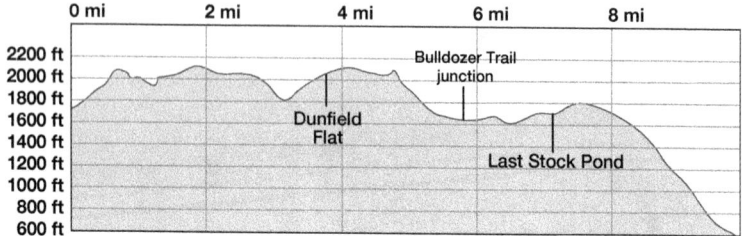

TRAIL 16 Cache Creek Ridge Trail Profile

and wire gate. Again, take care to touch only the plastic handle when unhooking the single line and be sure to close the gate behind you.

Vegetation transitions back to open oak woodlands as the descent moderates and the trail comes to a broad flat marked by an abandoned yellow bulldozer and a four-way trail junction. ▶5 At this point, you are more than 5.75 miles from the trailhead. The trail to the right (actually a closed jeep trail) enters the Cache Creek Wilderness and drops down to a large bend and broad flat on the north side of Cache Creek called New Cacheville, a failed real estate venture. The road to the left leads to Brophy Canyon. Your route continues straight along Cache Creek Ridge.

From the bulldozer junction, continue along Cache Creek Ridge as it undulates gently to the southeast through scattered oaks. Pass through one last electric fence gate. Again, be sure to close the gate behind you, as this section of the ridge seems free of trail-churning cattle. The trail climbs to a modest high point on the ridge and then drops down to a saddle and passes the last and most natural-appearing stock pond. At this point, you are slightly more than 7.0 miles from the trailhead. To your right, you can look down into Cache Creek Canyon to a large promontory in the bend of the creek called **Buck Island**.

Cache Creek Ridge Trail | TRAIL 16

From the pond, the trail climbs 200 feet to the last high point on the ridge, with an elevation of about 1800 feet. ▶6 Continue southeast as the undulating ridge becomes the dividing line between oak woodlands on your right and chaparral on your left. About a mile beyond the last stock pond, the Cache Creek Ridge Trail begins to descend in earnest toward the confluence of Cache and Bear creeks. About 0.75 mile from your destination, the trail leaves the ridgetop and turns north briefly before dropping down into an oak-wooded draw. You'll come to a T intersection. The road to the right pops over the ridge and down toward Cache Creek, upstream of your destination.

Your route continues straight as the descent steepens before reaching ▶7 a small flat on **Bear Creek** just upstream of the confluence with Cache Creek. Follow Bear Creek downstream, and cross before you reach the deeper water near the confluence. Wading is likely except during high-flow conditions. Continue downstream on the east side of Bear Creek to the flat rocky bar at the confluence of Cache and Bear creeks. A road climbs up to Hwy 16 and the parking area where you left your car, ▶8 nearly 10 miles from your starting point.

Stream

MILESTONES

▶1	0.00	Judge Davis Trailhead on Hwy 20
▶2	1.36	Judge Davis and Cache Creek Ridge Trails junction, veer left
▶3	1.64	At T junction at grassy saddle, go right and up the hill
▶4	2.48	Dunfield Flat Trail junction, go right
▶5	5.78	Bulldozer four-way trail junction, go straight
▶6	7.10	Last stock pond on the ridge, go straight
▶7	9.89	Bear Creek crossing, just upstream of Cache Creek confluence
▶8	9.90	Hwy 16 parking area above Bear/Cache Creeks confluence

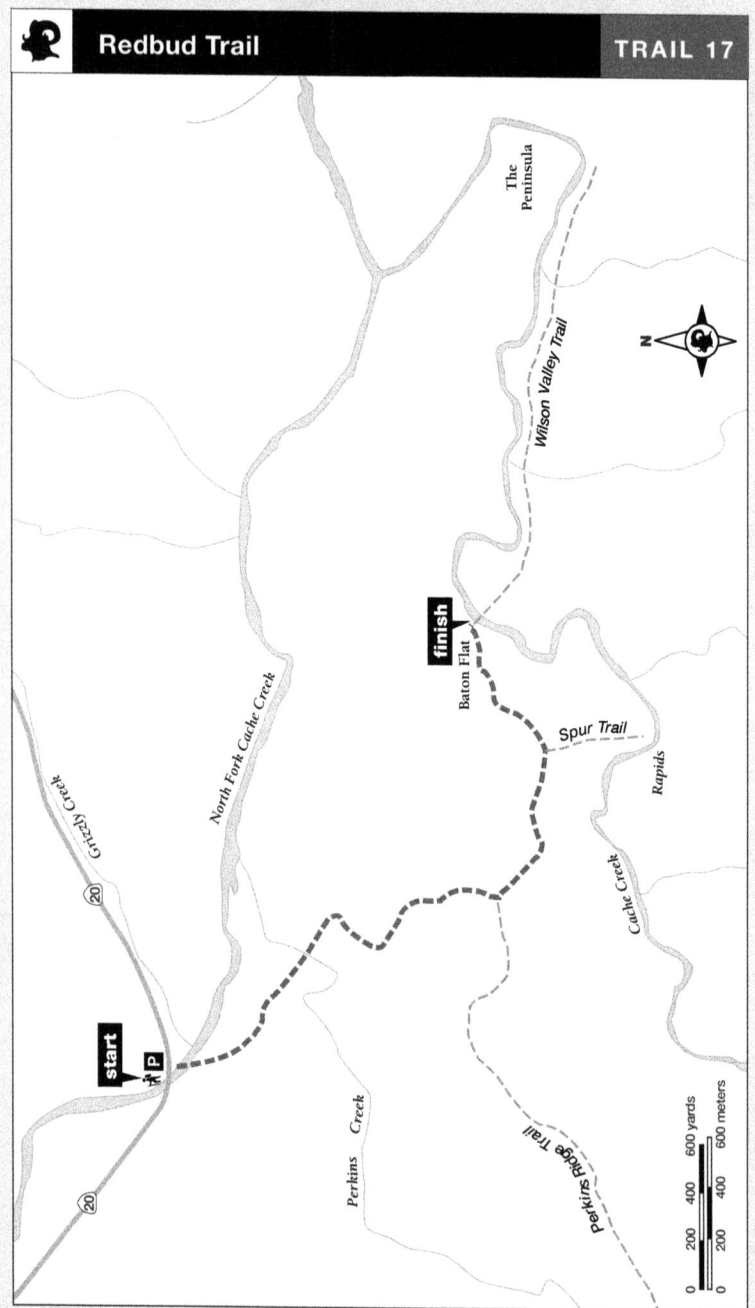

TRAIL 17 The Coast Range

Redbud Trail: Cache Creek Wilderness

The Cache Creek Wilderness and Wild & Scenic River are some of California's newest protected wild areas. Ironically, much of this area wasn't accessible to the public just 25 years ago. The large chunk of public land managed by the BLM was opened to the public when that agency and the California Department of Fish and Game worked together to acquire public lands that would allow trailheads to be developed along highways 20 and 16. Today, the magnificent oak woodlands, meadows, chaparral, and white-water rapids of the Cache Creek area are available for the public to enjoy. Tule elk, deer, bald eagles, bears, and river otters abound in this area, along with the rare adobe lily. The area is also rich in Native American cultural heritage. The Redbud Trail is one of the primary access trails to the newly designated Wilderness and Wild & Scenic River. Its trailhead is also the starting point for the class II+ wilderness white-water run for kayaks and small rafts.

Best Time

The Redbud Trail is accessible year-round, but spring is the best time to visit, for the cooler days and the outstanding wildflower displays. Hot temperatures, dry conditions, and annoying trailside stickers and foxtails make summer visits challenging.

Finding the Trail

From Sacramento, go north 24 miles on I-5 to the city of Woodland. Take the Hwy 16—Esparto exit.

TRAIL USE
Hike, Horse

LENGTH
4.02 miles, 2–3 hours

VERTICAL FEET
±470

DIFFICULTY
- 1 2 **3** 4 5 +

TRAIL TYPE
Out & Back

SURFACE TYPE
Dirt

FEATURES
Dogs Allowed
River
Canyon
Meadow
Wildflowers
Birds
Wildlife
Great Views
Photo Opportunity
Camping
Secluded

FACILITIES
Vault Toilets

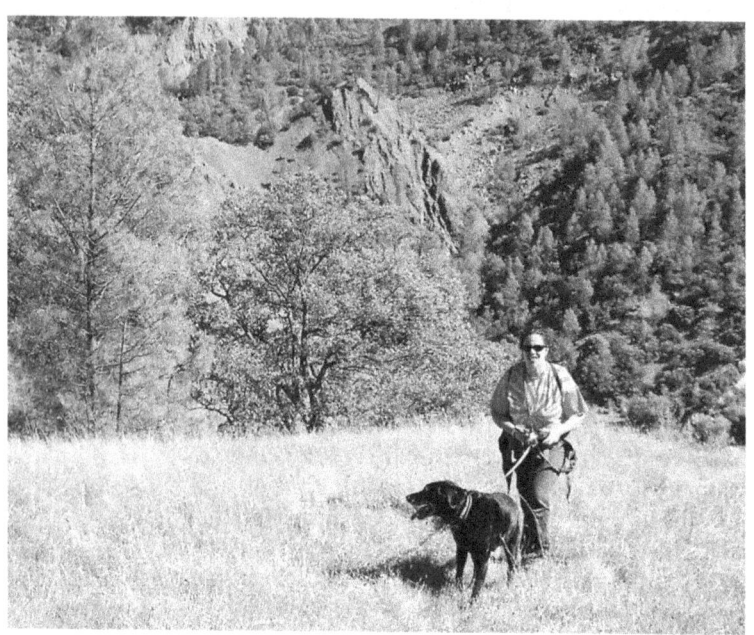

Dogs and people *enjoy the Redbud Trail's access to the Cache Creek Wilderness.*

Turn left and drive over I-5 and continue southeast for 3.1 miles on Hwy 16 to its intersection with Main St. Turn right and continue west approximately 10 miles on Hwy 16 to its intersection with Interstate 505. Cross over I-505 and continue west on Hwy 16 approximately 38 miles, driving through the small towns of Esparto and Capay, past the incongruous sprawl of the Cache Creek Casino in the middle of the otherwise bucolic Capay Valley, through the even smaller towns of Guinda and Rumsey, through Cache Creek Canyon and the three Yolo County Parks, and finally, along Bear Creek. Approximately 38 miles after crossing I-505, Hwy 16 dead-ends at Hwy 20. Turn left and drive west on Hwy 20 for approximately 12.5 miles. Just after crossing a bridge over the North Fork Cache Creek, turn left at the sign that says CACHE CREEK MANAGEMENT AREA.

Redbud Trail — TRAIL 17

Drive 0.3 mile to where the access road dead-ends at the Redbud Trailhead parking area.

Logistics

The Cache Creek area is popular for hunting. If the sight of well-armed people and the sound of guns disturb you, you may want to avoid this area during deer-, elk-, and turkey-hunting seasons. This trail enters the newly designated Cache Creek Wilderness. Mountain bikes and motorized vehicles are prohibited in the wilderness.

Although the route to Baton Flat is ideal for a short day hike, day visitors or backpackers may want go beyond Baton Flat to explore Wilson Valley and the truly wild canyons of Cache Creek farther downstream.

Trail Description

From the Redbud Trailhead parking area, ▶1 go through a locked gate and walk southeast along a gravel road used to access private inholdings downstream on the North Fork Cache Creek. The road cuts through a large meadow, which provides important tule elk habitat—but the formerly native grassland is overrun by non-native star thistle. Hopefully, the BLM and the Department of Fish and Game will continue to take steps to control or eliminate the thistle and restore the meadow's habitat value.

A brown fiberglass wand marks the start of the Redbud Trail proper, which diverges from the road to the right. ▶2 The trail soon crosses the seasonal streambed of **Perkins Creek**. Just after you cross the creek bed, a spur trail meanders off through the oaks and into the meadow on the left, but your route goes straight, climbs briefly, and begins to traverse the wooded slope above the meadow.

Almost immediately, the trail passes samples of the trail's namesake vegetation—redbud—which blooms a gorgeous reddish-purple color in the early spring.

🌿 Meadow

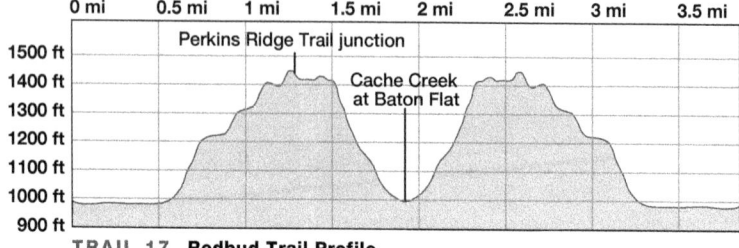

TRAIL 17   Redbud Trail Profile

The Redbud Trail begins a relatively gentle ascent through blue, live, and scrub oaks, as well as gray pine, skunkbush, manzanita, chamise, and the ever-present (at this elevation) poison oak. Trillium, with its dark green leaves veined in white, may be seen along this section of the trail in the spring. At one point, the trail goes through a stand of old-growth manzanita over 10 feet tall. Periodic views to the north include the North Fork meadow and the Baton Flat's "badlands" cliffs to the west, which are colored a remarkable bluish gray by their soft serpentine soils.

As it reaches the edge of a deeply incised gully, the trail turns to the southwest, and begins to ascend a steep side ridge. The trail climbs straight uphill for about 0.33 mile and then turns to the southeast again as it cuts across the head of the gully. It then continues its traverse of the wooded slope and crosses a couple of smaller drainages.

The trail reaches a ridgetop saddle and the junction with the **Perkins Ridge Trail**. ▶3 Turn left and proceed a short distance along the ridgetop. From here, you get your first good view of the main stem of **Cache Creek** and its rugged canyon. A rocky inner gorge in this segment is known by expert kayakers as the "The Jams." Fortunately, this is upstream of the confluence of the main stem and the North Fork, so less-skilled kayakers putting in at the Redbud Trail will live to paddle another day.

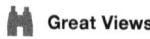 **Great Views**

Redbud Trail | TRAIL **17**

A couple of spur trails proceed down the side ridges on the right. The second use-trail actually leads to a seldom-visited bend in Cache Creek just upstream of Baton Flat, complete with bedrock mortar grinding holes. But the **Redbud Trail** continues west past these informal spur trails and then bends northwest as it drops steeply off the ridge and descends to another saddle. From there, the trail's descent moderates as it drops down toward a large, open meadow framed by looming eroded serpentine cliffs at **Baton Flat**.

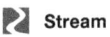 Stream

At Baton Flat, ▶4 the trail meets up again with the jeep road that it left in the meadow at the North Fork. Go right and walk the short distance to the bank of Cache Creek. Those enjoying a short day hike will stop here for lunch before ▶5 retracing their steps back to the trailhead.

Day hikers looking for a longer trip or backpackers seeking an overnight stay may ford Cache Creek and walk 4.0 more miles to Rocky Creek and Wilson Valley. Cache Creek may be difficult to ford at Baton Flat during winter/spring flows or during summer irrigation releases from upstream dams. But most of the time, the Baton Flat crossing can be done by using stepping stones.

Stream

MILESTONES

- ▶1 0.00 Redbud Trailhead off Hwy 20
- ▶2 0.30 Leave road, veer right on Redbud Trail
- ▶3 1.35 Junction with Perkins Ridge Trail, turn left
- ▶4 2.01 Baton Flat, retrace steps back to trailhead
- ▶5 4.02 Return to Redbud Trailhead

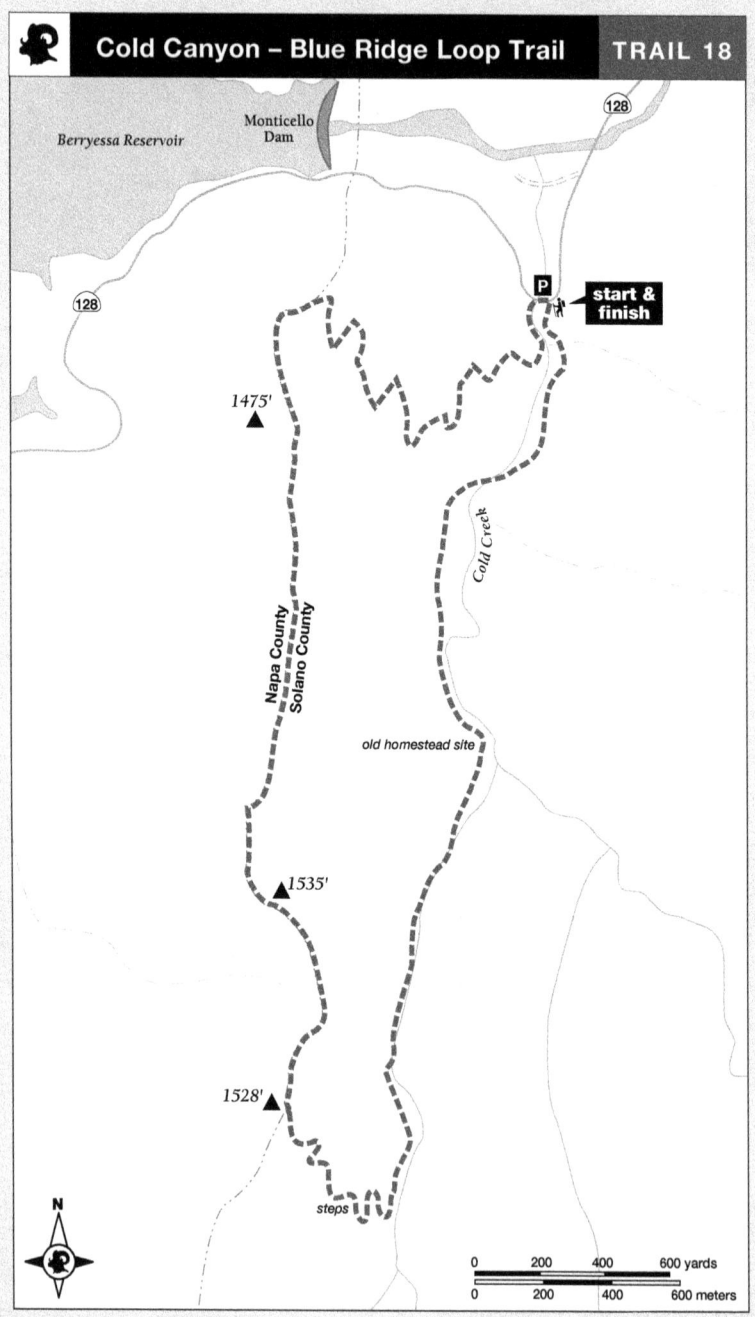

TRAIL 18 The Coast Range

Cold Canyon–Blue Ridge Loop Trail: Stebbins UC Reserve

This is the signature hike for residents of Davis and others who live in the Putah Creek watershed. People looking for an easy round-trip ramble with the family that is less than 2.0 miles long with only a 300-foot elevation gain may go out and back to the old homestead site in the Stebbins Cold Canyon Reserve, which is owned and managed by the University of California. But those looking for more of a physical challenge can go beyond the reserve to complete a demanding loop nearly 5.0 miles in length that climbs more than 1200 feet to the top of Blue Ridge. Along the way, hikers who brave the more challenging loop option will enjoy views of Berryessa Reservoir and much of the Coast Range.

Best Time

The hills are green and the wildflowers outstanding in the spring. Late fall and winter are also cool enough to do this loop. Only the hardiest hikers visit this trail in the summer and then only in the early morning.

Finding the Trail

From Sacramento, drive 29 miles west on Interstate 80 to its intersection with Interstate 505 in Vacaville. Drive 11 miles north on I-505 to the Winters/Hwy 128 exit. Take the Winters exit, turn left, go over the freeway, and drive approximately 11 miles east on Hwy 128. Just after the highway crosses over Putah Creek, it begins to climb toward Monticello Dam. You will come to a big bend in the road with a parking area on the right. Park here. The trailhead is just across the road.

TRAIL USE
Hike, Run

LENGTH
4.9 miles, 3.5–5 hours

VERTICAL FEET
±1200

DIFFICULTY
- 1 2 3 4 **5** +

TRAIL TYPE
Out & Back
Loop

SURFACE TYPE
Dirt
Rock

FEATURES
Child Friendly
Canyon
Meadow
Stream
Wildflowers
Birds
Wildlife
Historic
Great Views
Photo Opportunity
Steep

FACILITIES
None

> You reach a false summit with nice rocky perches favored by raptors.

Logistics

The UC Natural Reserve System offers guided hikes in the Stebbins Cold Canyon Reserve. For the current schedule of guided hikes, visit http://nrs.ucdavis.edu/stebbins/guides/guide_schedule.htm.

Trail Description

From the parking area on Hwy 183, ▶1 carefully look both ways for traffic and then cross the highway to the unmarked gated trailhead on the east side of the creek. Go through the gate, past a sign marking an uphill side trail on your left and continue straight past an information kiosk with a map. About 200 yards past the kiosk, another spur trail heads down to the creek on your right. Continue straight on the Cold Canyon Trail through a typical Coast Range low-elevation forest of live and blue oaks, buckeye, laurel, and gray pine. Native bunchgrass, yerba santa, toyon (Christmasberry), and coyote bush line the trail. The tread is often uneven due to rocks, and soon it ascends a series of hand-built steps to avoid a steep bank sloping down to the creek. A bit over 0.5 mile from the parking area, the trail crosses **Cold Creek**, ▶2 which is easily negotiated most any time except during high flows caused by heavy rains.

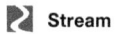 Stream

After crossing the creek, the trail continues its moderate ascent up Cold Canyon on the west side of the creek. Sections of this trail are heavily eroded as it makes its way under a thick canopy of oak, laurel, and manzanita. Eventually, the trail breaks out of the forest and you can see ahead the confluence of Cold Creek with a side canyon coming in from the southeast.

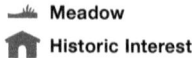
Meadow
Historic Interest

Continue on the trail to a small open meadow where retaining walls and foundations mark an old homestead ▶3. This is an excellent lunch spot for those who are doing the easy, out-and-back part of this walk. A spur trail on the left drops down toward

Cold Canyon–Blue Ridge Loop Trail | TRAIL 18

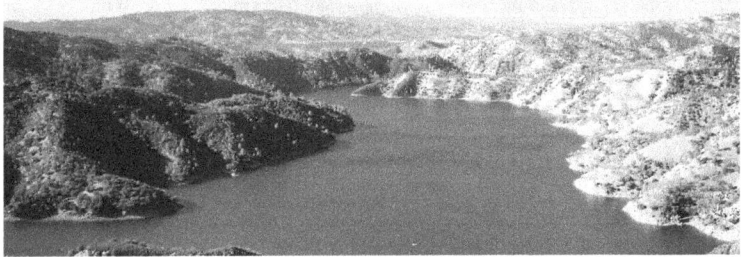

Berryessa Reservoir *from the top of the ridge on the Cold Canyon Loop Trail*

Cold Creek, where another foundation marks the spot of the homestead's former "cold house," where victuals were kept near the cool creek bed.

Continue up the main trail from the homestead. Since fewer people go beyond the homestead, the trail roughens and narrows, and is overgrown with brush in some segments. Then the trail steepens as it ascends farther up-canyon through thick brush and scrub oak, with a healthy understory of poison oak. Nearly 1.7 miles from the trailhead, your route drops down by Cold Creek again. The trail parallels the creek bed a short distance and then abruptly turns right and ascends a series of steep steps climbing the canyon's western slope. ▶4 Take a deep breath and prepare for a 400-foot climb in a bit over 0.25 mile.

 Caution

 Steep

Climbing a series of steps cut into the canyon's western slope, the trail negotiates some short switchbacks through a live-oak forest. The route crosses a rough wooden bridge spanning a seep and then continues its steep climb up another series of steps and switchbacks. Vegetation soon changes from live and scrub oak to toyon, coyote bush, and buckbrush. The trail ascent moderates somewhat and then reaches a brushy saddle where it reaches a Y intersection. The left branch is indistinct and may be little more than a deer trail. The Cold Canyon/Blue Ridge loop trail veers right and heads due north to climb ▶5 a knob (elevation 1528 feet) on **Blue**

 Summit

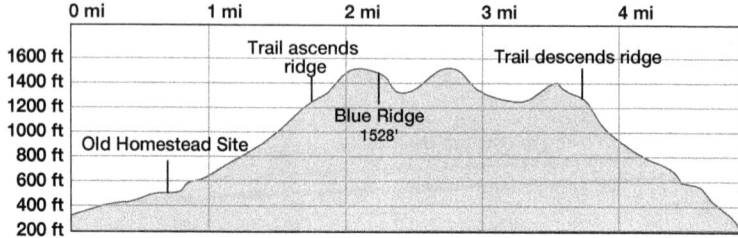

TRAIL 18 Cold Canyon–Blue Ridge Loop Trail Profile

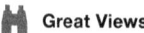 Great Views

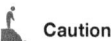 Caution

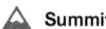 Summit

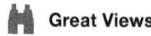 Great Views

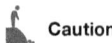 Caution

Ridge, which provides the first view of Berryessa Reservoir to the northwest, with Mt. Konocti near Clear Lake on the horizon.

After catching your breath, proceed north on the trail past a 2.0-mile marker along the increasingly rocky, brushy, and uneven top of Blue Ridge. The ridgetop trail pops down and up a couple of times before dropping down to a low point at about 1300 feet. From there, the trail begins another steep climb and comes to a sloping rock buttress. People seeking to avoid the uninviting rock slope—it's not quite a cliff—have created a path to the right that wanders off and dead-ends in the brush. Fortunately, the short, sloping buttress is easily negotiated with some hand and footholds and the exposure is minimal. Soon you reach the rocky summit of this high point in the ridge, which tops out at about 1535 feet. Find a handy rock to sit on, catch your breath, eat lunch, and enjoy the expansive views in all directions.

From this high point, the trail descends on rocky and uneven tread to 1250 feet, past a sign delineating the Cold Canyon Reserve boundary and public land managed by the BLM. The trail levels briefly, but then the tread virtually disappears as the route works its way over jumbled bedrock and boulders punctuated by heavy brush. Take care to avoid twisting an ankle in this segment.

Past mile marker 2.75, the trail tread reappears and walking becomes easier. At the 3.0-mile marker,

Cold Canyon–Blue Ridge Loop Trail   TRAIL 18

the trail ascends the last high point on Blue Ridge. You reach a false summit, and then continue north and uphill to the actual third high point of about 1429 feet. An arm of **Berryessa Reservoir** is directly below. From there, ▶6 the trail descends steeply past the 3.25-mile marker, sometimes requiring scrambling across sloping rock shelves. At the end of the ridge, the trail finally reaches relatively firm soil but its descent steepens as it drops into **Cold Canyon** in earnest.

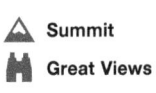

Summit

Great Views

The descent becomes so steep that it can be difficult to negotiate if it's wet. The trail continues its downhill plunge through blue oaks and brush. As of 2007, this segment of trail was being rebuilt with switchbacks so it should be easier to hike in the future. Eventually, the trail meets up with an old jeep trail ▶7 that switchbacks in a more stately fashion down into the canyon and then levels out as it proceeds north toward the highway. Side trails drop off to the right to cross Cold Creek and reconnect with the first segment of your loop, but it is easier to proceed north on the jeep trail to a gate at Hwy 183. ▶8 Carefully cross the highway, and turn right to follow the shoulder back to the parking area.

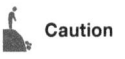

Caution

MILESTONES

- ▶1 0.00 Parking area
- ▶2 0.60 Cold Creek crossing
- ▶3 0.82 Old homestead site
- ▶4 1.72 Trail begins climb to Blue Ridge
- ▶5 2.00 1500-foot summit of Blue Ridge
- ▶6 3.73 Trail begins descending Blue Ridge
- ▶7 4.78 Trail connects with old jeep trail
- ▶8 4.90 Return to parking area

CHAPTER 3

Sierra Foothills

19. North Yuba River Trail
20. Humbug Creek–South Yuba Trails: South Yuba Wild & Scenic River
21. Empire Mine State Historic Park Loop Trails
22. Shingle Falls Trail: Spenceville Wildlife Area
23. Stevens Trail: North Fork American Wild & Scenic River
24. Codfish Falls Trail: Auburn State Recreation Area
25. American Canyon Trail: Auburn State Recreation Area
26. Western States Trail: El Dorado Canyon
27. Western States–Riverview Trails: Auburn State Recreation Area
28. Olmstead Loop Trail: Auburn State Recreation Area
29. Cronan Ranch Loop: South Fork American River
30. Marshall Gold Discovery State Historic Park Loop

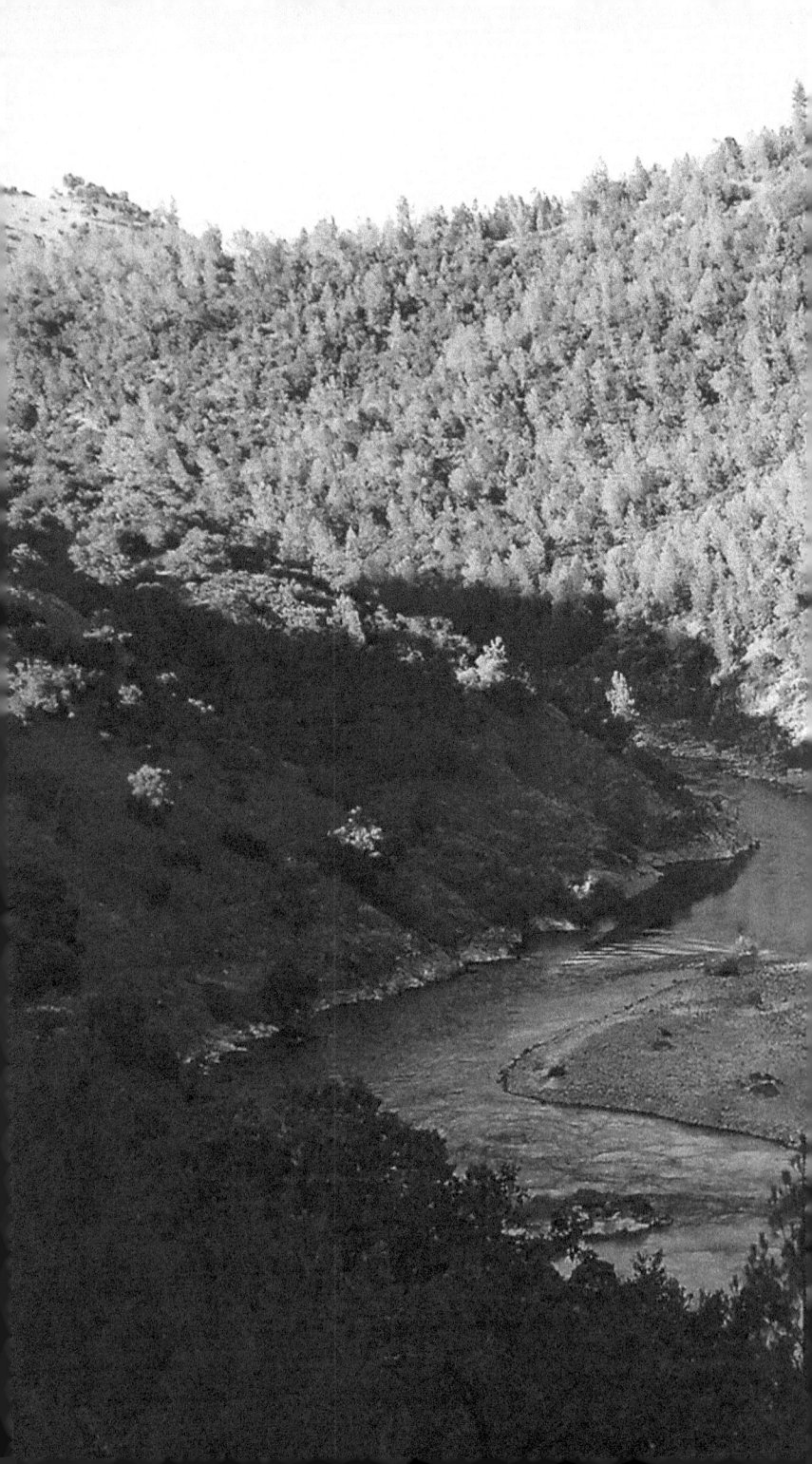

AREA OVERVIEW

Sierra Foothills

About 30 years ago, a new "gold" rush started in the Sierra foothills. Except this time, people are relocating to the Mother Lode not in search of gold, but to enjoy its rural nature, historical value, and the foothill ridges and river canyons covered in blue oak forests, meadows, and chaparral. Fortunately, federal, state, and non-governmental agencies have been working to acquire public lands in the Sierra foothills and Coast Range to protect open space from development and to provide year-round recreation opportunities in this fast growing region.

Maps and Permits

USGS 7.5-minute quad maps best identify topography and physical features. Since many of the trails newly established for hiking, biking, and equestrian use follow old road and jeep trails systems, many are still accurately depicted on the USGS maps. Some specific areas have trail maps published by the managing agency and are found at outdoor recreation equipment stores and/or on the Internet. These are listed in the appendix, as are the specific USGS quads for each trail.

Modest parking fees are charged at the State Parks featured in this chapter. Because many of the areas with featured trails were established to preserve wildlife and their habitat, dogs are prohibited or at least required to be on leash.

Overleaf and opposite: *The Riverview segment of the Western States Trail provides outstanding views of the North Fork American River (Trail 27).*

AREA MAP

Sierra Foothills

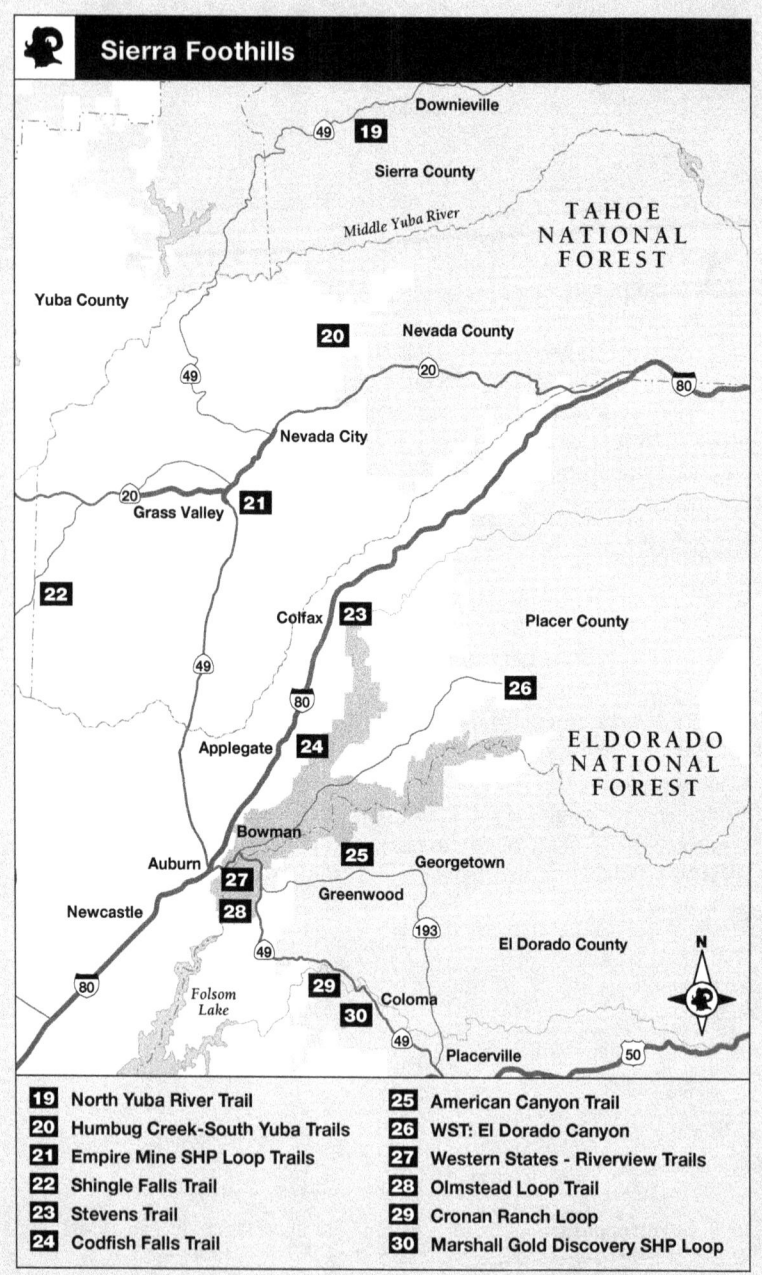

19 North Yuba River Trail	25 American Canyon Trail
20 Humbug Creek-South Yuba Trails	26 WST: El Dorado Canyon
21 Empire Mine SHP Loop Trails	27 Western States - Riverview Trails
22 Shingle Falls Trail	28 Olmstead Loop Trail
23 Stevens Trail	29 Cronan Ranch Loop
24 Codfish Falls Trail	30 Marshall Gold Discovery SHP Loop

TRAIL FEATURE TABLE

Sierra Foothills

TRAIL	Difficulty	Length	Type	USES & ACCESS	TERRAIN	FLORA & FAUNA	OTHER
19	4	7.5	Point-to-Point	Hiking, Running, Biking, Dogs	River/Stream, Waterfall, Canyon	Wildflowers, Fall Colors	Historic, Great Views, Camping, Photo
20	4	6.82	Point-to-Point	Hiking, Running, Biking, Dogs	River/Stream, Waterfall, Canyon	Wildflowers, Fall Colors	Historic, Great Views, Steep, Camping, Photo
21	3	4.47	Loop	Hiking, Horses, Running, Biking, Child Friendly, Fee, Dogs	River/Stream, Canyon	Wildflowers	Historic, Geologic, Photo
22	3	4.9	Loop	Hiking, Horses, Running, Biking, Dogs	River/Stream, Waterfall, Meadow, Canyon	Wildflowers, Birds, Wildlife	Historic, Great Views, Photo
23	5	7.0	Out & Back	Hiking, Biking, Dogs	River/Stream, Waterfall, Canyon	Wildflowers, Fall Colors	Historic, Great Views, Steep, Camping, Photo
24	2	2.8	Out & Back	Hiking, Child Friendly	River/Stream, Waterfall, Canyon	Wildflowers	Great Views, Photo
25	4	5.74	Out & Back	Hiking, Horses, Running, Biking, Dogs	River/Stream, Waterfall, Meadow, Canyon	Wildflowers, Fall Colors	Historic, Great Views, Steep, Photo
26	4	5.6	Out & Back	Hiking, Running, Biking, Dogs	River/Stream, Canyon	Wildflowers	Historic, Great Views, Steep, Secluded, Camping
27	3	4.2	Point-to-Point	Hiking, Horses, Running, Biking	River/Stream, Canyon	Wildflowers, Birds, Wildlife	Historic, Great Views, Photo
28	4	8.5	Loop	Hiking, Horses, Running, Biking, Dogs	River/Stream, Waterfall, Meadow, Canyon	Wildflowers, Fall Colors, Birds, Wildlife	Great Views, Geologic
29	3	4.9	Loop	Hiking, Horses, Running, Biking, Child Friendly, Dogs	River/Stream, Meadow, Canyon	Wildflowers, Birds	Great Views
30	3	3.6	Loop	Hiking, Running, Fee	River/Stream, Canyon	Fall Colors, Wildlife	Historic, Great Views, Steep, Photo

Legend

USES & ACCESS
- Hiking
- Horses
- Running
- Biking
- Child Friendly
- Handicap Access
- $ Fee
- Permit Required
- Dogs Allowed

TYPE
- Loop
- Out & Back
- Point-to-Point
- V Variable

DIFFICULTY
- 1 2 3 4 5 +
less ← → more

TERRAIN
- River or Stream
- Waterfall
- Lake
- Wetland
- Meadow
- Canyon
- Mountain

FLORA & FAUNA
- Wildflowers
- Fall Colors
- Birds
- Wildlife

FEATURES
- Historic Interest
- Geologic Interest
- Great Views
- Steep
- Secluded
- Camping
- Photo Opportunity

TRAIL SUMMARIES

Sierra Foothills

TRAIL 19
Hike, Run, Bike
7.5 miles, Point to Point
Difficulty: 1 2 3 **4** 5

North Yuba River Trail 163
Explore one of the Sierra's longest segments of free-flowing rivers as you walk along this relatively easy trail. Spectacular views of the North Yuba's rapids and canyon slopes abound. The trail also crosses three major creeks as they cascade down into the canyon, and offers glimpses of the area's Gold Rush heritage.

TRAIL 20
Hike, Run, Bike
6.8 miles, Point to Point
Difficulty: 1 2 3 **4** 5

**Humbug Creek–South Yuba Trails:
South Yuba Wild & Scenic River** 169
The South Yuba is everyone's favorite swimming river. This trail begins along Humbug Creek in Malakoff Diggins State Park, drops steeply downhill past a scenic Humbug Creek Falls, and then accesses a less-visited portion of the South Yuba River, providing nice views of the river canyon and access to two semi-developed campsites.

TRAIL 21
Hike, Run, Bike, Horse
4.5 miles, Loops
Difficulty: 1 2 **3** 4 5

**Empire Mine State Historic Park
Loop Trails** 177
Explore the old tailings piles, stamp-mill foundations, and other historic aspects of the Empire Mine State Park on these relatively easy loop trails. At the end of your walk, you can visit the mouth of the mine's ominous 5000-foot-deep shaft and its associated buildings, including the palatial English-style manor and rose garden of the mine's former owner.

Shingle Falls Trail:
Spenceville Wildlife Area 185

Visit one of the tallest waterfalls in the Sierra foothills and explore the little-known Spenceville Wildlife Area. This trail meanders along scenic Dry Creek and climbs up through oak woodlands and meadows spangled with wildflowers, to the edge of a deep, rocky gorge and spectacular 100-foot-high Shingle Falls.

TRAIL 22

Hike, Run, Bike, Horse
4.9 miles, Loop
Difficulty: 1 2 **3** 4 5

Stevens Trail:
North Fork American Wild &
Scenic River 191

This forgotten historic Gold Rush trail was rediscovered by a Boy Scout in 1969 and has become a favorite spring or fall hike for Sacramentans. The trail descends on a relatively gentle grade more than 1000 feet to the North Fork American Wild & Scenic River, while providing great views of the canyon. This hike's ultimate destination includes one of the most inviting pools you'll find for swimming in the warm summer months.

TRAIL 23

Hike, Bike
7.0 miles, Out & Back
Difficulty: 1 2 3 4 **5**

Codfish Falls Trail:
Auburn State Recreation Area 197

This is a great spring hike for the family. It's short and flat, but rich in wildflowers and views of the North Fork American River, and includes one of the prettiest little waterfalls in the Sierra foothills. The many languid pools of the North Fork beckon to swimmers in the summer.

TRAIL 24

Hike
2.8 miles, Out & Back
Difficulty: 1 **2** 3 4 5

TRAIL 25

Hike, Run, Bike, Horse
5.74 miles, Out & Back
Difficulty: 1 2 3 **4** 5

**American Canyon Trail:
Auburn State Recreation Area** 201

One of the best hikes in the Auburn State Recreation Area, the American Canyon Trail provides access to the scenic Middle Fork American River, as well as cascades created by American Canyon Creek. The trail packs in a lot of variety, from deep forest, lush riparian habitat, and oak/chaparral, with a sprinkling of Gold Rush mining sites.

TRAIL 26

Hike, Run, Bike
5.6 miles, Out & Back
Difficulty: 1 2 3 **4** 5

**Western States Trail:
El Dorado Canyon** 207

The beautiful stream flowing through El Dorado Canyon is the destination of this relatively steep segment of the Western States Trail. Following an historic route used to supply Gold Rush mines, the trail provides incredible views of the nearly vertical canyon slopes of the North Fork of the Middle Fork American River and offers a nice campsite as well as opportunities for swimming and fishing at the bottom. But be prepared for the climb back out.

TRAIL 27

Hike, Run, Bike, Horse
4.2 miles, Point to Point
Difficulty: 1 2 **3** 4 5

**Western States–Riverview Trails:
Auburn State Recreation Area** 213

This section of the Western States Trail starts in the city of Auburn and makes its way downhill through the canyon of the North Fork American River, past the now-abandoned Auburn Dam site, and across the historic "No Hands" Bridge. The trail provides great views of the river canyon and visits a pretty tributary waterfall. Toward the end, you can drop down to the river for a refreshing dip.

Olmstead Loop Trail:
Auburn State Recreation Area 221
This Olmstead Loop Trail circumnavigates a large Sierra foothill meadow as it makes its way through oak woodlands, chaparral, and low-elevation pines. This area is rich in wildlife, offers dramatic overlooks of the North Fork American River canyon, crosses two streams, and provides access to a scenic cascade on Knickerbocker Creek.

TRAIL 28
Hike, Run, Bike, Horse
8.5 miles, Loop
Difficulty: 1 2 3 **4** 5

Cronan Ranch Loop:
South Fork American River 229
The recently aquired Cronan Ranch Regional Trails Park provides a rare opportunity to hike on public lands along the South Fork American River. This easy loop trail provides a nice ramble through oak and riparian woodlands and foothill grasslands. You'll find a spectacular spring wildflower display and opportunities to view wildlife. The loop trail also offers direct access to the South Fork, which is one of California's most popular white-water rivers.

TRAIL 29
Hike, Run, Bike, Horse
4.9 miles, Loop
Difficulty: 1 2 **3** 4 5

Marshall Gold Discovery
State Historic Park Loop 235
Marshall Gold Discovery State Park is the site of the event that changed California forever. The Monroe Ridge and Monument trails provide access to many of the park's diverse historic and interpretive sites, and offer nice views of the Coloma Valley and the South Fork American River.

TRAIL 30
Hike, Run
3.6 miles, Loop
Difficulty: 1 2 **3** 4 5

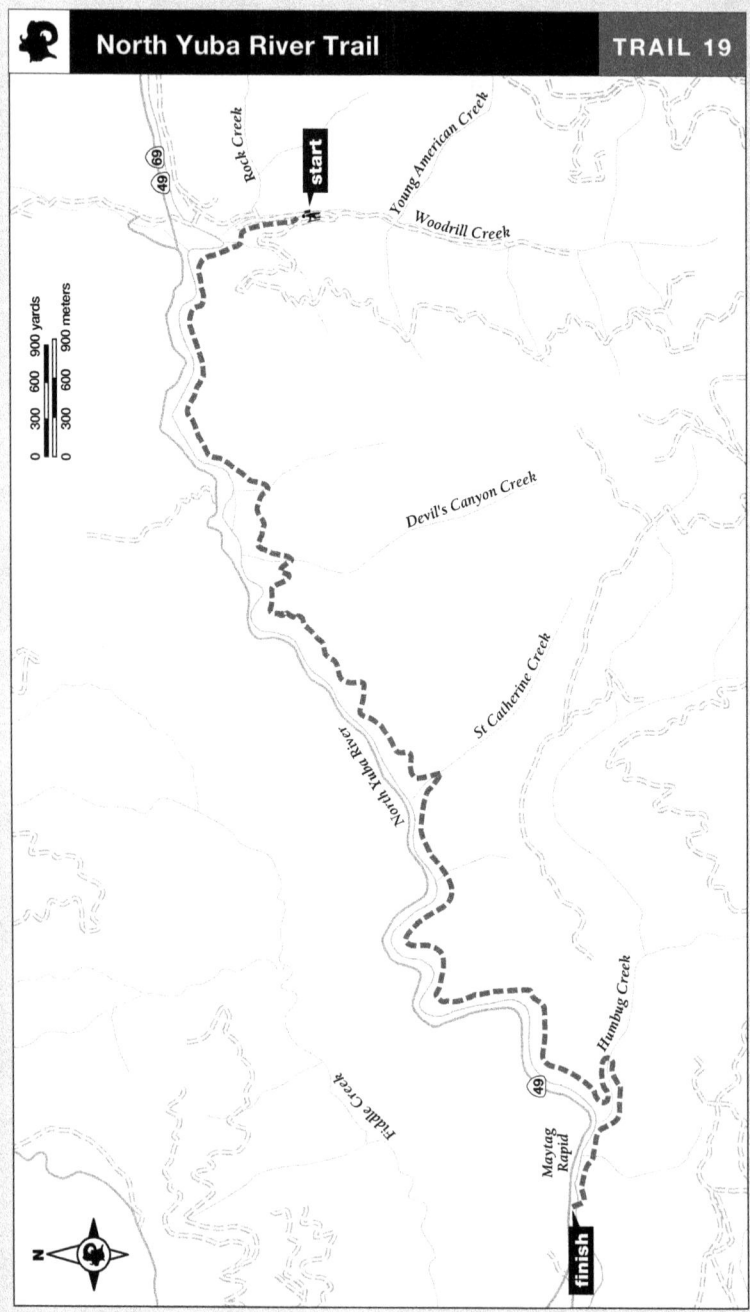

TRAIL 19 Sierra Foothills

North Yuba River Trail

The section of the North Yuba River that this trail parallels is one of the longest free-flowing river segments in the Sierra. Large rapids make the North Yuba a favorite run for expert white-water boaters. Although Hwy 49 parallels the opposite river bank, the highway is largely unobtrusive from much of the trail. Two scenic tributaries with cascades, the diverse low-elevation forest, and the river's rich Gold Rush history make this a great trail to visit virtually any time of the year.

Best Time

This relatively low-elevation trail (beginning at 2700 feet and ending at 2300 feet) is snow free most of the winter, but can be quite wet and icy due to its north-facing aspect. Although its forest overstory offers some shade during the hot summer months, spring and fall are the best times to hike this trail.

Finding the Trail

Drive 34 miles east from Sacramento on Interstate 80. Take the Hwy 49 exit in Auburn and turn left; drive north 24 miles on Hwy 49 to Nevada City. Just past the downtown Nevada City exit, turn left to continue north on Hwy 49. After descending into and then climbing out of the South Yuba and the Middle Yuba River valleys, Hwy 49 finally crosses the North Yuba River about 32 miles north of Nevada City. Beyond the North Yuba bridge, the highway turns east. Continue east 1.0 mile to the Rocky Rest area, on your right. This is the end trailhead for

TRAIL USE
Hike, Run, Bike
LENGTH
7.5 miles, 4–5 hours
VERTICAL FEET
-400
DIFFICULTY
- 1 2 3 **4** 5 +
TRAIL TYPE
Point to Point
SURFACE TYPE
Dirt

FEATURES
Dogs Allowed
River
Streams
Waterfall
Canyon
Fall Color
Wildflowers
Camping
Historic
Great views
Photo Opportunity

FACILITIES
Vault Toilets

> At one point, you have to carefully inch your way around a large tree root-ball sticking out over the trail.

this trip. To go to the beginning trailhead, continue east on Hwy 49 another 6.5 miles to the Goodyears Bar turnoff. Turn right, cross the North Yuba River again, and drive slowly through the small community of Goodyears Bar approximately 0.5 mile. The starting trailhead will be on your right.

Logistics

This is a great trail to visit with friends in a second car, so you can do a point-to-point 7.5 mile hike with a short car shuttle. Alternative trips include there and back from Goodyears Bar to St. Catherine Creek (7.0 miles round-trip) or there and back from Rocky Rest to Humbug Creek (1.5 miles round-trip). Hikers may camp at Rocky Rest and other nearby campgrounds, or stay in the bed and breakfast in Goodyears Bar to allow more time to explore the trail and enjoy the river.

Trail Description

From the upper trailhead just south of the small community of **Goodyears Bar**, ▶1 the trail begins on the west side of Forest Road 300 and climbs easily through Douglas firs and cedars. After you negotiate a short switchback, there is a sign that says NORTH YUBA TRAIL: ST. CATHERINE CREEK—3.5, ROCK REST TRAILHEAD—7.5. Continue north past the sign. The trail zigzags into a side canyon and crosses a small stream. As it climbs out of the side canyon, it rounds the end of a ridge, providing a view of the hamlet of Goodyears Bar. It then enters the **North Yuba River canyon** proper and turns west. Shortly thereafter, the trails crosses an abandoned mining ditch and continues west, dropping down briefly along the river.

After paralleling the river a short distance, the trail begins climbing and then switchbacks upward

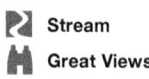
Stream
Great Views

North Yuba Trail   TRAIL 19

to cross a landslide on narrow and temporary tread. At one point, you have to carefully inch your way around a large tree root-ball sticking out over the trail. Passing seasons, yearly erosion, and the vagaries of Forest Service trail maintenance may have changed this situation by the time you hike the trail. After crossing the landslide, the trail switchbacks down and continues west along the river.

Even though Hwy 49 is located just across the river, it is seldom noticeable along this trail segment. Trailside vegetation changes to ferns and willows as the trail crosses several seeps and two large springs. As the trail dips in and out of side drainages, subtle differences in slope aspect change the overstory from a shady Douglas fir forest to a sunnier live oak forest. Moist side canyons transition to black oak and big leaf maple. In the wetter season, mushrooms and heart-shaped trillium can be found along the trail.

West of the landslide, the trail drops down to a large alluvial flat along the river, incised by braided seasonal streambeds. At the west end of the flat, the trail switchbacks upward, crosses a small perennial creek, and enters a live oak forest with tree trunks luxuriant in lichen.

About 2.2 miles west of Goodyears Bar, ▶2 the trail drops into a larger side canyon fed by **Devils Canyon Creek**. The creek can be easily crossed by rock hopping during most of the year, but care should be taken when the creek is swollen by rain. After crossing the creek, the trail climbs a switchback and returns to the North Yuba canyon. As it heads west, the trail passes above a riverside flat shaded by large ponderosa pines—a nice place for camping except for the visible highway just across the river.

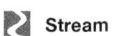 Stream

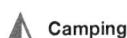 Camping

The trail drops downward to avoid a large rock outcrop and then switchbacks upward. After a short, steep pitch, the trail climbs well above the highway on the other side of the canyon. Unfortunately, this

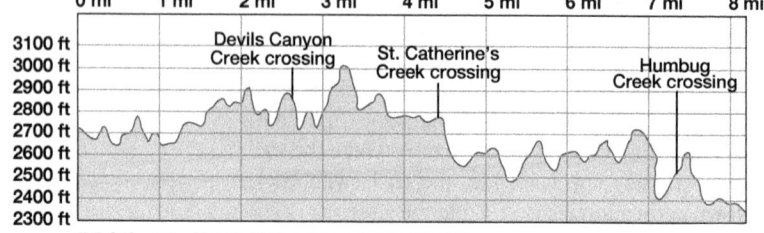

TRAIL 19 **North Yuba River Trail Profile**

means that traffic noise from the highway becomes more noticeable. Continuing westward, the trail zigzags in and out of a barely perennial canyon tributary, and then crosses another seasonal stream, this one decorated with large rounded stones clothed in emerald green lichen.

Stream

With little fanfare, the trail turns south and drops down to a footbridge crossing ▶3 **St. Catherine Creek**, about 3.5 miles from your starting point. At this largest tributary crossing yet, the creek banks have large rocks that provide an opportunity to rest and eat lunch. After crossing the footbridge over St. Catherine Creek, the trail climbs out of the side-canyon and then drops down close to the North Yuba River. A concrete pylon enclosing a river gauge is visible across the river just above a large rapid.

West of the stream gauge, the trail begins a long but easy climb traversing the canyon slope. The trail ultimately turns to the northwest as it begins to negotiate the first of two large bends in the river, which add more than 3.0 miles to the trail's length. After rounding the first large bend, the trail continues west through an extensive black oak grove, traverses a rocky slope covered in live oaks, and crosses two large seeps flowing down bedrock cliffs. The trail then negotiates the second large river bend.

Stream

West of the second bend, the trail drops down two switchbacks and crosses ▶4 **Humbug Creek** over a sturdy footbridge. Here you are about 6.75

North Yuba Trail — TRAIL 19

miles from your starting point and less than 1.0 mile from your destination. Humbug Creek cascades over a series of bedrock shelves upstream and downstream of the footbridge. An excellent swimming hole is downstream of the bridge on the right, at the foot of a particularly beautiful cascade.

After leaving Humbug Creek, the trail continues west and parallel to a large bedrock outcrop on the North Yuba River that forms **Maytag Rapid**. The North Yuba River downstream from Goodyears Bar is an experts-only class IV–V white-water run. Really a waterfall, class V Maytag Rapid is considered the toughest rapid on this section of the North Yuba and is not to be trifled with. Hikers visiting this section of the trail on any May weekend day may be treated to the thrilling view of rafts and kayaks negotiating (or not) this dangerous drop.

Downstream of Humbug Creek and Maytag Rapid, the trail follows the edge of the river, providing several opportunities to access the river. Lichen-covered rocks once stacked along the trail by gold miners create eerie-looking walls and foundations reminiscent of ancient ruins.

About 0.75 mile downstream of the Humbug Creek crossing, the trail turns right and crosses a large footbridge spanning the North Yuba River. ▶5 Cross the bridge to the Rocky Rest parking area and campsites next to Hwy 49.

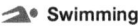 Waterfall

Swimming

River

MILESTONES

- ▶1 0.00 Goodyears Bar Trailhead
- ▶2 2.20 Devils Canyon Creek, continue west
- ▶3 3.50 St. Catherine Creek, continue west
- ▶4 6.75 Humbug Creek, continue west
- ▶5 7.50 Rocky Rest Trailhead

Sierra Foothills

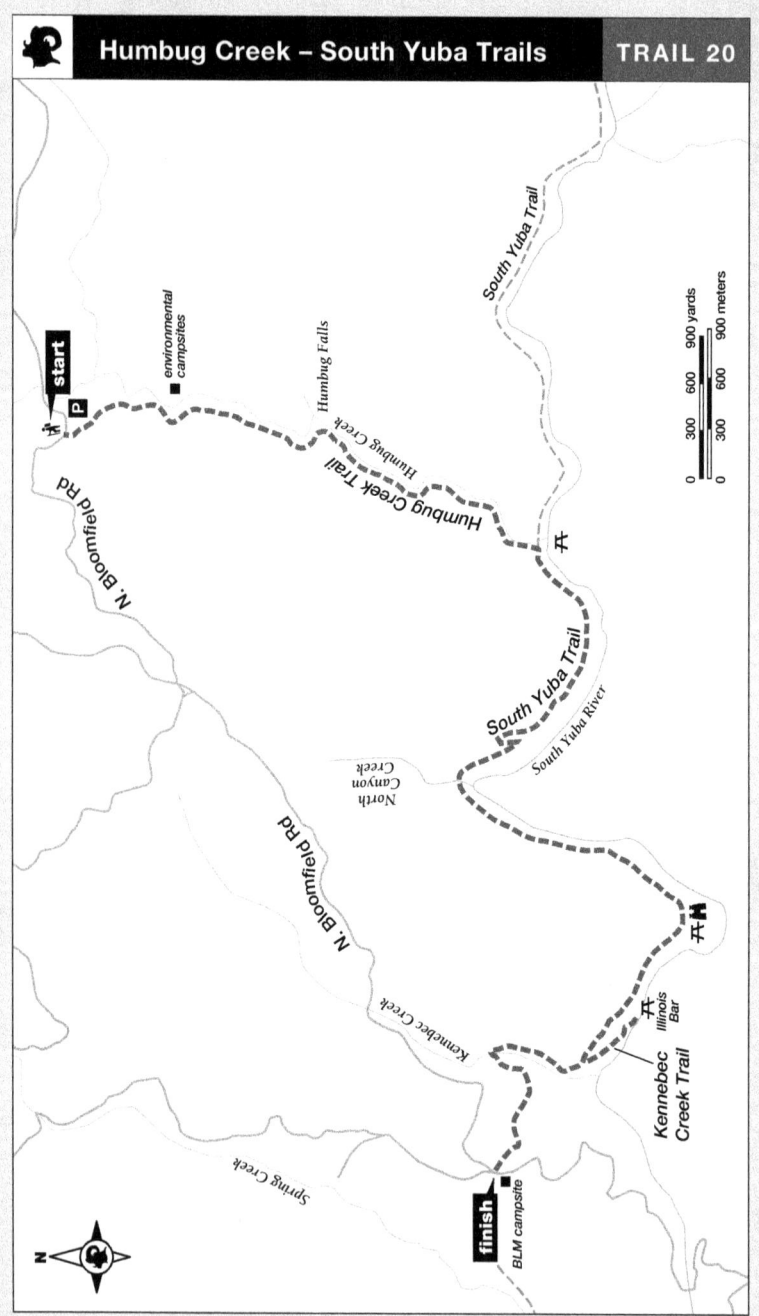

TRAIL 20 Sierra Foothills

Humbug Creek–South Yuba Trails: South Yuba Wild & Scenic River

Everyone's favorite swimming river in the summer, the South Yuba River also offers colorful springtime wildflowers and autumnal foliage as well. This trail passes by some ideal semi-developed campsites (with pit toilets and picnic tables) along the South Yuba, and the Humbug Creek segment features a dramatic waterfall that has carved its way through a bedrock slot. Add the facts that the entire area is rich in Gold Rush history and its trails are accessible nearly year-round, and the South Yuba River and Humbug Trails pretty much cover all bets.

Best Time

The optimal hike time is spring for the wildflowers, fresh green oak leaves, an inspiring waterfall, and the roaring river. Fall is nice with gold and red autumnal colors, but the river and creeks have low flows. Because at 2000–3000 feet in elevation the trails are generally below the snowline, they can be wet in winter, but outstanding on sunny days. Summer's heat is mitigated by the fact that you can go swimming in the cool waters of the South Yuba.

Finding the Trail

Drive 34 miles east from Sacramento on Interstate 80. Take the Hwy 49 exit in Auburn and turn left to drive north on Hwy 49 for 24 miles to Nevada City. Just past downtown Nevada City, turn left to follow Hwy 49, and within 0.25 mile turn right on North Bloomfield Road. Drive north on North Bloomfield Road for about 0.5 mile to the intersection with

TRAIL USE
Hike, Run, Bike
LENGTH
6.82 miles, 4–5 hours
VERTICAL FEET
-1000 / +600
DIFFICULTY
- 1 2 3 **4** 5 +
TRAIL TYPE
Point to Point
SURFACE TYPE
Dirt

FEATURES
Dogs Allowed
River
Streams
Waterfall
Canyon
Wildflowers
Fall Color
Camping
Historic
Great Views
Photo Opportunity
Steep

FACILITIES
Toilets
Picnic Tables

The South Yuba River is good for a quick, refreshing dip.

Lake Vera Road. Turn right to continue on North Bloomfield Road as it drops down to the South Yuba River, crosses the Edwards Crossing Bridge, and then climbs up San Juan Ridge for about a mile to the intersection of North Bloomfield Road and Grizzly Flat Road. Turn right to follow North Bloomfield and then immediately turn right again onto the BLM South Yuba Campground access road. Turn left into the South Yuba Trailhead parking area.

If you are doing a car shuttle or wish to begin an out-and-back hike at the Humbug Creek Trailhead, continue past the BLM South Yuba River Campground turn-off on North Bloomfield Road, 5.3 miles before Malakoff Diggins State Park. Look for a sign on the right that says HUMBUG TRAIL. Parking off the road is limited, but use is generally light. Take the time to drive 1.5 miles farther east on North Bloomfield Road to visit the park's headquarters and museum.

Logistics

If you are hiking with companions and have a second car, this trip makes a good one-way hike with a short car shuttle. Otherwise, you can hike there and back either from the South Yuba River Trailhead or the Humbug Creek Trailhead.

Trail Description

At the Humbug Trailhead, ▶1 a sign says HUMBUG TRAIL, ENVIRONMENTAL CAMPSITES—0.5, HUMBUG CREEK—1.25, SOUTH YUBA NATIONAL TRAIL—2.7. From the trailhead, your route—a former road—drops down along a seasonal tributary of **Humbug Creek** through Douglas firs, black oaks, and dogwoods. Within minutes, the trail reaches Humbug Creek proper on the left and the first of many flooded mine shafts on your right. Some of these shafts are seeping

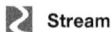 Stream

Humbug Creek–South Yuba Trails | TRAIL 20

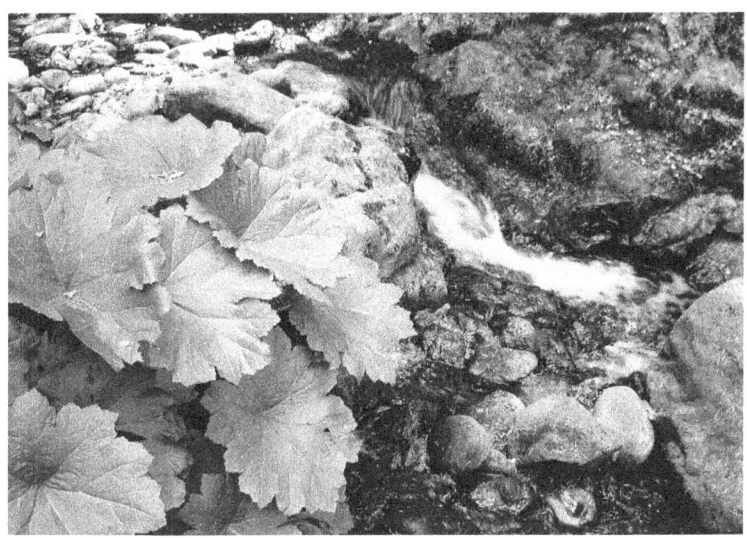

Indian rhubarb grows along Humbug Creek.

orange-colored water into Humbug Creek. Drinking is not advisable.

The trail continues its gentle downward trend past the Park's "Environmental Campsites," located on a creek-side bench. Either the bears or the campers didn't like the smell from the pit toilets because at least one has been turned over and torn apart. The trail crosses another tributary of Humbug Creek and then connects with an old jeep road coming in from the right. Continue your downward trek to the left on the Humbug Trail while enjoying periodic views of Humbug Creek.

After crossing another side stream, the trail becomes a single track and its descent steepens. The tread gets rockier and undulates up and down a bit. Just past its confluence with **Pan Ravine**, the trail enters Humbug Creek's rocky inner gorge. There are a couple of opportunities to drop down to the creek, which is lined with Indian rhubarb. Two short downward switchbacks on the main trail

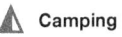 Camping

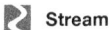 Stream

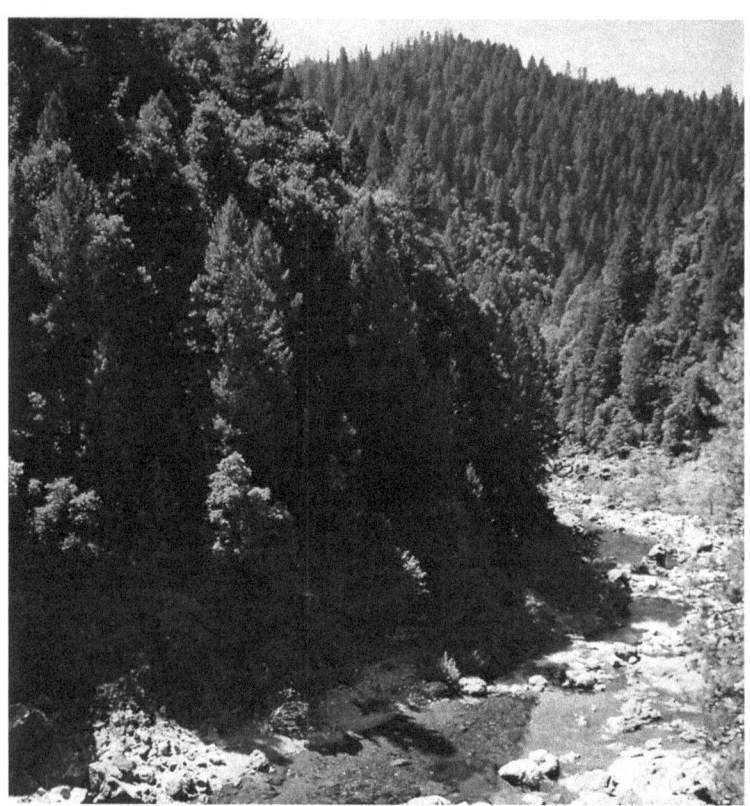

The South Yuba River *is a scenic feature of the Humbug Creek–South Yuba Trail.*

Waterfall

bring you to the top of inspiring **Humbug Falls** on your left. You can get a better view of the falls a little farther down the trail. The falls consists of a series of sinuous cascades and potholes carved by water in the metamorphic rock. It is most spectacular in the spring but slows to a trickle in the fall.

Below the waterfalls, the trail gets steeper and rockier. Hikers will have to scoot over sloping bedrock in some areas. The thick forest overstory continues, but changes from the formerly dominant Douglas fir to live oak, with a sprinkling of big leaf maple, cedar, ponderosa pine, and fir. The trail

Humbug Creek–South Yuba Trails TRAIL **20**

levels out briefly and then drops down one last steep pitch before reaching the junction of the **South Yuba Trail**, a bit over 2.0 miles from the trailhead.

Just below the junction is the Humbug Picnic Area on a shady bench above the **South Yuba River**. The site has a pit toilet with two picnic tables. The bench consists of mining debris—sediment and cobbles—washed down from the **Malakoff Diggins** and other old hydraulic mines. This debris clogged rivers in the foothills and the Great Valley in the late 1800s, causing flooding and polluting the water, prompting one of the first environmentally based lawsuits and subsequent legal decisions by a California court. The ruling ended this destructive mining practice in the Sierra foothills. Since then, the South Yuba has been eroding away the debris, leaving these high benches along the river as a testament to an age when miners moved mountains.

Below the bench and near its confluence with Humbug Creek, the South Yuba flows through smooth bedrock with pools ideal for swimming (although you might want to swim upstream of the Humbug Creek confluence to avoid any mining pollution the creek may be contributing to the South Yuba River).

From the trail junction above the picnic site, turn right ▶2 and follow the **South Yuba River Trail** downstream (west). The trail remains fairly high above the river, with limited access points and only occasional views up and down the canyon. Relatively level at first in its westward trek, the trail soon begins a steady climb through a forest of live oaks and then turns northward into the tributary canyon of **North Canyon Creek**. It then drops downward via three switchbacks and crosses seasonally flowing North Canyon Creek itself, ▶3 about 1.33 miles from the Humbug Trail junction.

From the North Canyon Creek crossing, the trail climbs up two switchbacks and then levels

- Camping
- Historic Interest
- Geologic Interest
- River
- Swimming
- Canyon
- Stream

Sierra Foothills 173

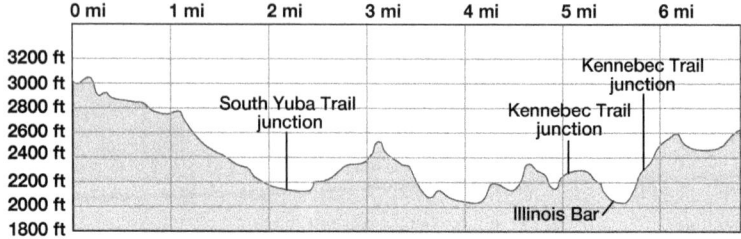

TRAIL 20 Humbug Creek–South Yuba Trails Profile

out. Soon, the trail reaches a junction with the North Canyon Spur Trail (not noted on any current maps), which leads downward to the left. Continue westward on the South Yuba River Trail. Beyond the North Canyon spur junction, hikers are treated to a dramatic downstream and upstream view of the South Yuba River as the river negotiates a large bend.

Great Views

The trail continues through a forest of live oak, laurel, buckeye, and redbud, and begins to climb gradually and then level out again. At one point, the trail crosses an open area of metamorphic basement rock, and soon thereafter reaches the Overlook Point picnic area on the left, signaled by the presence of a dilapidated picnic table shaded by live oaks and set close to a rough trail that leads to a river overlook. ▶4 At this point, you have walked a bit less than 1.25 mile from the North Canyon Creek crossing.

Beyond the Overlook Point picnic area, the South Yuba River Trail continues in a northwesterly direction through the now ubiquitous live-oak forest. In less than 0.75 mile, you will reach a junction with the **Kennebec Creek Trail**. ▶5 Turn left to follow the Kennebec Creek Trail down to Illinois Bar on the South Yuba River. This spur trail drops steeply downhill on an old mining road about 0.25 mile to reach the Illinois Bar campsite. Also a remnant of old hydraulic mining debris, this flat bench above the river has four picnic tables and a pit toilet.

Camping

Historic Interest

Humbug Creek–South Yuba Trails | TRAIL 20

From the bench, you can make your way down to the cobbled bar along the river. The river runs shallow in this area but a suitable swimming hole may be found just downstream.

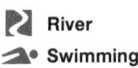
River
Swimming

After a refreshing dip, climb steeply back up the Kennebec Creek Trail, ▶6 stopping to admire the hand-built rock retaining wall along the trail (and to catch your breath). Sooner than anticipated, you reach the junction with the South Yuba Trail. From here, it is about 1.0 mile to the trailhead at the BLM Campground, so take another deep breath, ▶7 turn left, and continue climbing up the South Yuba Trail, which at this point is still following the old Kennebec Creek mining road.

Soon the trail leaves the South Yuba River Canyon behind and continues its moderate climb into the side canyon carved by Kennebec Creek. The trail reaches a junction, where the old Kennebec Road goes straight and the South Yuba Trail veers left and crosses perennial Kennebec Creek. The trail then resumes its moderate ascent through fir and oak forest to an unsigned junction. The South Yuba Trail continues straight to Edwards Crossing. ▶8 Turn right to follow the spur trail to ▶9 the nearby South Yuba River Trailhead.

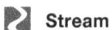
Stream

MILESTONES

- ▶1   0.00   Humbug Creek Trailhead
- ▶2   2.18   Junction with the South Yuba Trail, turn right
- ▶3   3.56   North Canyon crossing, continue straight
- ▶4   4.79   Overlook picnic site, continue straight
- ▶5   5.27   Junction with Kennebec Trail, turn left
- ▶6   5.55   Illinois Bar on the South Yuba River, turn back
- ▶7   5.83   Junction with the South Yuba River Trail, turn left
- ▶8   6.58   Turn right on spur trail to BLM Campground Trailhead
- ▶9   6.82   South Yuba River Trailhead at BLM Campground

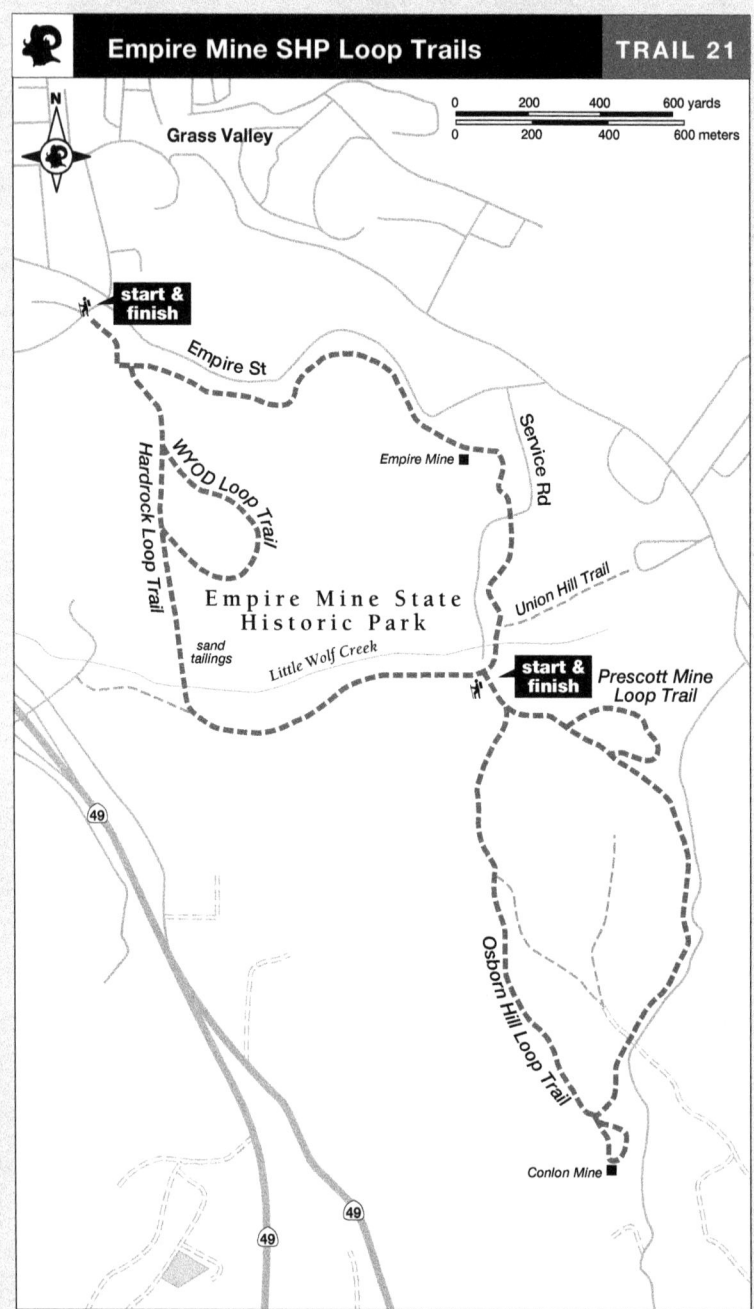

TRAIL 21 Sierra Foothills

Empire Mine State Historic Park Loop Trails

Visiting Empire Mine State Park is almost like a stroll back through time. Many of the mine buildings and equipment remain, as well as the palatial grounds and extensive rose garden of the mine's former owner. You can easily spend much of the day simply visiting the mine's infrastructure, including the mouth of the mine's ominous 5000-foot-deep shaft, but the park also boasts an extensive trail system, with a series of loops that feature old tailings piles, abandoned mine shafts, stamp-mill foundations, and a pleasant walk through a mixed oak and conifer forest. This is an ideal family outing, offering a wide variety of walking options and a fun and educational glimpse of California's mining history.

Best Time

Spring wildflowers and fall color make these two seasons the preferred time to visit. Elevations in the park range from 2600 to 2900 feet, so summer visits can be hot, and winter months are often snow free.

Finding the Trail

From Sacramento, drive 35 miles east on Interstate 80 to Auburn. Take the Hwy 49 exit in Auburn and drive 22.6 miles north to Grass Valley. Take the Empire St./Empire Mine State Park exit and turn right onto Empire St. Drive approximately 1.0 mile to the Penn Gate Trailhead parking area, on the right. The Empire Mine State Park visitors center is on Empire St. another 0.7 mile east of the Penn Gate parking area.

TRAIL USE
Hike, Run, Bike, Horse
LENGTH
4.47 miles, 2–3 hours (both loops)
VERTICAL FEET
±75
DIFFICULTY
- 1 2 **3** 4 5 +
TRAIL TYPE
Loop
SURFACE TYPE
Dirt

FEATURES
Dogs on Leash
Child Friendly
Parking fee
Stream
Canyon
Fall Color
Historic
Interpretive
Photo Opportunity
Geological Interest

FACILITIES
Vault Toilets

> The Work Your Own Diggings (WYOD) Mine got its name from the mine's practice of leasing portions to individual miners.

Logistics

Parking is free at the Penn Gate Trailhead parking area. The Hardrock Loop Trail is also accessible from the visitors center, but a $3 entrance fee is charged. Paying the fee is worth it because you can visit the museum, browse the bookstore, explore mine buildings and equipment, and marvel at the English-style manor and garden house and the beautiful rose garden. For a nominal fee, you can buy a brochure that provides historical information about key points along the park's trails.

Trail Description

Hardrock Loop Trail

From the **Penn Gate Trailhead** parking lot, ▶1 proceed southeast along an access road that provides the route for the **Hardrock Loop Trail**. Almost immediately, you come to the remains of the **Pennsylvania Mine**, the first of many former mines acquired by the expansionist Empire Mine. The two mushroom-shaped concrete buildings once housed the Penn Mine's transformers, and nearby foundations supported its compressor house and head frame. Also at the Pennsylvania Mine site, you'll see a junction from where a trail leads off to the left. This is the trail from the visitors center that will take you back to the Penn Gate Trailhead.

Proceed down the Hardrock Trail/road through a pleasant open forest of second-growth ponderosa pine, with a sprinkling of cedars and sugar pine. Less than 0.5 mile from the trailhead, the **Work Your Own Diggings** (WYOD) loop trail leads off to the left. ▶2 This 0.39-mile loop takes you to the top of the tallest tailings pile in the park and to the edge of a recovering wetlands area called the Sand Tailings. Hikers have the option to take the WYOD loop or continue on the Hardrock Trail.

Empire Mine State Historic Park Loop Trails | TRAIL 21

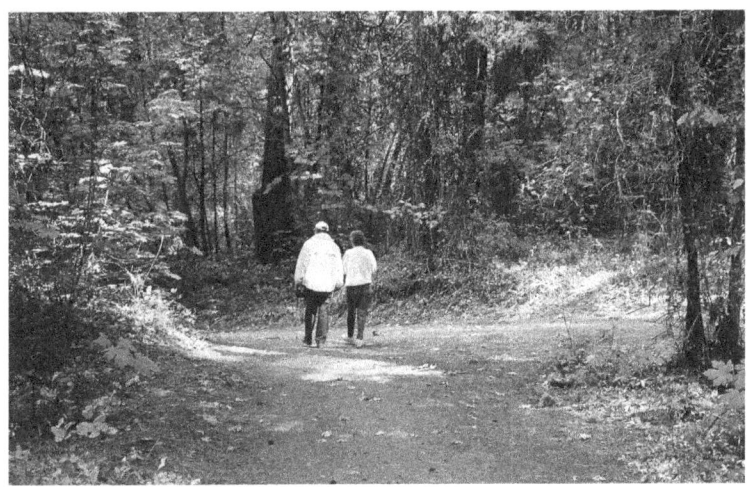

The extensive trail system *around the Empire Mine adds opportunities to explore several old mine sites.*

After the second junction with the WYOD Loop Trail, the Hardrock Trail splits, with the road veering to the right and the briefly single-track Hardrock Trail veering to the left. The single track then proceeds across an earthen berm called the Sand Dam, which was originally a trestle from where Pennsylvania Mine ore cars dumped waste rock. The slurry that accumulated behind the berm created the Sand Tailings. Just after crossing the berm, the Hardrock Trail crosses a ditch used to reroute **Little Wolf Creek** around the Sand Tailings.

🏠 Historic Interest

After rejoining the road, the Hardrock Trail begins a gentle climb parallel to Little Wolf Creek. Here, the forest is dominated by black oak and big leaf maple, promising excellent fall color. The trail goes over a barely noticeable hill and drops down to the junction with the ▶3 **Osborn Hill Loop Trail**.

▶ Stream

Adding the Osborn Hill Trail Loop is a good choice for those who want to stretch their legs and get a bit more of a workout than what is provided by the 2.37-mile Hardrock Loop. The spur trail loops

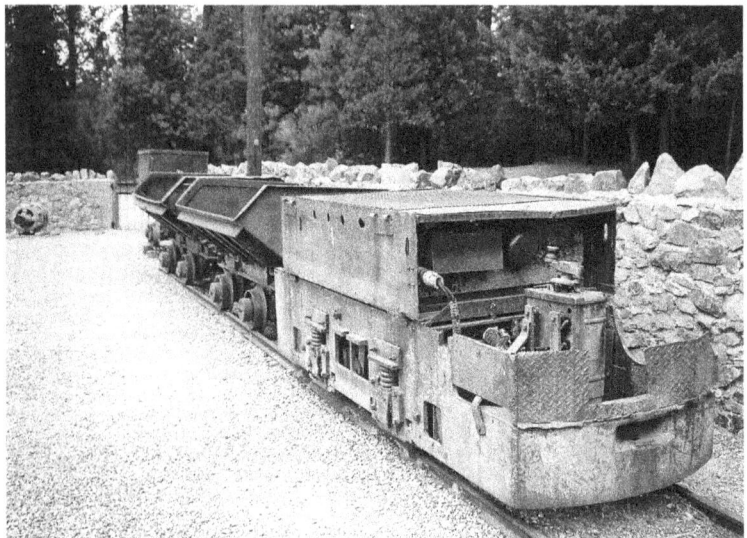

Take the time *to view the Empire Mine's collection of machines after hiking the trails.*

around Osborn Hill through a thick ponderosa pine and Douglas fir forest, and visits three abandoned mines (see trail description, below).

At the junction with Osborn Hill Loop Trail, proceed straight on the Hardrock Trail, which immediately drops down into a shallow gully and crosses **Little Wolf Creek**. The trail fords the creek, which is reduced to a trickle in late summer or early fall, and then climbs steeply back out of the gully.

▶ Stream

A three-way junction heralds the Union Hill Trail to the right, a service road straight ahead, and the Hardrock Trail to the left. In 2007, the Hardrock Trail beyond the junction was closed because it crosses the Empire Mine's primary tailings pile, and the soil was being tested for heavy metals. So go straight on the service road, ▶4 which curves east around the tailings pile and the large open area that has been bulldozed flat to store debris and equipment. As the service road passes the open area, the Empire Mine yard is visible to your left. Turn left off

Empire Mine State Historic Park Loop Trails | TRAIL 21

the service road and walk down into the mine yard, where you can peer into the many remaining buildings, survey mining equipment, and look down into the main shaft of the Empire Mine. Walk through the yard to the visitors center. ▶5

Go through the visitors center to its front entrance. To your right are restrooms and the visitors center parking lot. From the entrance, turn left to follow the Empire St. Trail back to the Penn Gate Trailhead. For nearly 0.25 mile, this trail follows the stone wall surrounding the nearly surreal grounds of the English-style manor house and large rose garden of the mine's former owner, William Bowers Bourne Jr. At times, the trail is barely a few feet wide as it threads its way between the wall and busy traffic on Empire St. As the trail curves around a corner in the wall, hikers should carefully negotiate a sharp left turn to avoid getting too close to oncoming traffic on Empire St.

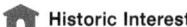 Historic Interest

Eventually, the Empire St. Trail leaves the walled gardens behind and drops back from the street into the now ubiquitous second-growth pine forest with its pungent understory of mountain misery. The trail crosses a park service road and comes to an unsigned fork. Go left to follow the Empire St. Trail, which connects with the Penn Gate Trail next to mushroom-shaped concrete compressor buildings of the Pennsylvania Mine. ▶6 Turn right and make your way back to the parking area.

Osborn Hill Loop Trail

From the Hardrock Trail junction, ▶1 turn right on the Osborn Hill Loop Trail, which climbs a short hill. ▶2 Almost immediately, you will reach a Y junction, veer left, and then climb a short but steep section past the Prescott Mine tailings pile on your right. Another trail junction offers the opportunity to follow the 0.25 mile-long Prescott Mine Loop Trail ▶3 on your left or continue on the Osborn Hill Loop Trail on your right. ▶4 The Prescott Mine

Loop shortly rejoins the Osborn Hill Loop in an area of former mining pits, mounds, and gullies. Also at this point, the unsigned Powerline Trail leads off to the right. Continue straight on the Osborn Hill Loop Trail

Soon, the Osborn Trail begins to parallel the park boundary fence. On the other side of the fence is Osborn Hill Road. Occasional access points allow entry through the fence from the road. A cleared power line right-of-way marks the junction with the Osborn Crosscut Trail on the right. Continue straight along the Osborn Hill Loop Trail, which continues to parallel the park boundary fence. More mounds and gullies mark the unsigned remains of the Betsy Mine.

After passing a gate that provides access from Osborn Hill Road, the trail reaches the junction ▶5 with the **Conlon Mine Spur Trail**. A sign says CONLON MINE—0.1 MILE. Turn left to follow the Conlon Mine Spur Trail, which leads through a stand of black oaks to the mine's tailing pile. An unmarked trail goes to the top of the pile on the left, but you should continue straight to the mine's concrete foundation, which marks the former site of its stamp mill. The foundation makes a handy bench where you can eat lunch and speculate about the 750-foot-deep mine shaft somewhere beneath your feet.

🏠 **Historic Interest**

From the first concrete foundation, the Conlon Spur then circles to the left and comes to the foundations that formerly supported the mine's headworks. A fenced-off area to the left marks the mine shaft entrance. Visitors should stay away from all fenced-off areas to avoid falling into mine shafts. The spur trail climbs steeply to the top of the tailings pile and then follows the pile crest to close the loop and reconnect with the ▶6 Osborn Hill Loop Trail.

From the junction of the Osborn Hill and Conlon Mine trails, turn left. At this point, the

Empire Mine State Historic Park Loop Trails | TRAIL **21**

Osborn Hill Loop Trail is a road. Shortly, you come to a picnic bench, which offers another good lunch spot if you didn't stop at the Conlon Mine. A break in the trees offers a teasing glimpse of Grass Valley. Beyond the picnic bench, a confusing proliferation of formal and informal use-trails lead off from the Osborn Hill Loop Trail to the left, including one marked SCENIC VISTA. A short walk down this trail through a thick field of manzanita will likely reveal the vista to be obscured by brush, so you may want to skip it. On the Osborn Hill Loop Trail, another trail leads right to the ubiquitous tailings pile, which marks the Daisy Hill Mine, but by now, you will want to get back to explore the granddaddy of them all—the Empire Mine—by proceeding north ▶7 back to the junction with the Hardrock Trail.

MILESTONES

Hardrock Loop Trail

- ▶1 0.00 Start at Penn Gate Trailhead
- ▶2 0.39 WYOD Loop Trail
- ▶3 1.65 Osborn Hill Loop Trail
- ▶4 1.80 Straight at three-way junction
- ▶5 2.05 Visitors Center
- ▶6 2.75 Return to Penn Gate Trailhead

Osborn Hill Loop Trail

- ▶1 0.00 Start at Hardrock Loop Trail
- ▶2 0.10 Loop Junction
- ▶3 0.25 Prescott Loop Trail
- ▶4 0.52 Return to Osborn Hill Loop Trail
- ▶5 0.93 Conlon Mine Spur Trail
- ▶6 1.08 Return to Osborn Hill Loop Trail
- ▶7 1.72 Return to Hardrock Loop Trail

Shingle Falls Trail

TRAIL 22

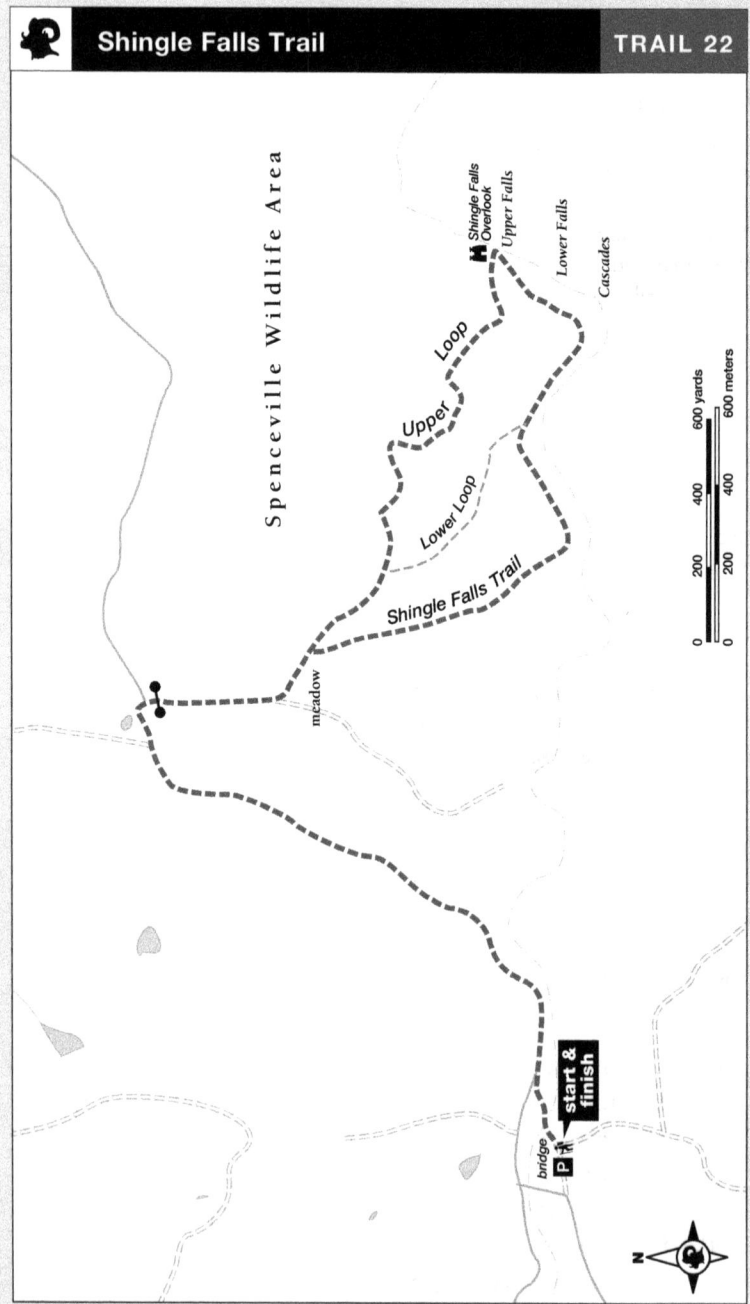

TRAIL 22 Sierra Foothills

Shingle Falls Trail: Spenceville Wildlife Area

This trail features one of the area's best waterfalls in the Sierra foothills. The little-known Spenceville Wildlife Area is directly east of Beale Air Force Base and the town of Marysville. This is classic Sierra foothill country, with verdant oak woodlands, open meadows, and jungle-like riparian habitat. It's all green splendor in the spring, but a bit dry and plagued with stickers the rest of the year. During spring flows, Shingle Falls (also know as Fairy Falls) forms a spectacular 100-foot-high falls. Much of the hike follows gated roads, but some single-track loop trail options add visual and topographical diversity.

Best Time

Spring is best for wildflowers, meadows, and thundering falls. Hot summer days are definitely not the best times for this low-elevation trail.

Finding the Trail

From Sacramento, drive 22 miles east on Interstate 80 to Hwy 65 in Roseville. Drive north 21 miles on Hwy 65 to the town of Wheatland. Turn right on Main Street, which becomes Spenceville Road after .5 mile. From Wheatland, drive 6.0 miles east on Spenceville Road, then turn right on Camp Far West Road. (Note: Spenceville Road between Wheatland and the Spenceville Wildlife Area is closed to public use where it enters Beale Air Force Base, requiring the detour on Camp Far West Road). Drive 2.6 miles on Camp Far West Road. Just before reaching Camp Far West Dam, turn left to continue on Camp Far West

TRAIL USE
Hike, Run, Bike, Horse
LENGTH
4.9 miles, 2–4 hours
VERTICAL FEET
±259
DIFFICULTY
- 1 2 **3** 4 5 +
TRAIL TYPE
Loop
SURFACE TYPE
Dirt

FEATURES
Dogs Allowed
Waterfall
Stream
Canyon
Meadow
Wildflowers
Birds
Wildlife
Historic
Great Views
Photo Opportunity

FACILITIES
None

> During spring runoff, you have your fill of the negative ions produced by Shingle Fall's spray.

Road (not to be confused with Blackford–Camp Far West–McCourtney Road, which crosses a bridge over the dam spillway). Camp Far West Road turns to gravel after 2.0 miles. Proceed another 2.0 miles on Camp Far West Road and turn right onto Spenceville Road. Proceed 2.0 miles to the trailhead parking area on the left, just before the road ends at Dry Creek.

Logistics

Although the Spenceville Wildlife Area and the Shingle Falls Trail are found in few trail books, this area and trail are popular with knowledgeable local hikers, mountain bikers, and equestrians. You will definitely share the trail with others on spring weekends, but it's well worth the sharing.

Trail Description

From the trailhead parking lot, ▶1 proceed across the small bridge over Dry Creek. The large barren hill in front of you is the tailings pile of the old Spenceville Mine, a still-toxic reminder of the area's Gold Rush heritage.

Once across the bridge, turn right and proceed east on the closed road through blue oak woodlands. The road follows Dry Creek for nearly 0.5 mile. A path branches off to the right and proceeds across a small meadow to a beach on **Dry Creek.** Pass the footpath by and continue up the road as it turns north and goes up a tributary gully. As the trail climbs up the gully, the oaks thin out and hikers on sunny days will miss the shade.

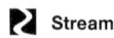 Stream

The road soon reaches the head of the gully. A green gate on the left and a sign announce the junction with the **North Valley Trail.** Pass this side trail by and continue 100 feet on the road to a white gate; ▶2 turn right before the gate onto another road

Shingle Falls Trail TRAIL 22

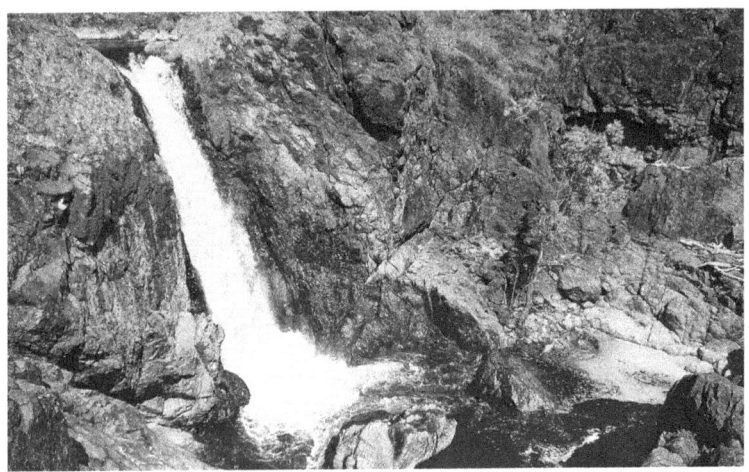

Upper Shingle Falls *is even more spectacular than the lower falls.*

blocked by a rusty third gate. At this point, you are 1.2 miles from the trailhead.

Proceed through the pedestrian way to the right of the third gate and continue on the road as it proceeds south and slowly climbs a ridge for more than 0.25 mile. A jeep trail continues up the ridge, but the **Shingle Falls Trail** veers to the left as it continues to follow the road, which crosses a cattle guard that long ago lost its fence line. From the cattle guard, you can see that the road circles a small meadow, while a cutoff trail traverses across the meadow and reconnects with the road at a multiple-trail junction.

≛ Meadow

Proceed around the meadow on the road to its nearby trail junction, which is signless except for a small plate prohibiting mountain bikes. At this point, you have a choice whether to take the Upper Loop Trail on the far left, the Lower Loop Trail on the middle left, or continue straight on the road. All three routes eventually lead to Shingle Falls. The best course probably is to turn sharp left up the

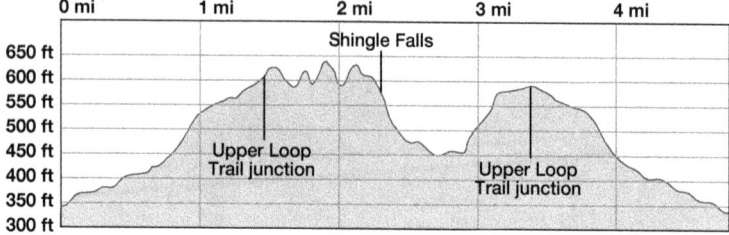

TRAIL 22 Shingle Falls Trail Profile

Upper Loop Trail, ▶3 which climbs steeply at first through the oaks but then quickly levels off.

The Upper Loop Trail traverses a heavily wooded ridge and soon connects with and follows an old mining ditch, which was probably used to supply water to the Spenceville Mine. The trail then parallels the ditch through oak woodlands, roughly following the 600-foot-elevation contour line. Along the way, the trail drops in and out of three gullies carved by small seasonal tributaries of Dry Creek. Continuing its eastward traverse, the Upper Loop Trail reconnects with the road, now little more than a jeep trail, about 0.33 mile from where you left it at the multi-trail junction.

Waterfall

Veer left on the jeep trail and proceed eastward ▶4 less than 0.25 mile to the **Shingle Falls** overlook. The jeep trail ends at a small rocky promontory overlooking Dry Creek just upstream of the falls. An old "donkey" engine that apparently was part of a small tractor is cemented into the rock at the edge of the cliff. It was probably used to pump water up from Dry Creek into the mine ditch. From the engine, a footpath ▶5 drops down to a chain link fence on the rocky rim with a great view of the 100-foot-high Shingle Falls. One of the highest waterfalls in this region of the Sierra foothills, Shingle Falls really thunders during spring runoff, but is reduced to a veil-like trickle later in the year.

Great Views

Continue down the path along the lip of the inner gorge. As you continue downstream, ▶6 the path provides views of a smaller but still impressive lower waterfall and then a series of smaller cataracts downstream. Some steep spur trails go down to the water's edge below the lower falls, but these are only advisable for the sure-footed and the poison-oak resistant.

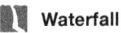 Waterfall

About 0.25 mile downstream from Shingle Falls, the pathway reconnects with the jeep trail. Veer left and continue downstream. Soon you pass a junction on the right for the Lower Loop Trail. Continue straight on the jeep trail. The jeep trail transforms into the road as the terrain evens out. The road continues downstream about 0.5 mile, providing occasional access to Dry Creek, before it turns north and proceeds up a gully.

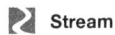 Stream

Nearly a mile from the Shingle Falls, the road closes the loop by reaching ▶7 the Upper and Lower Loop Trails Junction. From the junction, continue north on the road to retrace your steps to the rusty gate and ▶8 follow the road 1.5 miles back to the trailhead.

MILESTONES

- ▶1 0.00 Start at trailhead at the end of Spenceville Road
- ▶2 1.20 White gate, turn right
- ▶3 1.50 Upper/Middle Loop Trails junction, turn sharp left on Upper Loop Trail
- ▶4 2.25 Connect with jeep trail, continue east on jeep trail
- ▶5 2.40 Shingle Falls overlook, drop down to the right and follow fence/gorge rim
- ▶6 2.52 Reconnect with jeep trail/road, continue west (downstream)
- ▶7 3.37 Return to road junction with Upper Loop/Middle Trails, retrace your steps
- ▶8 4.87 Return to trailhead

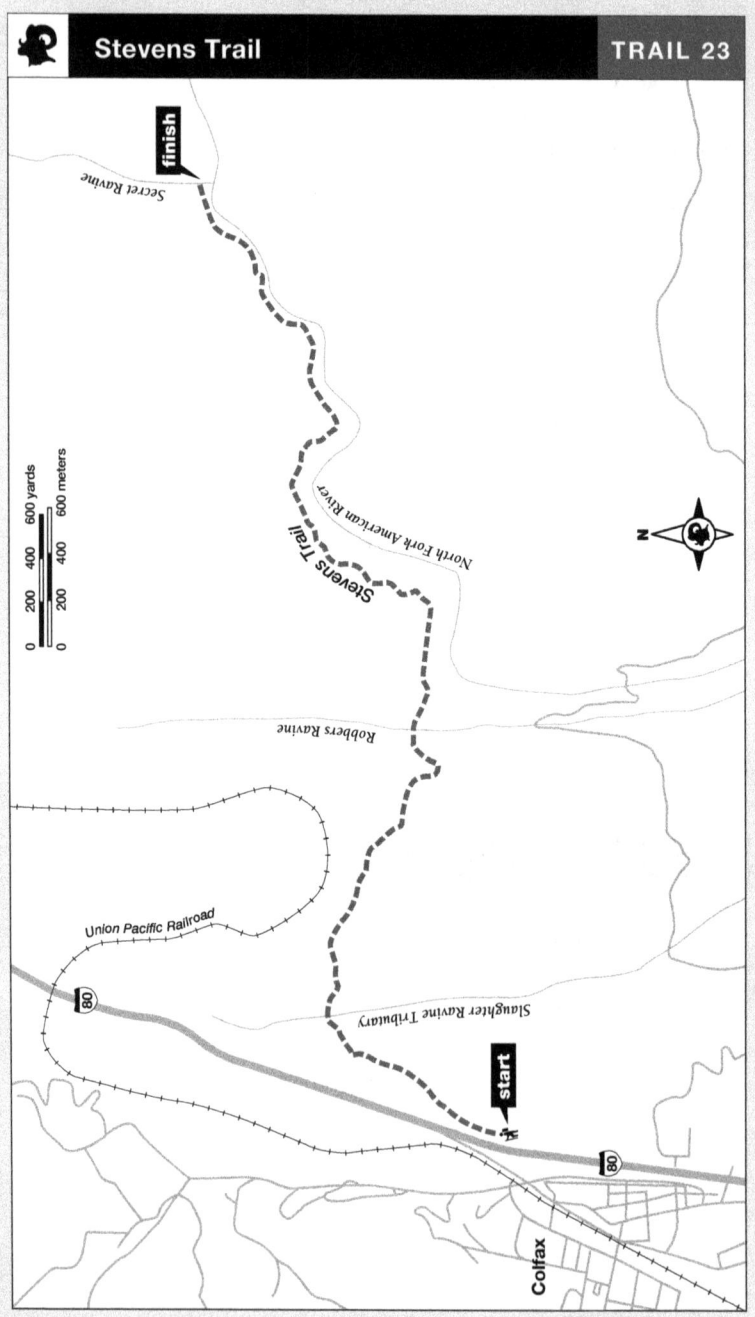

TRAIL 23 Sierra Foothills

Stevens Trail: North Fork American Wild & Scenic River

The Stevens Trail is one of the most popular Sierra foothills hikes for Sacramentans. Even though it is a path rich in history, it was virtually unknown until the late 1960s, when a Boy Scout rediscovered it. Now maintained and managed by the BLM, the trail provides year-round opportunities to visit the North Fork American Wild & Scenic River. Starting in the pines near Colfax, the trail drops more than 1000 feet down into a rugged canyon clothed in live oak and chaparral, providing magnificent views of one of California's most scenic Wild Rivers. This former Gold Rush toll road once connected the mining town of Iowa Hill with the railroad town of Colfax and is on the National Register of Historic Places.

Best Time

This is a year-round trail, snow-free except after the most intense winter storms. Spring provides an outstanding display of wildflowers. It can be quite hot in the summer, so it is best hiked in the early morning or evening. Fall brings its own muted color display of gold, tan, brown, and rust as the trees, grasses, and shrubs prepare for winter. Hikers should be aware of potential high water when crossing small creeks during winter and spring, and take care when they get down to the much larger North Fork American River. Bring plenty of water with you in the summer.

TRAIL USE
Hike, Bike
LENGTH
7.0 miles, 3–5 hours
VERTICAL FEET
±1100
DIFFICULTY
- 1 2 3 4 **5** +
TRAIL TYPE
Out & Back
SURFACE TYPE
Dirt

FEATURES
Dogs Allowed
River
Streams
Canyon
Waterfall
Wildflowers
Camping
Historic
Great Views
Photo Opportunity
Steep

FACILITIES
None

Finding the Trail

A segment of the trail features handmade rock retaining walls that hold the path in place against the steep slope.

From Sacramento, drive east 51 miles on Interstate 80 to the town of Colfax. Take the Colfax/Hwy 174 exit and turn left onto North Canyon Way, a frontage road that parallels I-80 eastward. Drive 1.6 miles east on North Canyon Way to the Stevens Trail parking lot, on the left. The parking lot is marked with a BLM sign saying STEVENS TRAIL.

Logistics

The trailhead parking lot is small and can be crowded on spring weekends. If you need to park along North Canyon Way, be sure to not block residential driveways. The BLM sign at the trailhead indicates that the North Fork American River is 4.5 miles, but at least one mapping program indicates it is 3.5 miles (7.0 miles round-trip).

Trail Description

From the parking area, ▶1 proceed east through a blackberry bramble shaded by live oaks. The trail quickly drops down through the forest for about 0.5 mile and then crosses a seasonal tributary to **Slaughter Ravine**.

Just after the stream crossing (where you may or may not find a board in place to keep your feet dry), the trail connects with a dirt road that leads to ▶2 **Robbers Ravine**. A trail post advises you to turn right and follow the road upward along a relatively open and sunny slope for about 0.25 mile. Unseen just upslope from the road is the historic but still in use Cape Horn segment of the Union Pacific Railroad's primary east/west line. The construction of the rail line around the sheer 1000-foot-high cliffs of Cape Horn in 1866 was considered a major engineering feat of the Central Pacific Railroad in its drive east to build the transcontinental railroad.

Historic Interest

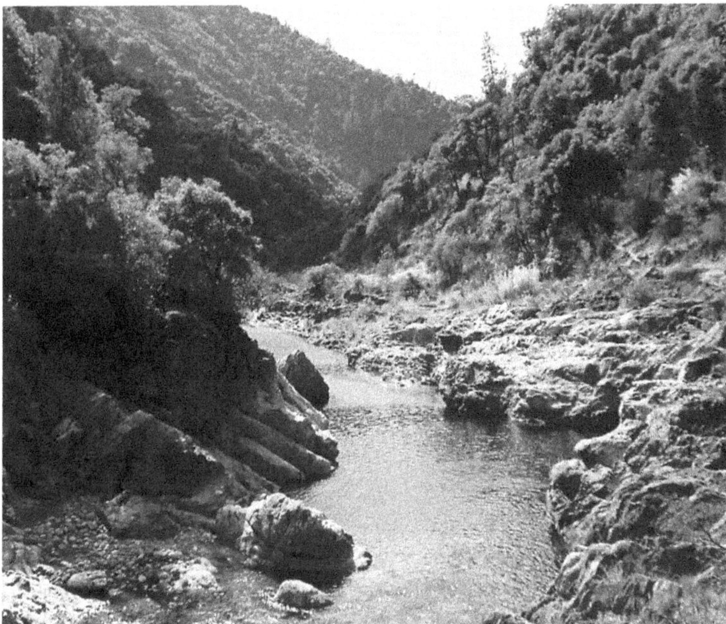

Stevens Trail | TRAIL 23

The North Fork American Wild & Scenic River *flows at the bottom of the Stevens Trail.*

▶3 The trail/road reaches a saddle. Robbers Ravine Road splits off to the right, while your trail/road goes straight over the saddle for another 100 feet, where a trail post indicates the beginning of the single-track **Stevens Trail** on your left. Turn left here.

The trail begins its downward journey into the **North Fork American River** canyon through a shady forest of ponderosa pine, live oak, laurel, and old-growth manzanita. A bit over 0.25 mile down from the saddle, the trail splits at a post that advises mountain bikes to go right and hikers to go left. Taking the left trail, your route goes through a recently burned area and past a rock outcrop that provides the first scenic view downstream of the North Fork American River, with the Colfax–Iowa Hill Road and bridge visible in the distance.

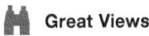 **Great Views**

Sierra Foothills 193

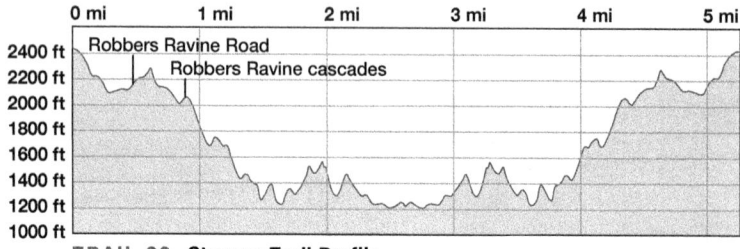

TRAIL 23 Stevens Trail Profile

Waterfall

Shortly past the rock outcrop, the trail drops steeply down into the rocky gorge of **Robbers Ravine**. Seasonal flows create spectacular cascades over huge boulders in the bottom of the ravine, but it can be dry as a bone in the late fall. After negotiating the rocky crossing, the trail climbs out of the ravine, reconnects with the mountain bike trail on the right, and heads into the open southwest-facing slopes of the North Fork American River. The trail continues traversing the canyon slope dotted with live oaks and pines, crosses the foot of a talus field, and then winds its way past rocky cliffs and an old mine-shaft entrance. Although some may be tempted to explore the shaft, smart hikers should stay away and live to hike another day.

Caution

Historic Interest

The next trail segment features handmade rock retaining walls that hold the path in place against the steep slope. These walls were built by Truman Allen Stevens, who arrived in California in 1859. Stevens operated a ranch in Iowa Hill (which at the time was a major mining metropolis) and a livery stable in Colfax (then known as Illinoistown). He built the trail and bridge crossing the North Fork and charged a toll to the miners who used it. Use of the trail declined after 1890, and the route was all but forgotten until Eric Kiel rediscovered and recharted the trail in 1969 as a Boy Scout project.

The trail continues down its historic tread, rounds a ridge, and enters the North Fork canyon

Stevens Trail

proper. There are stunning views up- and down-canyon of the river, which flows about 500 feet below. After making its way eastward around a large river bend, the trail drops down into a small tributary drainage, where water seeps over a large mossy boulder into a grotto lined with giant ferns. Soon thereafter, you reach the first of several spur trails that lead steeply down to the river. Hikers should continue eastward on the Stevens Trail for about another 0.75 mile to ▶4 the confluence of Secret Ravine and the North Fork.

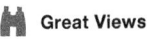 Great Views

The Stevens Trail crosses Secret Ravine Creek where it flows perennially through a lush gully shaded by alders. The trail ends on the other side of the creek in a flat, open area that provides an excellent lunch or camp spot overlooking the North Fork. Rock retaining walls and an apple tree upstream suggest that this may have been where the trail toll booth was located. Foundations for the suspension bridge that once crossed the river are found nearby. Just downstream of the Secret Ravine confluence, the North Fork empties into a large, emerald-green pool. Swimmers willing to work their way downstream over the rocky shelves along the river will enjoy this pool in the summer and fall months.

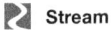 Stream

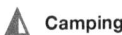 Camping

Swimming

To return to the trailhead, ▶5 retrace your steps back up the Stevens Trail's moderate grade to Colfax.

MILESTONES

- ▶1 0.00 Trailhead
- ▶2 0.61 Robbers Ravine Road
- ▶3 0.87 Saddle
- ▶4 3.50 Secret Ravine and North Fork American River
- ▶5 7.00 Return to Trailhead

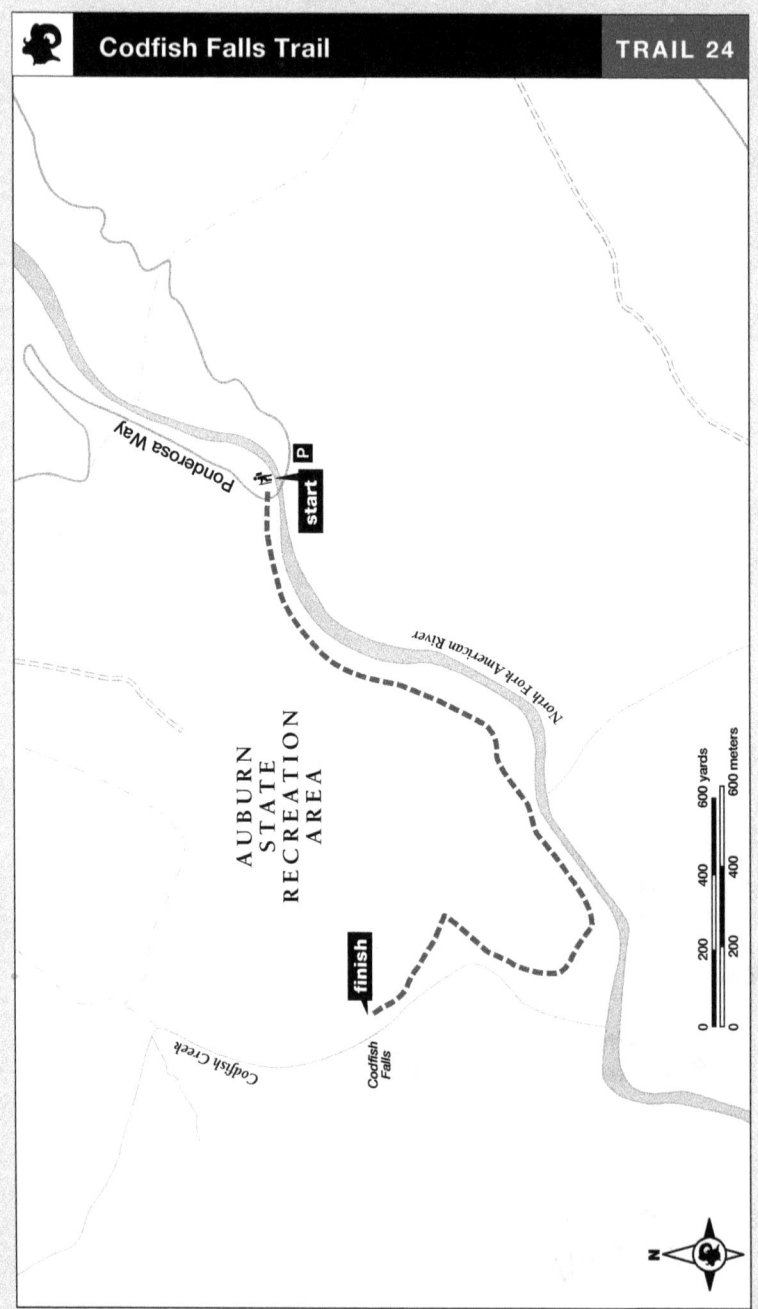

TRAIL 24 Sierra Foothills

Codfish Falls Trail: Auburn State Recreation Area

This is an excellent walk for families with children. It packs a lot of scenery into a short, easy hike along the beautiful North Fork American River, with pretty Codfish Falls as the destination. The spring wildflower display is wonderful, and the languid pools of the North Fork invite you to cool off from the summer heat. It's a perfect half-day trip just a short drive from Sacramento.

Best Time

Spring is best for the wildflowers. Summer mornings or later afternoons are good, particularly if you like to swim. The trail is accessible year-round, although the lower section of unpaved Ponderosa Way can be rough for low-slung sedans.

Finding the Trail

From Sacramento, drive approximately 46 miles east on Interstate 80, past Auburn, and take the Weimar Crossroads exit. Turn right on Ponderosa Way. Head west on Ponderosa Way, go over the railroad tracks, and then the road becomes quite curvy. A bit over 3.0 miles from the freeway, the blacktop ends and Ponderosa Way becomes graded dirt as it begins to drop down into the North Fork American River canyon. Unless you have a high-clearance vehicle, this portion of the road may be impassable during heavy rain periods in the winter and spring. Ponderosa Way becomes quite narrow as it switchbacks down into the canyon and eventually reaches the Ponderosa Way Bridge across the North

TRAIL USE
Hike
LENGTH
2.8 miles, 1–3 hours
VERTICAL FEET
±100
DIFFICULTY
- 1 **2** 3 4 5 +
TRAIL TYPE
Out & Back
SURFACE TYPE
Dirt

FEATURES
Dogs on Leash
Child Friendly
Waterfall
Stream
River
Canyon
Wildflowers
Great Views
Photo Opportunity

FACILITIES
None

Fork in about 5.62 miles. Park in the small parking area before the bridge, or if it's full, cross the bridge to another small parking area on the north side. Be sure to take valuables with you or lock them out of sight in your trunk, as this parking area has been the target of vandals in the past.

> Small children need to be supervised during a short section of trail with a steep drop-off.

Logistics

You may need a high-clearance vehicle for Ponderosa Way during rainy periods in the winter and spring.

Trail Description

The trail, which begins from the north side of the **Ponderosa Bridge,** ▶1 heads west and drops down to a sandy beach on the **North Fork American River,** follows the base of the canyon slope and then climbs up into the oaks trees and scrub. Although the trail goes up and down in some sections, it stays pretty much level, as there is less than a 100-foot elevation difference between the trailhead and Codfish Falls. The trail continues westward and downstream through clumps of blue oaks, brush, and an overstory of ponderosa, gray pines, and small Douglas firs. Occasional open grassy areas along the trail are dotted with spring wildflowers and provide nice views of the river.

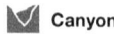
Canyon

A steep slope on the left separates the trail from the river along much of its length. There are some spur trails leading left down to inviting bedrock slabs along the river, but most of these informal routes are quite steep and eroded. At one point, the trail narrows with a steep drop down to the river on the left, but fortunately the trail itself remains flat and easy to negotiate. If you are hiking with small children, it's a good idea to take their hands or even pick them up and carry them past the short section with the steep drop-off.

River

In a bit under a mile, the trail reaches the wide mouth of ▶2 **Codfish Creek Canyon**, where it enters the larger canyon of the North Fork. At this point, the trail turns north and heads into Codfish Creek Canyon through a thicket of Douglas firs, which close overhead. Depending on the season, this trail segment may be frequented by mosquitoes, so be sure to bring some bug juice. A couple of trail junctions on the left announce spur trails leading down to wide floodplain of Codfish Creek, but the route to the falls continues straight and to the north. The trail dips briefly in and out of a seasonally flowing tributary and then climbs briefly up to as-yet-unseen but soon-heard **Codfish Falls**.

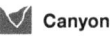 Canyon

Abruptly, the trail reaches the falls, ▶3 which tumbles over a 50-foot-high cliff composed of dark metamorphic rock. There is another fall above, but the rocks are wet and slippery, and climbing to the upper falls is only for the experienced or foolish. Large boulders provide an ideal lunch spot at the foot of the main falls, which sleets over a broad slab of rock.

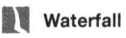 Waterfall

After enjoying the falls, retrace your steps to the trailhead. ▶4 For a side visit, take one of the spur trails that drop down to the right to Codfish Creek and explore the cobbled floodplain where it meets the North Fork American River. Just downstream of the confluence is a shallow pool that provides a nice cooling-off option for summer hikers.

▲• Swimming

MILESTONES

- ▶1   0.00   Ponderosa Way Bridge trailhead
- ▶2   1.00   Codfish Creek canyon
- ▶3   1.50   Codfish Falls
- ▶4   3.00   Return to trailhead

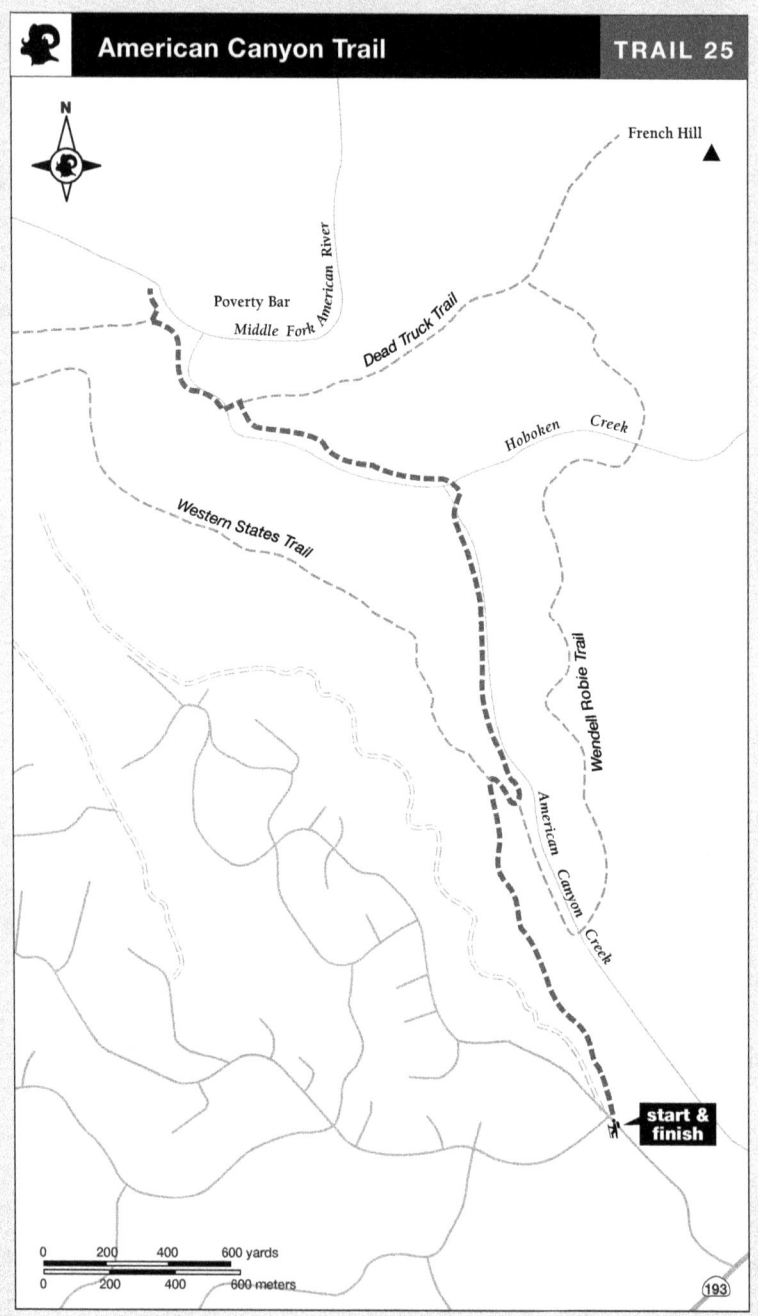

TRAIL 25 Sierra Foothills

American Canyon Trail: Auburn State Recreation Area

This is one of the best all-around hikes in the Auburn State Recreation Area, which provides outdoor recreation for more than a million visitors annually. The well-graded route includes segments of the Western States National Recreation Trail and descends 1100 feet down American Canyon, which contains a small tributary of the Middle Fork American River. American Canyon's northeast facing slopes are clothed in a dense oak forest, and the canyon bottom is covered with lush riparian vegetation. This almost tropical habitat contrasts sharply with the much drier and brushy southwest-facing slopes found later in the hike. Alert visitors may observe examples of our Gold Rush heritage. Hikers will also enjoy the canyon's inner gorge, which is filled with scenic cascades and waterfalls as they make their way to the Middle Fork, a worthy destination in its own right.

Best Time

Ranging from 1700 to 600 feet in elevation, this is a year-round foothill trail. Best times are spring and fall. Summer afternoons can be quite warm, so you may want hike in the morning. Muddy trail conditions and stream crossings can be challenging during the rainy season.

Finding the Trail

From Interstate 80 in Auburn, take the Hwy 49 exit and proceed south 3.8 miles to the small town of Cool (this segment of the highway goes through

TRAIL USE
Hike, Run, Bike, Horse
LENGTH
5.74 miles round-trip, 3–5 hours
VERTICAL FEET
±1100
DIFFICULTY
- 1 2 3 **4** 5 +
TRAIL TYPE
Out & Back
SURFACE TYPE
Dirt

FEATURES
Dogs on Leash
River
Stream
Canyon
Meadow
Waterfalls
Wildflowers
Fall Color
Historic
Great Views
Photo Opportunity
Secluded

FACILITIES
None

Look for a ditch along part of the trail and a small rock dam in an upslope gully. They are reminders of the region's gold mining heritage.

downtown Auburn and then drops down and climbs out of the deep American River canyon). Turn left on Hwy 193 and proceed approximately 6.0 miles east to the junction on the left with Sweetwater Trail on the left, which may or may not be signed. The road on the opposite side of Hwy. 193, Pilgrim Court, is signed. Turn left on Sweetwater Trail and proceed 300 feet to the trailhead; turn out on the right just before the gated entrance to the Auburn Lake Trails development.

Logistics

Trailhead parking accommodates only two or three cars, but this trailhead isn't that heavily used. There is more parking along Sweetwater Trail, closer to Hwy 193. Trail names in this region can be confusing at times, particularly since some of the trails have multiple names, and sign makers, cartographers, and trail guide writers appear to have had different opinions as to which trails are which. In addition, some of the trail signs display clearly incorrect mileage estimates, so bring along a good, up-to-date map (the 1998 Auburn State Recreation Area map by Sowarwe–Werher Maps and Guides is the best available).

Trail Description

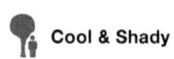
Cool & Shady

From the turnout at the trailhead, ▶1 proceed down an old road (now closed to vehicles), which is heavily shaded by live oak trees. The well-graded former roadbed promises a relatively easy climb out of the canyon on your return trip. About 0.1 mile from the trailhead, an unmarked spur climbs to the left. Continue straight.

Within 0.66 mile, you will reach the intersection with the **Wendell Robie Trail**. ▶2 A sign says WESTERN STATES TRAIL 1.3 MILES. Turn right and go

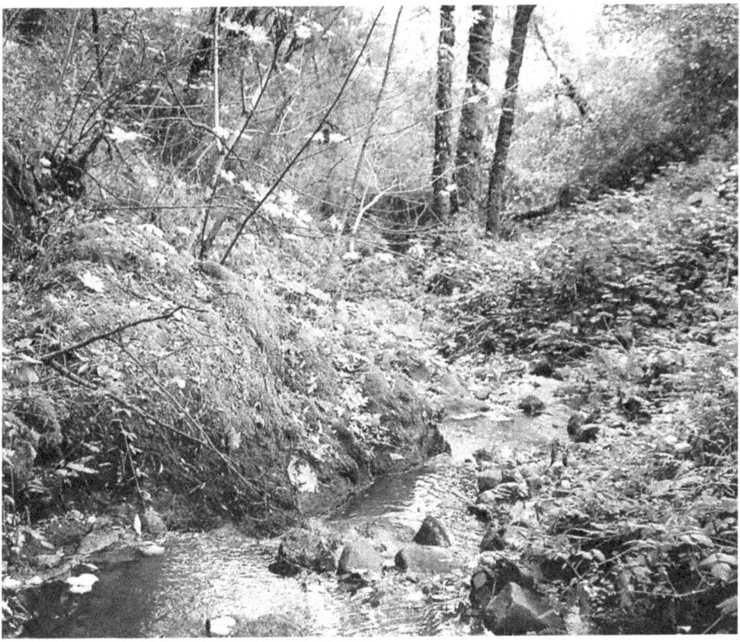

American Canyon Trail | TRAIL **25**

Rich, jungle-like habitat *along American Canyon Creek*

farther down into American Canyon via a couple of short switchbacks. 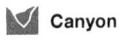 Canyon

In a little bit more than 0.1 mile, you come close to the bottom of American Canyon and the intersection of the Wendell Robie Trail with the **American Canyon Trail**. ▶3 Here too a trail sign says WESTERN STATES TRAIL 1.3 MILES (to give an example of a misleading trail sign). Take the trail on the left and proceed down-canyon. Below is the sound of **American Canyon Creek**, hidden by its dense riparian forest.

This nearly level trail segment follows the slope above the canyon bottom for a bit more than 0.5 mile before it drops down to cross American Canyon Creek. ▶4 The small stream and its overhanging trees, lush streamside vegetation, and green mossy rocks almost seem designed by a master Japanese 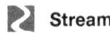 Stream

Sierra Foothills 203

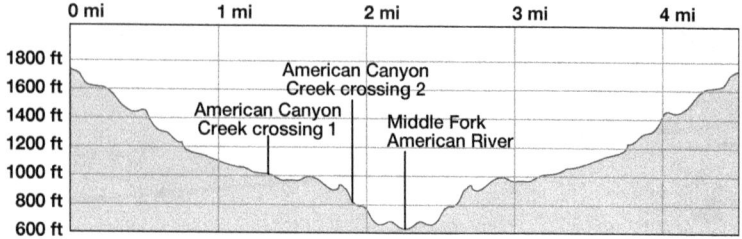

TRAIL 25 American Canyon Trail Profile

gardener. Rocks offer a dry crossing for most of the year except during periods of high runoff. Right after the first stream crossing, you will also cross **Hoboken Creek**, a small tributary of American Canyon Creek.

From the stream crossings, the trail proceeds down-canyon again, this time on the much dryer southwest-facing slope, occasionally breaking out of the sparser live oak forest and picking its way through some rocky areas. A ditch along part of the trail and a small rock dam in an upslope gully are reminders of the region's gold mining heritage.

About 0.5 mile after the stream crossings, the trail intersects with the **Dead Truck Trail**, which heads straight up the ridge on your right (which perhaps explains why the truck died). ▶5 Proceed left downhill on the American Canyon Trail through a small dry meadow. The trail switchbacks to the left as it again heads downhill toward American Canyon Creek.

About 0.33 mile from the Dead Truck Trail intersection, your route crosses American Canyon Creek for the second time. ▶6 Again, rocks provide a dry crossing most of the year. From the crossing, the trail traverses northward along the canyon slope, but the creek has some serious elevation to lose in order to reach its confluence with the Middle Fork less than 0.25 mile away. Over the ages, this segment of American Canyon Creek has chiseled its

Stream

way through bedrock, forming a series of scenic cascades and waterfalls. The upper cascade is fairly accessible from the trail but the questionable deer paths to the lower falls lead down steep, unstable, and slippery slopes.

Waterfall

A bit over 0.25 mile from the second crossing of American Canyon Creek, the American Canyon Trail intersects with the Tevis Cup segment of the **Western States Trail** (the separate portion of the WST that is the preferred route of the Tevis Cup Trail Ride, a competitive equestrian event). ▶7 Turn right and follow the Tevis segment down toward the Middle Fork American River.

River

In less than 0.25 mile, a short trail breaks to the left and leads directly to a large gravel bar on the south bank of the Middle Fork. ▶8 The bar offers a variety of lunch spots. Just upstream and across the river is **Poverty Bar**. Imagine this large gravel bar in 1849, when it was the site of a small town housing more than 10,000 gold miners.

Historic Interest

At this point, you will have dropped 1100 feet over 2.87 miles. Weather permitting, take a quick dip in the cold, clear water of the Middle Fork before retracing your steps ▶9 and tackling the moderate climb out of the canyon.

Swimming

MILESTONES

- ▶1 0.00 Trailhead
- ▶2 0.67 Western States–Wendell Robie Trail intersection, turn right
- ▶3 0.79 Wendell Robie–American Canyon Trail intersection, turn left
- ▶4 1.35 American Canyon Creek—upper crossing
- ▶5 1.85 Dead Truck Trail intersection, turn left
- ▶6 2.00 American Canyon Creek—lower crossing
- ▶7 2.27 American Canyon Creek–Tevis Trail intersection, turn right
- ▶8 2.87 Middle Fork American River
- ▶9 5.74 Retrace steps to trailhead

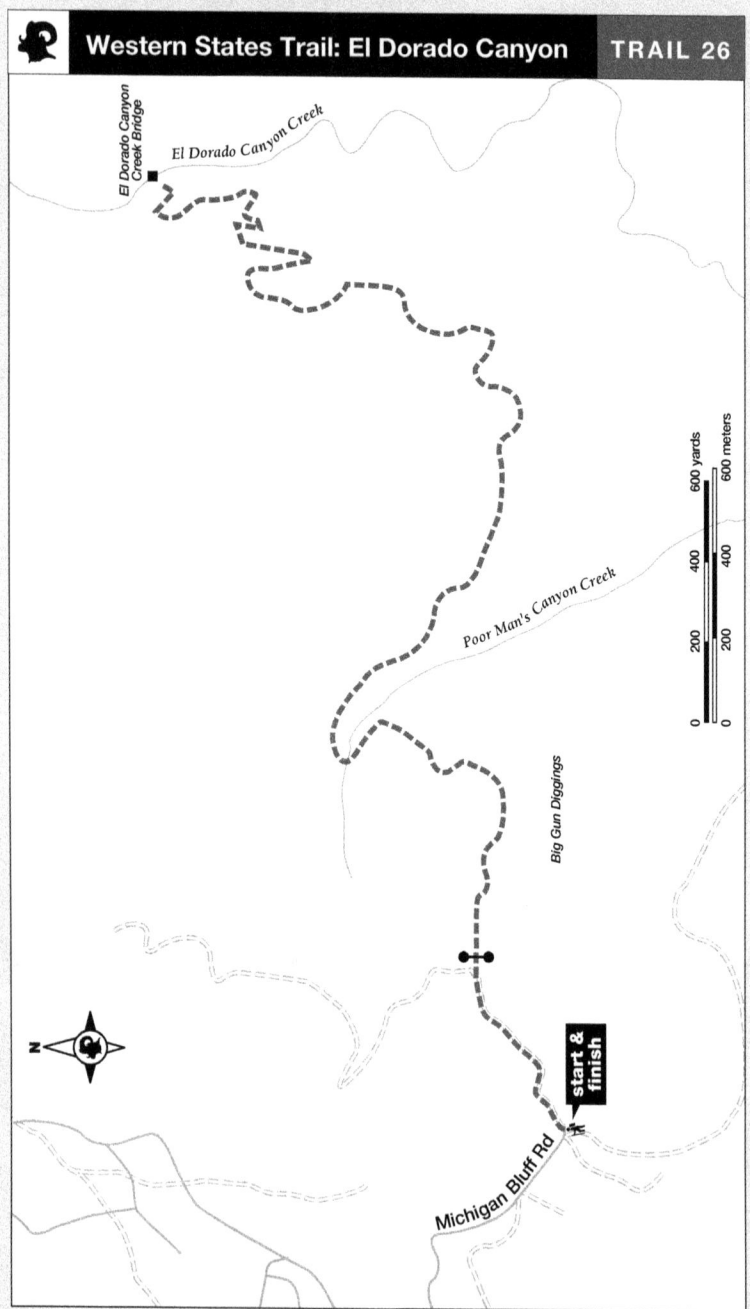

TRAIL 26 Sierra Foothills

Western States Trail: El Dorado Canyon

Unlike its more popular sections lower in the foothills, this segment of the **Western States Trail** is off the beaten track. Its topography is steeper and the mid-elevation vegetation more diverse than the WST in the lower Sierra foothills. Also, the trail played an important role in Gold Rush history and provides magnificent views of and access to a roadless area being proposed for wilderness protection. The stream flowing through **El Dorado Canyon** is quite scenic and offers opportunities for fishing and camping.

Best Time

Except when the strongest winter storms hit the Sierra, this trail is accessible pretty much year-round. It's at its best in the spring and the fall. The canyon's plethora of black oaks are particularly attractive when fall brings out their burnt-orange color. Summer can be quite hot, so plan on hiking this trail in the early morning.

Finding the Trail

From Sacramento, drive 36 miles east on Interstate 80 to Auburn. Take the Foresthill Road–Secret Ravine exit, turn right on Foresthill Road, and proceed through the stoplight and across the Foresthill Bridge. Drive 18 miles northeast on Foresthill Road through the town of Foresthill. Continue northeast on Foresthill Road 3.2 miles to Michigan Bluff Road, then turn right. Drive 2.3 miles southeast on Michigan Bluff Road. At a **Y** intersection with

---

TRAIL USE
Hike, Run, Bike
LENGTH
5.6 miles, 3–6 hours
VERTICAL FEET
±1600
DIFFICULTY
- 1 2 3 **4** 5 +
TRAIL TYPE
Out & Back
SURFACE TYPE
Dirt

FEATURES
Dogs Allowed
Stream
Canyon
Fall Color
Camping
Secluded
Historic
Great Views
Steep

FACILITIES
None

This first section of the Western States Trail drops steeply downward through thick manzanita on the edge of the "Big Gun Diggings," promising a challenging climb back.

Chicken Hawk Road, veer right and drive 0.5 mile to the end of the pavement in the small community of Michigan Bluff. Park at the end of the pavement, taking care not to block any private roads or driveways.

Logistics

This portion of the WST is used for competitive events such as the Western States Endurance Run and the Tevis Cup Ride. It is a good idea to avoid the trail during the events by checking with the Foresthill Ranger Station (Tahoe National Forest) at (530) 367-2224. As you slog your way up the steeper sections of this trail, it is amazing to think that people participating in the Western States Endurance Run actually run up the trail in their 100-mile journey between Squaw Valley and Auburn. In addition, motorized use of this trail is allowed, so be sure to avoid motorbikes on some of the more narrow sections of trail.

Trail Description

Historic Interest

Your hike begins in the historic town of **Michigan Bluff**. Formerly known as Michigan City, this gold mining town and its hydraulic mining operation (the "Big Gun Diggings") were bankrolled by railroad tycoon Leland Stanford (who would later become Governor of California). Water cannons chewed away the hillsides so successfully, it undermined the town, which in 1893 was relocated to its present site and was renamed Michigan Bluff. Because of its rich Gold Rush heritage, the El Dorado Canyon segment of the Western States Trail is on the National Register of Historic Places. It was built as a toll road in 1850 to carry supplies from Michigan Bluff to the Deadwood and Last Chance mining camps. Look for the National Register monument and historic

Western States Trail | TRAIL 26

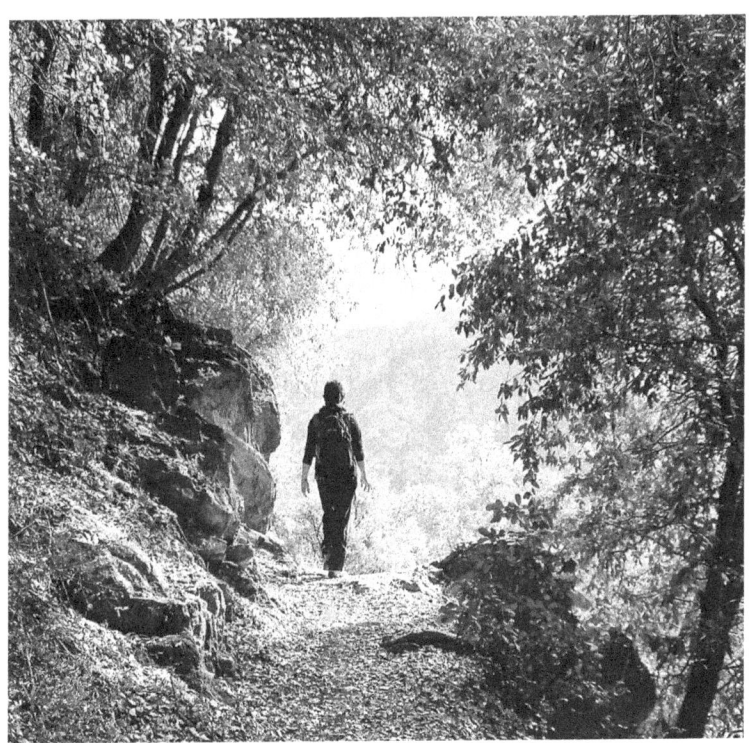

Live oaks *frame the trail down into El Dorado Canyon.*

interpretive sign on the left, or north side of the road at pavement's end on Michigan Bluff Road. There is no parking available at the trailhead so park here.
▶1 Turn left and walk up the gravel road. You will soon come to a **Y** intersection with a green gate on the left. Walk around the gate and continue up the road.

In slightly more than 0.25 mile, you will reach the **Western States Trail** trailhead on the right. ▶2 A sign says EL DORADO CANYON—2.5 MILES. Turn right and proceed down the trail through old-growth manzanita over 6 feet high punctuated by ponderosa and gray pines, and black oaks. This first section of the trail drops steeply downward through thick

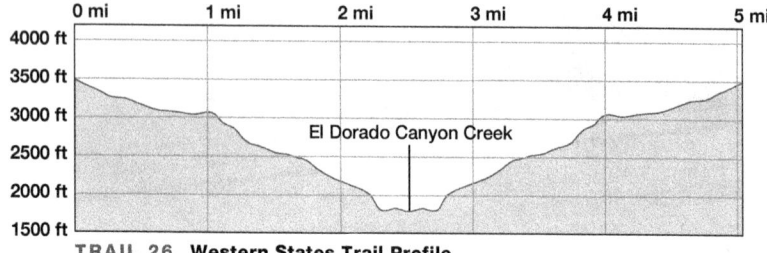

TRAIL 26 Western States Trail Profile

manzanita on the edge of the "**Big Gun Diggings**," promising a challenging climb back.

After dropping steeply for about 0.25 mile, the trail's descent moderates somewhat and enters a small drainage, drops quickly down two short switchbacks and crosses a seasonal creek. The manzanita understory thins and diversifies with bay laurel and other shrubs, and the overstory becomes dominated by Douglas fir and black and live oaks. The trail climbs out of the small drainage, turns the corner around the end of a ridge and then drops down another switchback into a larger drainage. Hikers will hear the sound of water emanating from the drainage below.

Stream

Soon, the trail reaches perennial **Poor Man's Canyon Creek**. After an easy crossing, continue straight on the trail, ▶3 which climbs out of the side drainage and rounds subsidiary ridges dropping down from Chicken Hawk Ridge above. As the trail rounds the ridges, expansive views are provided across the steep North Fork of the Middle Fork American River canyon. Protruding metamorphic bedrock streaked with quartz is common along this stretch of the trail. The trail crosses a second seasonal drainage and rounds one last side ridge with a great view and then drops down into **El Dorado Canyon** proper.

Great Views

Canyon

A bit over 2.0 miles from your car, the Western States Trail crosses a mine access road dropping down from left to right. ▶4 Continue straight across the road and follow the trail as it descends more steeply into El Dorado Canyon. The environment becomes moister and the Douglas firs and oaks grow larger. Maples and ferns join the understory. The trail continues steeply downhill through three switchbacks and crosses the mining road a second time. Continue straight across the road on the Western States Trail, which negotiates one last switchback and meets up with the mining road again at the bottom of lushly vegetated El Dorado Canyon.

 Steep

Cross the road and proceed to the footbridge across El Dorado Canyon Creek, which is lined with alders, maples, and Indian rhubarb. There is a great swimming hole directly below the bridge, and the creek is big enough to support a small trout fishery. Creekside boulders and bedrock shelves provide good places to rest, eat lunch, and appreciate the view. Just west of the footbridge, there are a couple of large flats suitable for camping, surrounded by the rock piles indicative of past mining. After crossing the creek, the trail climbs steeply uphill to the historic mining camp site of Deadwood, but day hikers should plan on turning back at this point ▶5 to allow plenty of time for the long climb back out of the canyon.

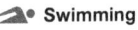 Swimming

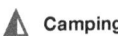 Camping

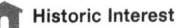 Historic Interest

Retrace your steps back up the WST to the trailhead ▶6 and end of Michigan Bluff Road.

MILESTONES

▶1	0.00	End of Michigan Bluff Road, turn left
▶2	0.28	WST Trailhead, turn right
▶3	1.85	Poor Man's Canyon Creek, continue straight
▶4	2.10	First mining road crossing, continue straight
▶5	2.80	El Dorado Canyon bridge, turn back
▶6	5.60	Retrace steps back to car

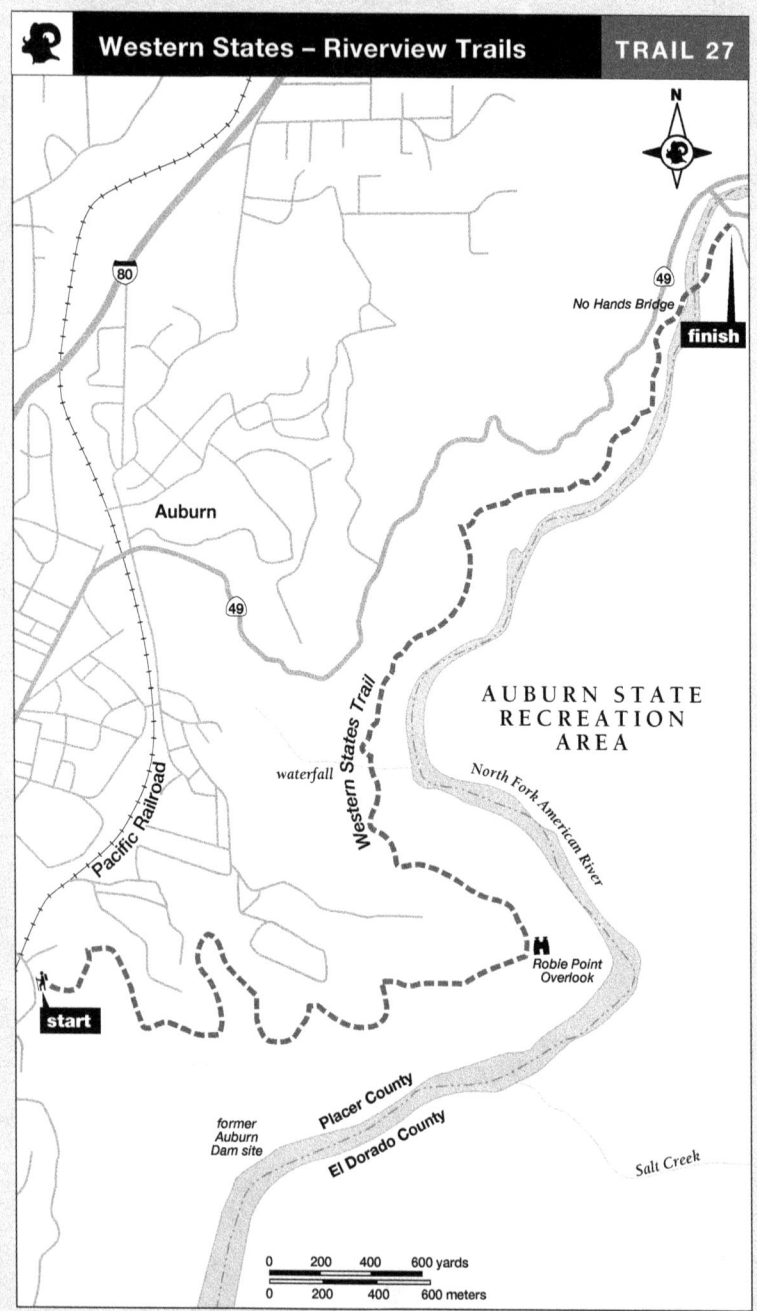

TRAIL 27 Sierra Foothills

Western States–Riverview Trails: Auburn State Recreation Area

The Western States Trail begins near Lake Tahoe and ends in Auburn and is used for two famous competitive events—the Western States Endurance Run (for ultramarathon runners) and the Tevis Cup Ride (for equestrians). This last section of the trail—from Auburn to the Hwy 49 Bridge—provides a unique glimpse of the site of the former Auburn Dam, as well as great views of the North Fork American River. The trail also crosses a couple of scenic side creeks, one with a pretty but seasonal waterfall. Part of the trail follows the route of the abandoned Mountain Quarries Railroad and crosses the graceful and historic Mountain Quarries (also known as the No Hands) Bridge. Unless you want to retrace your steps uphill, arrange this hike as a point-to-point trip with a car shuttle.

Best Time

This is a year-round, relatively low-elevation trail that goes from 1300 to 650 feet in elevation. It can get quite hot on summer afternoons. Fall–Spring is the best time for this trail.

Finding the Trail

From Sacramento, drive 34 miles east on Interstate 80 to Auburn. Take the Old Auburn exit, go straight on Maple St. After climbing a hill, Maple crosses Lincoln St. and becomes Auburn-Folsom Road. Shortly past Lincoln, the Auburn-Folsom Road curves south and crosses High St. Shortly after you go through the High St. intersection, turn left on

TRAIL USE
Hike, Run, Bike, Horse
LENGTH
4.2 miles, 2–3 hours
VERTICAL FEET
-650
DIFFICULTY
- 1 2 **3** 4 5 +
TRAIL TYPE
Point to Point
SURFACE TYPE
Dirt

FEATURES
Dogs on Leash
River
Stream
Waterfall
Canyon
Wildflowers
Birds
Wildlife
Historic
Great Views
Photo Opportunity

FACILITIES
None

> If the 500-foot-high Auburn Dam had been completed, all this area would have drowned under the reservoir created behind the dam.

Sacramento St. Soon thereafter, turn left on Pacific Ave., drive past Railhead Park on the left and the American River Canyon/Auburn Dam Overlook Park on your right. Immediately after Overlook Park, turn right into the dirt parking lot for the Western States Trailhead. To drop off a car at the Hwy 49 trailhead, drive east another 0.25 mile on Interstate 80 to the Hwy 49 exit, turn right. Follow the Hwy 49 signs through town. After crossing Lincoln, Hwy 49 drops steeply down into the North Fork American River canyon. Once you reach the river, turn right to follow Hwy 49 across the North Fork bridge. Park on the right immediately after the bridge for the Western States Trail trailhead. To get to the upper trailhead in Auburn from the highway bridge, retrace your drive back to Auburn, turn left on Lincoln, and then right on Auburn-Folsom Road. From there, follow the first set of directions.

Logistics

Call the Auburn State Recreation Area at (530) 885-4527 to make sure you are not planning your hike during the Western States Endurance Run, Tevis Cup Ride, or any other competitive events that use the trail. The first 2.0 miles of the trail follow a maze of former roads (used for the foundation construction of the Auburn Dam) and link with a number of side routes that lead up to Auburn and down to the river. To avoid following the wrong trail, pay particular attention to trail and road junctions, and follow the occasional WST (Western States Trail) markers where available.

Trail Description

A sign at the trailhead says COOL—7.3, POVERTY BAR—13, R.A.C.—16.2. ▶1 Proceed down the trail, which follows a former road, and immediately enter a cool gully shaded by live oaks with a thick understory of blackberry brambles. Cross a seasonal stream and follow the trail out of the side gully into the **North Fork canyon** proper. Vegetation changes to a much lighter overstory of live oaks punctuated by large manzanita. Through the brush, you get your first glimpses of the former **Auburn Dam** site.

Authorized by Congress in 1965, work on the dam foundation ground to a halt in 1975 due to earthquake safety concerns and rising costs. Attempts to resume construction of the dam have been rejected by Congress three times. Much of the visible site consists of the dam's massive foundation on the opposite canyon wall and the barren cobblestone area of the riverbed that was the site of a 200-foot-high coffer dam that diverted the river into an upstream diversion tunnel to allow for construction of the Auburn Dam foundation in the riverbed. The coffer dam blew out in a spectacular fashion in the 1986 flood.

Just past the WST mile 0.5 marker, the trail leaves the former road it has been following and becomes a single path that bends into another side canyon. A trail junction on the right leads downward. Proceed straight ahead. Cross another seasonal stream that hosts croaking frogs. Above, you'll see houses overlooking the canyon.

The trail winds its way out of the side canyon and comes to a road junction on the left that climbs up to Auburn. Proceed ahead on the **Western States Trail**, which drops and then climbs briefly. Again the trail turns into the North Fork canyon proper, and the sunny aspect favors gray pines, scrub oak, and more manzanita. You get another good view of the dam site, particularly of the upstream diversion tunnel through which the North Fork flows. A restoration project scheduled for completion in 2008 will close the diversion tunnel and restore the North

Canyon

Fork riverbed, as well as provide public river access to the former dam site and restored river.

Soon after passing the WST mile 1.0 marker, the single path trail reaches a wide switchback on a former road. Unfortunately, the previously reliable WST markers seem to be missing, and it is tempting to veer right and down the road, but veer left and go up the road instead. Soon after you leave the single track to follow the road, there is a trail junction on the left. Continue straight on the road, which dips in and out of another side canyon. Shortly after passing the WST mile 1.5 marker, another road junction leads up to your left to the top of **Robie Point**. Continue straight.

▶2 The Western States Trail reaches an expansive overlook of the canyon as the river bends around the outlying ridge dropping down from Robie Point. Here, you have a perfect opportunity to stop and rest, and to view the devastated Auburn Dam site downstream on your right and the wild North Fork canyon on your left.

Great Views

From the overlook, continue east (upstream) on the Western States Trail, which dips up and down as it traverses the canyon wall through the oak, pines, and chaparral. Your route continues past an uphill road junction on the left. As you come around a canyon bend and begin once again to enter a side canyon, Hwy 49 and the high Foresthill Bridge (not your destination) come into view upstream.

Soon, your route reaches another junction. The road you have been following heads uphill toward Hwy 49, but the Western States Trail breaks off and drops down to the right on a single track closed to mountain bikes. Veer right to follow the trail as it drops down toward a tributary stream in the bottom of the side canyon, which is darkly shaded by an oak forest with a lush riparian understory. After a few switchbacks, the trail passes a rocky pool that

Stream
Cool & Shady

Western States–Riverview Trails TRAIL 27

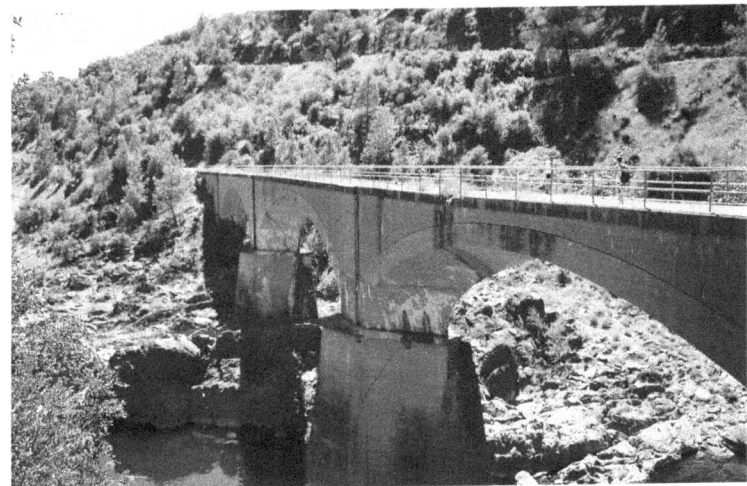

The Riverview segment *of the Western States Trail crosses the historic No Hands Bridge.*

gathers spring waters on the left and then crosses a larger seasonal stream.

After crossing the stream, the trail switchbacks uphill to meet up with the old Mountain Quarries Railroad grade at a concrete buttress. The buttress formerly held one end of a railroad trestle that spanned the stream you just crossed. The Mountain Quarries Railroad hauled limestone from the Cool quarry 7.0 miles out of the North Fork canyon to the Central Pacific railhead in Auburn. The railroad spanned the various tributaries and the North Fork on eighteen trestles and one large triple-arch concrete bridge. Service ended in 1939, and the rails were torn up and recycled in 1941 for the war effort, but most of the grade remains, providing a nicely graded route for the Western States Trail.

Just beyond the trestle buttress, you pass the mile 2.5 marker as the trail continues to follow the railroad grade east. Look for occasional piles of old railroad ties along the trail. Soon after you pass yet another road junction, which heads left uphill toward Hwy 49, the railroad grade is eroded away

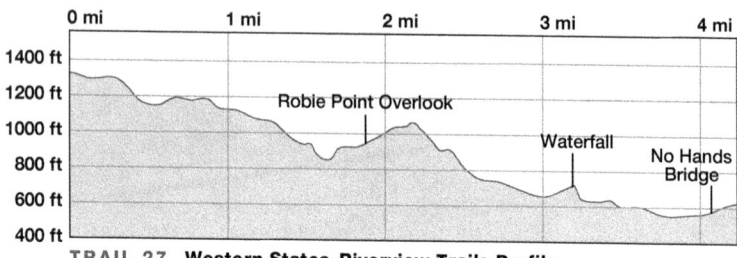

TRAIL 27 **Western States–Riverview Trails Profile**

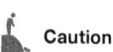
Caution

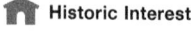
Waterfall

🏠 Historic Interest

👀 Great Views

and the trail briefly becomes single track again, but then picks up the grade and continues east.

The Western States Trail reaches another side canyon and drops steeply to the bottom, down a series of steps constructed in the steep slope. ▶3 The trail crosses the tributary at the foot of a scenic waterfall. Stop here for a final rest before pushing on to climb up out of the side canyon and back to the railroad grade. When you resume your hike, almost immediately the trail drops into one last side canyon and then climbs quickly back to the railroad grade, this one marked by a concrete buttress with the year 1921 carved into it. At this point, a spur trail drops steeply down on the right, through the poison oak and scrub to the river, while the Western States Trail continues straight along the grade.

After going around a canyon bend, hikers will catch their first sight of the graceful arches of the Mountain Quarries Bridge. Built by 800 workers at a cost of $300,000, it was the longest concrete triple-arch bridge in the world when it was completed in 1912. Since it was intended for railroad use, the bridge originally had no sides or handrails, thereby earning the local moniker of "No Hands" Bridge. Standing 150 feet over the North Fork, the bridge has withstood numerous natural floods and two human-made ones, including the 1964 collapse of the Hell Hole Dam upstream and the 1986 blowout of the Auburn coffer dam downstream. Now the

Western States–Riverview Trails | TRAIL 27

route of the Western States Trail, the bridge was added to the National Register of Historic Places in 2004.

As you follow the mellow grade on its way to the bridge, a spur road branches to the left and climbs the hill to Hwy 49. Soon thereafter, another spur road drops you right down to the river. Use this spur road if you want to cool off in the river before ending your trek. It's worth the relatively short hike back up to the railroad grade to stand under the stately arches of the No Hands Bridge and appreciate historic architecture that was both functional and beautiful.

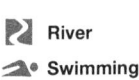
River
Swimming

From the spur road that leads down to the river at the foot of the bridge, continue on the Western States Trail to the actual No Hands/Mountain Quarries Bridge crossing. ▶4 Be sure to take the time to appreciate the expansive canyon views upstream and downstream. The Hwy 49 Bridge across the North Fork is just a few hundred yards upstream, so you know that you are quite near the end of your walk.

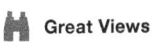
Great Views

After crossing the No Hands Bridge, your route intersects with one more trail junction, this one to the right and climbing straight up the canyon slope to Cool and the Olmstead Loop. From this intersection, ▶5 proceed straight on the Western States Trail to the trailhead parking area on Hwy 49.

MILESTONES

▶1	0.0	Start at Western States Trail staging area on Pacific Ave.
▶2	1.9	Robie Point overlook of North Fork American River
▶3	3.2	Side stream with waterfall
▶4	4.0	Mountain Quarries (No Hands) Bridge
▶5	4.2	Hwy 49 trailhead

Sierra Foothills

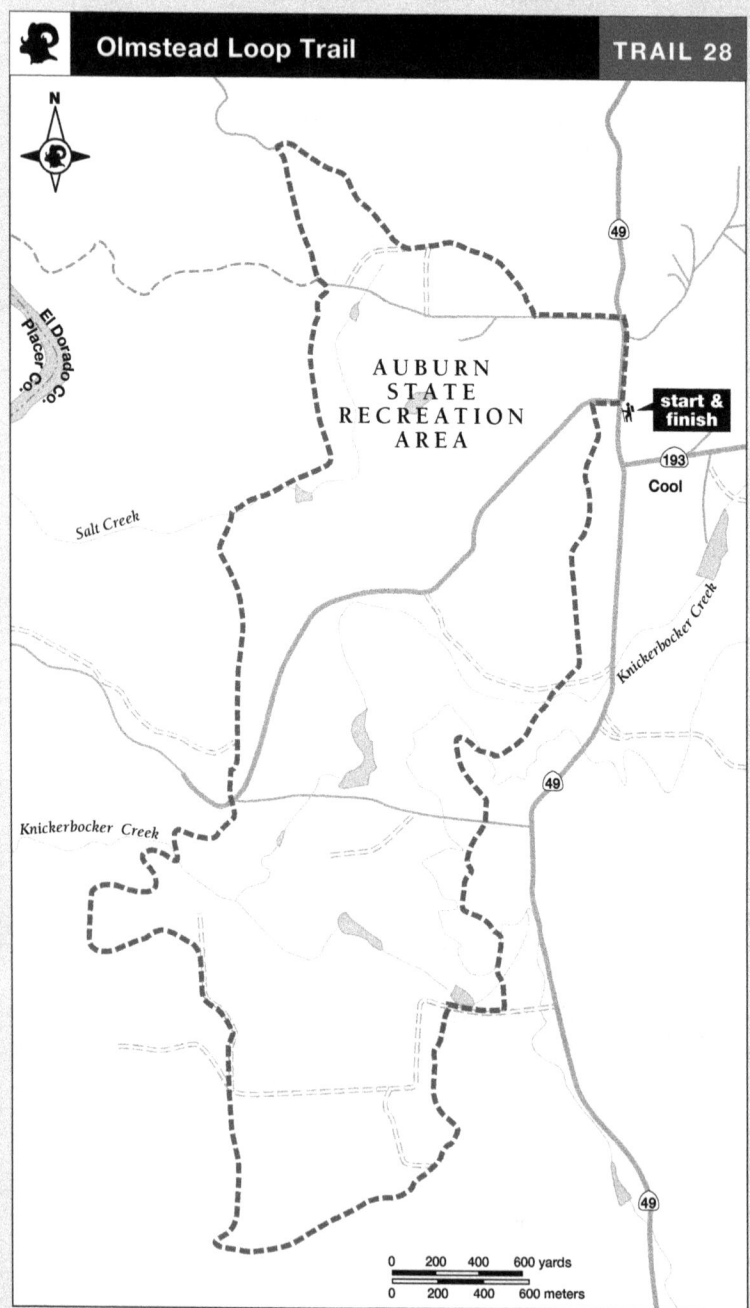

TRAIL 28 Sierra Foothills

Olmstead Loop Trail: Auburn State Recreation Area

Public land in the Sierra foothills is somewhat limited, and most of what is public is confined to river and creek canyons. The Olmstead Loop Trail (also known as the Knickerbocker Creek Trail) circles a chunk of public land in the Sierra foothills that encompasses a large meadow cut by a couple of small streams. This is a rare opportunity to hike through the rolling foothill countryside and explore oak woodlands and large grassy meadows, and to see wildflowers and wildlife on public lands. The Bureau of Reclamation acquired the entire area in the 1970s to partially mitigate the proposed drowning of the adjacent American River canyons and their extensive trail system by the construction of the Auburn Dam. But although the dam's construction was halted by safety concerns and escalating costs, the Olmstead Loop and its associated spur trails remain connected to the overall trail system in the Auburn State Recreation Area.

Best Time

Spring offers a fantastic display of wildflowers, the meadows are a lush green, and the new oak leaves are vibrant. Although the relatively low elevation makes this a year-round trail, it can be quite hot in the summer and wet and muddy in the winter. Take care when crossing even seasonal streams during high water in the winter and spring.

TRAIL USE
Hike, Run, Bike, Horse
LENGTH
8.5 miles, 4–6 hours
VERTICAL FEET
±350
DIFFICULTY
- 1 2 3 **4** 5 +
TRAIL TYPE
Loop
SURFACE TYPE
Dirt

FEATURES
Dogs on Leash
Stream
Canyon
Fall Color
Meadows
Wildflowers
Waterfalls
Birds
Wildlife
Great Views
Geologic Interest

FACILITIES
Porta-potty
Water

A small cascade just upstream of the Knickerbocker Creek crossing beckons to waders.

Finding the Trail

From Sacramento, drive east on Interstate 80 to the Hwy 49 exit in Auburn. Exit Hwy 49 and turn right (south); proceed on Hwy 49 through Auburn and into the American River canyon. The highway drops down into the canyon, crosses the American River, and then climbs back out of the canyon as you continue south. After climbing out of the canyon, you come to the small town of Cool. Just before entering the town and reaching the junction of highways 49 with 193, turn right at St. Florian Court, drive past the fire station, and find the Olmstead Loop parking lot, behind the fire station.

Logistics

The Olmstead Loop is a popular equestrian and mountain bike trail, so be prepared to share the trail with others. There are numerous other trails and roads that connect with the loop. Follow directions closely to avoid veering off on the wrong trail. Most of the loop follows dirt roads, although some segments narrow to a single track. A series of mileage posts run in a clockwise direction, but this hike follows the loop counterclockwise.

Trail Description

From the trailhead parking lot in Cool, ▶1 walk across the access street grandly named St. Florian Court and follow the trail briefly southeast along the fence to the highway. Turn left and walk a short distance northeast, parallel to the highway. The trail then turns left, to the northwest, and heads away from the highway and Cool. A sign saying AUBURN—7.3, POVERTY BAR—6.7, RAC [RUCK-A-CHUCKY]—9.9, DOGS ON LEASH reminds you that this loop trail connects with the much larger trail system of the Auburn State Recreation Area.

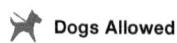
Dogs Allowed

Olmstead Loop Trail | TRAIL **28**

As the trail continues northwest away from the highway, it climbs a low hill. Soon the trail intersects with the **Quarry Trail** on your right. Continue straight ahead, along a fence line through rolling pastures and low hills studded with oaks. The Olmstead Loop leaves the fence line and veers right in a more northerly direction. It connects with the **Wendell Robie** segment of the **Western States Trail**, which comes in from the right. Continue straight, and within 100 feet the Western States Trail breaks away again to the right and the Olmstead Loop continues straight.

Shortly thereafter, you come to yet another trail junction, this one unsigned on your left. Veer right to stay on the Olmstead Loop, which crosses a meadow and then begins to gently climb through the oaks and an occasional gray pine. Another unsigned trail junction on your right provides a cutoff to the Western States Trail. The Olmstead Loop continues straight in a northerly direction as it reaches the top of a low hill studded with natural rock "tombstones" characteristic of the central Sierra foothills. Called "gravestone schist" by geologists, this metamorphosed volcanic rock was created undersea 140 million years ago and upended and changed by the mountain-building forces that formed the Sierra. Standing in the metaphorical geological graveyard, you see hints of the American River canyon through the trees, but actual vistas are blocked by vegetation.

Yet another trail junction heralds the connection of the Olmstead Loop with the **Training Hill Trail**, which drops steeply down to the right into the river canyon. ▶2 At the junction, the Olmsted Loop makes an abrupt left turn away from the canyon rim and leads off in a southwesterly direction. The trail immediately begins to drop gently down off the hilltop as it makes its way through oaks, gray pines, ceanothus, and manzanita. After passing the

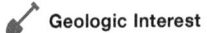

Meadow

Geologic Interest

Sierra Foothills

M7 post, the trail's descent steepens as it drops into the Salt Creek drainage.

The trail continues downward, past another unsigned trail junction on the left, and the tread becomes more eroded as it zigzags briefly downhill and then begins to parallel **Salt Creek** to the left, which feeds into a pond. ▶3 The trail crosses Salt Creek just below the pond. Although the creek is largely seasonal, care should be taken when crossing it during high water in the winter or spring.

After crossing Salt Creek, the Olmstead Loop climbs steeply out of the creek canyon. A path on your right marks the junction with the Coffer Dam Trail. Follow the Olmstead Loop to your left and continue climbing at a more moderate rate. Woodpeckers can be heard foraging in the nearby gray pines.

Past the M6 marker, the trail levels out and continues on a nearly level grade through scrub oak, gray pines, and coyote bush and other chaparral. At this point, the Olmstead Loop is circumnavigating a larger meadow system, which can be glimpsed through the brush and trees on your left. Soon you come to the four-way trail junction. A cutoff trail leads right and to north to the Coffer Dam Trail. The left trail leads to a paved road that your route will shortly cross. Continue straight on the Olmstead Loop in a southeasterly direction.

The trail enters a large open area on the edge of the meadow system and crosses a paved road. If you turn left on this road, you can follow it back to the trailhead in Cool (and thereby cut your loop trek in half). But you'll miss some of the prettiest parts of the loop trail, so cross the paved road and follow the Olmstead Loop Trail as it climbs over a low ridge and begins a moderate descent into the lower Knickerbocker Creek drainage through a thick oak-pine-scrub forest.

Olmstead Loop Trail | TRAIL **28**

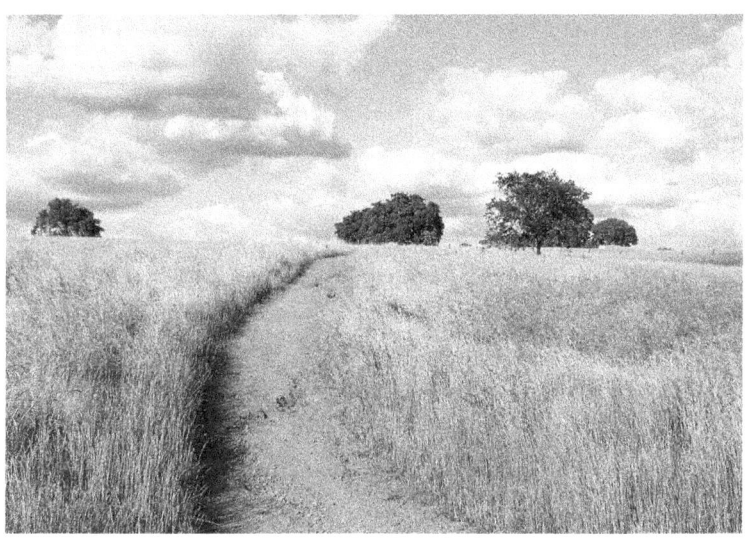

Rare public access *to the Mother Lode's foothill grasslands is one of the many nice features of the Olmstead Loop Trail.*

The Olmstead Loop crosses lower **Knickerbocker Creek** ▶4 on a seasonally installed wood footbridge. An inviting cascade is just upstream. Again, care should be taken when crossing Knickerbocker Creek during higher flows in the winter and spring.

A moderate climb out of the creek canyon leads the Olmstead Loop back into the oak savanna. The trail comes to the rim of the American River canyon. Several oak trees provide shade for those who want to eat their lunch with a view. Beyond the viewpoint, the trail makes a left turn at a fence line and then another left as it drops into a seasonal drainage. As it climbs out of the drainage, the trail enters a large meadow, where deer and coyotes play a deadly game of hide-and-seek. As the trail makes its way through the meadow, it briefly narrows into a single track.

Widening once again into a road, the trail cuts through a swath of live oak, blackberry brambles, and black walnut trees as it passes the M4 marker.

 Stream

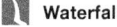 Waterfall

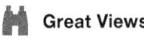 Great Views

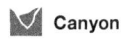 Canyon

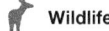 Wildlife

Sierra Foothills

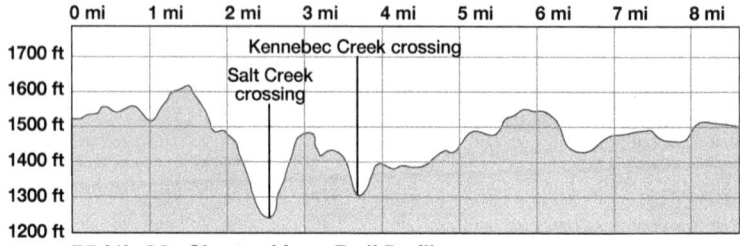

TRAIL 28 Olmstead Loop Trail Profile

Shortly thereafter, an unsigned trail junction leads off to the left, but the Olmstead Loop continues straight, past an old walnut orchard on the left. The trail drops gently down into another shallow drainage and then climbs back up through a sylvan glade of blue oaks.

The trail reaches its southwest corner of the loop ▶5 and makes a sharp left turn in a southeasterly direction. Four tall radio towers are visible beyond the tree line as the trail passes the M3 marker. It leaves the oak glade behind and enters an open pasture dotted with solitary oak trees.

Continuing southeast through open pasture and solitary oaks, the trail parallels a fence line marking the western boundary of the Auburn State Recreation Area. It passes an unsigned trail junction on the left, crosses a small seasonal drainage near the M2.5 marker, and then climbs over a low hill. Houses appear nearby on the right, and the trail again narrows to a single track as it begins to angle northward.

At the top of a low ridge, the trail bends to the northeast and gently descends through meadows broken by lines of oaks and blackberry brambles. You begin to hear and see traffic on Hwy 49 as the trail nears and then runs parallel to the highway. After passing the M2 marker, the trail reaches an unsigned trail junction to the left. The trail turns right at the junction then turns left as it follows

Olmstead Loop Trail — TRAIL 28

a tributary to upper Knickerbocker Creek. The creek overflows onto the trail at this point, turning the whole general area into a shallow pond. An unsigned road on the right leads to a gate on Hwy 49. Continue straight on the Olmstead Loop, which enters a live oak grove and then crosses the small tributary stream and wetland on a crude wood walkway. 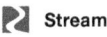 Stream

After leaving the stream and wetland behind, the Olmstead Loop climbs a low hill and crosses an irrigation ditch. The trail continues northeast through rolling pasture and woodlands frequented by quail and wild turkey, past an unsigned trail junction on the left at marker M1.5. Going through a gate, the trail climbs a rise, passes another unsigned trail junction on the left. The trail then goes past a school on the right facing Hwy 49. Just beyond the school, a gated road on the right leads to the highway. Wildlife

Shortly after the M1 marker, the trail crosses the irrigation ditch for a second time, then briefly parallels upper Knickerbocker Creek, ▶6 before crossing the creek on a wood walkway. Soon thereafter, the trail crosses one last road that leads to the left and the right, past a few houses on the right, and then drops down into a seasonal drainage, ▶7 before climbing back to the trailhead in Cool. 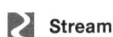 Stream

MILESTONES

- ▶1 0.00 Trailhead in Cool
- ▶2 1.40 Training Hill Trail junction, bear left
- ▶3 2.60 Salt Creek crossing
- ▶4 3.75 Lower Knickerbocker Creek crossing
- ▶5 5.40 Southeast corner of the loop, trail goes left
- ▶6 7.64 Upper Knickerbocker Creek crossing
- ▶7 8.51 Return to trailhead

Cronan Ranch Loop

TRAIL 29

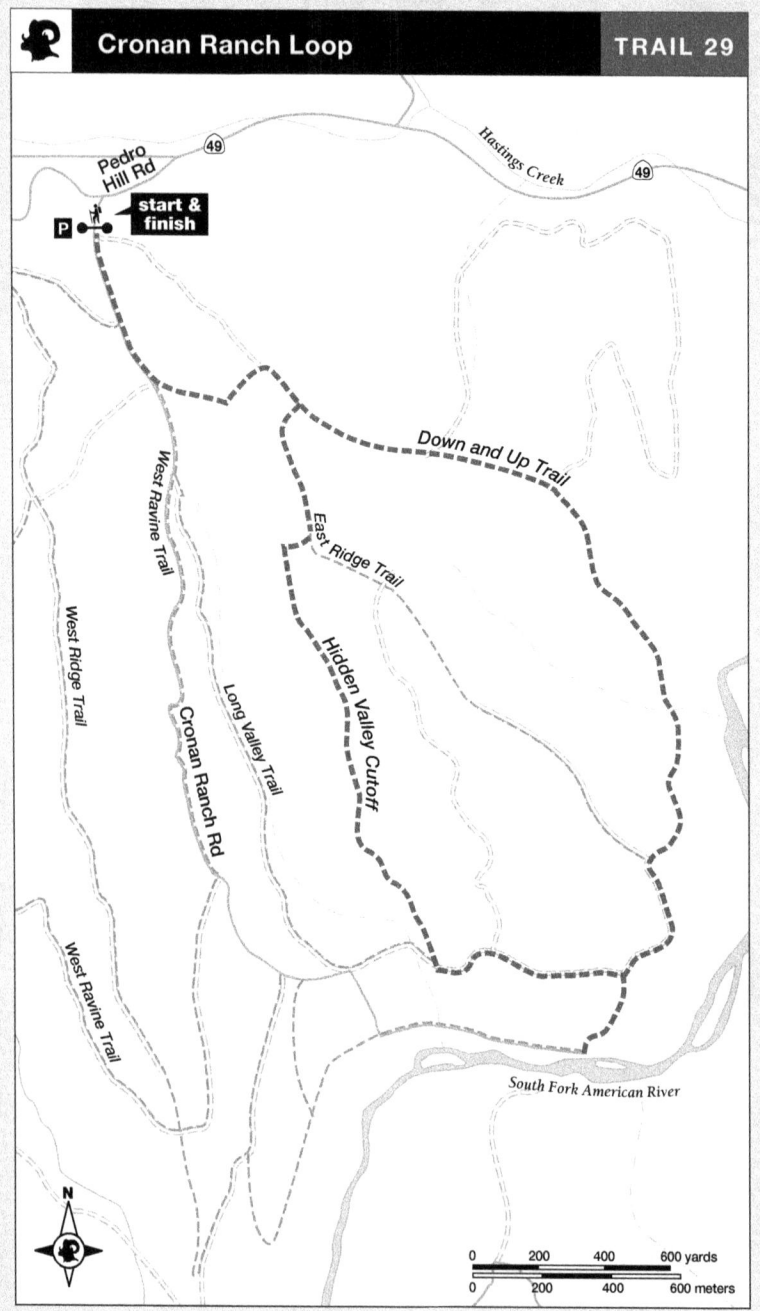

TRAIL 29 Sierra Foothills

Cronan Ranch Loop: South Fork American River

The South Fork American River in the Sierra foothills south of Placerville is one of California's most popular white-water rivers. The South Fork is where gold was discovered by Europeans in 1849, so the river is also rich in Gold Rush history. Not so long ago, public access along the South Fork was quite limited. The American River Conservancy and the BLM are acquiring land for public recreation and habitat purposes along the river. This easy loop trail, in the recently acquired Cronan Ranch Regional Trails Park, provides a nice ramble through oak and riparian woodlands and foothill grasslands, as well as direct access to the South Fork American River.

Best Time

This is a year-round, relatively low-elevation trail (600–880 feet). It can get hot on summer afternoons, so it is best walked in the mornings or evenings. Spring provides a remarkably colorful display of wildflowers, while summer evokes Kate Bush's folk song about the "rolling golden hills of California." Hikers should beware of high-water flows in the river during winter and spring.

Finding the Trail

From Sacramento, take Hwy 50 east to Placerville. Take Hwy 49 north from Placerville to Coloma. Start tracking your mileage after Hwy 49 crosses the South Fork bridge in Coloma. Approximately 5.1 miles north of the Hwy 49 bridge in Coloma, turn

TRAIL USE
Hike, Run, Bike, Horse
LENGTH
4.9 miles, 3–4 hours
VERTICAL FEET
±220
DIFFICULTY
- 1 2 **3** 4 5 +
TRAIL TYPE
Loop
SURFACE TYPE
Dirt

FEATURES
Dogs Allowed
Child Friendly
River
Canyon
Stream
Meadow
Wildflowers
Birds
Wildlife
Great Views

FACILITIES
Porta-potties

> Willow, alder and other riparian trees and shrubs dominate the trailside.

left on Pedro Hill Road. Within 100 yards, turn left into the Cronan Ranch Regional Park parking area.

Logistics

Do not leave valuables in your car, as the parking lot has been the target of vandals.

Trail Description

From the **Cronan Ranch Regional Trails Park** parking area, ▶1 proceed past the gate and hike up the road to a low grassy saddle. From the saddle, you get an expansive view of the park's upper grassy bowl, carved by coulees (shallow gullies) and surrounded by low oak covered ridges. From the saddle, the West Ravine Trail branches off to the right, but your route continues south and downhill from the saddle as the road drops toward the South Fork American River.

About 0.3 mile from the parking lot, ▶2 turn left on to a jeep road, which marks the beginning of the **Down and Up Trail**. This trail climbs gently up through the open savanna while meadowlarks provide musical (if seasonal) accompaniment and hawks cruise the thermals above. As the trail reaches a second low saddle, another jeep trail breaks off to the right and south—this is the **East Ridge Trail** ▶3 and your return route.

Birds

Continue southeast on the Down and Up Trail, as it drops into a shallow coulee and then climbs easily up to a third saddle. From here, you get your first view of the South Fork American River, appropriately to the south. Follow the trail as it narrows to a single track and drops more steeply into a gully lined with live oaks.

The gully deepens and, depending on the time of year, water may be flowing in its bottom. Soon, you reach an unmarked trail junction on the

Cronan Ranch Loop | TRAIL **29**

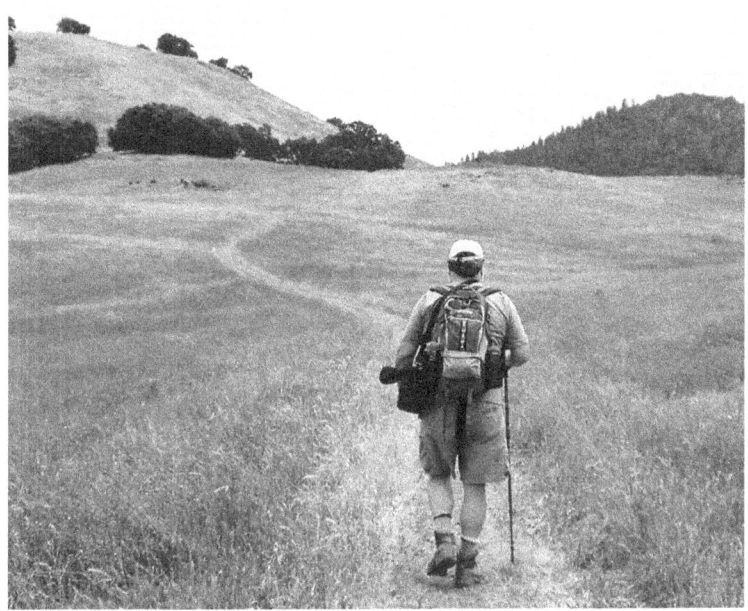

The upper segments of the Cronan Ranch trails wind through rolling grasslands.

left, which leads east toward Greenwood Creek. Continue south on the Down and Up Trail.

After crossing the seasonal stream, the Down and Up Trail climbs a steep but short pitch up a low ridge and begins to parallel the South Fork, which is heard but not seen through a screen of trees. The trail climbs over the low ridgetop and drops into another coulee. You reach another trail junction, where the East Ridge Trail branches off to the north (right), ▶4 but you should continue straight (west) on the Down and Up Trail.

About 0.2 mile later, you come to an unnamed trail junction, this one on the left. ▶5 Turn left to take this river access route down to the South Fork American River. Here, commercial outfitters have placed picnic tables and porta-potties for use

 River

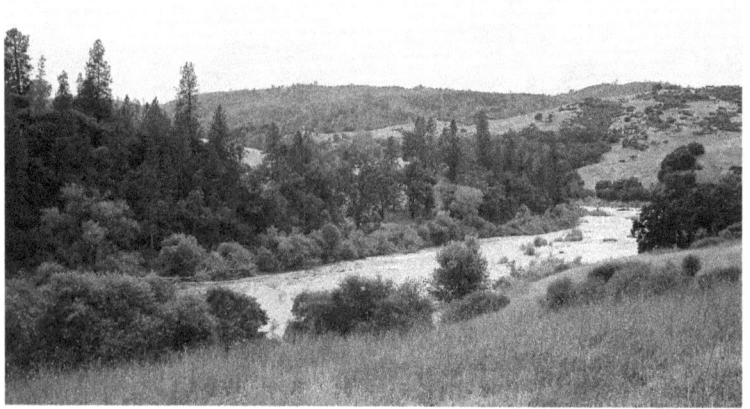

There are many ways to reach The South Fork American River *on the Cronan Ranch trail system.*

 Birds

by their rafting customers. Have lunch under the riverside trees and if it is summer, watch the rafters and kayakers float by. In the spring, yellow-breasted chats nest and forage in the riparian habitat and fill the air with an amazing repertoire of caws and whistles.

From your riverside lunch spot, ▶6 retrace your steps up the river access trail to the Down and Up Trail and turn left. ▶7 The trail continues its undulating path in and out of shallow, oak-covered coulees with some barren areas dominated by serpentine soils.

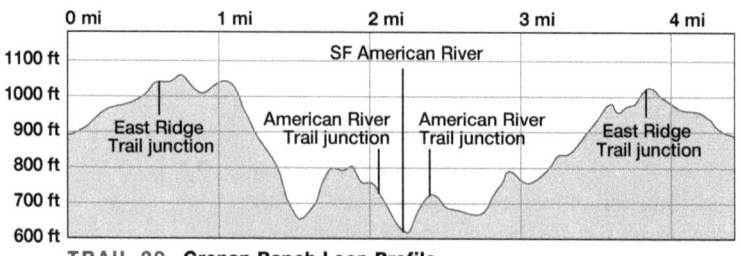

TRAIL 29 Cronan Ranch Loop Profile

Cronan Ranch Loop — TRAIL 29

In the bottom of yet another shallow and tree-lined coulee, you reach the junction with the **Hidden Valley Cutoff Trail**. Turn right ▶8 and begin climbing moderately through oak woodlands and savanna, accented by scenic rock outcrops. About 0.8 mile up the ridge, the Hidden Valley Cutoff Trail ends at the East Ridge Trail. ▶9 Turn left on the East Ridge Trail, which continues north, climbing gradually into the large grass-covered bowl from whence your hike started. About 0.2 mile from the Hidden Valley/East Ridge junction, you reach the junction of the East Ridge and Down and Up Trails. ▶10 Turn left and retrace your steps to the Cronan Ranch Road. ▶11 Turn right on the road and proceed back to ▶12 the trailhead parking area.

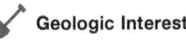 Geologic Interest

MILESTONES

▶1	0.0	Start at trailhead (from Cronan Ranch Parking Lot)
▶2	0.3	Down & Up Trail junction, turn left
▶3	0.9	Upper East Ridge Trail junction, continue straight on Down & Up Trail
▶4	2.1	Lower East Ridge Trail junction, continue straight on Down & Up Trail
▶5	2.3	River access trail junction, turn left
▶6	2.5	South Fork American River, retrace steps back to Down & Up junction
▶7	2.7	Return to Down & Up Trail, turn left
▶8	3.0	Hidden Valley Cutoff Trail junction, turn right
▶9	3.8	Hidden Valley/East Ridge trails junction, turn left
▶10	4.0	East Ridge/Down & Up trails junction, turn left
▶11	4.6	Cronan Ranch Road, turn right
▶12	4.9	Return to trailhead parking area

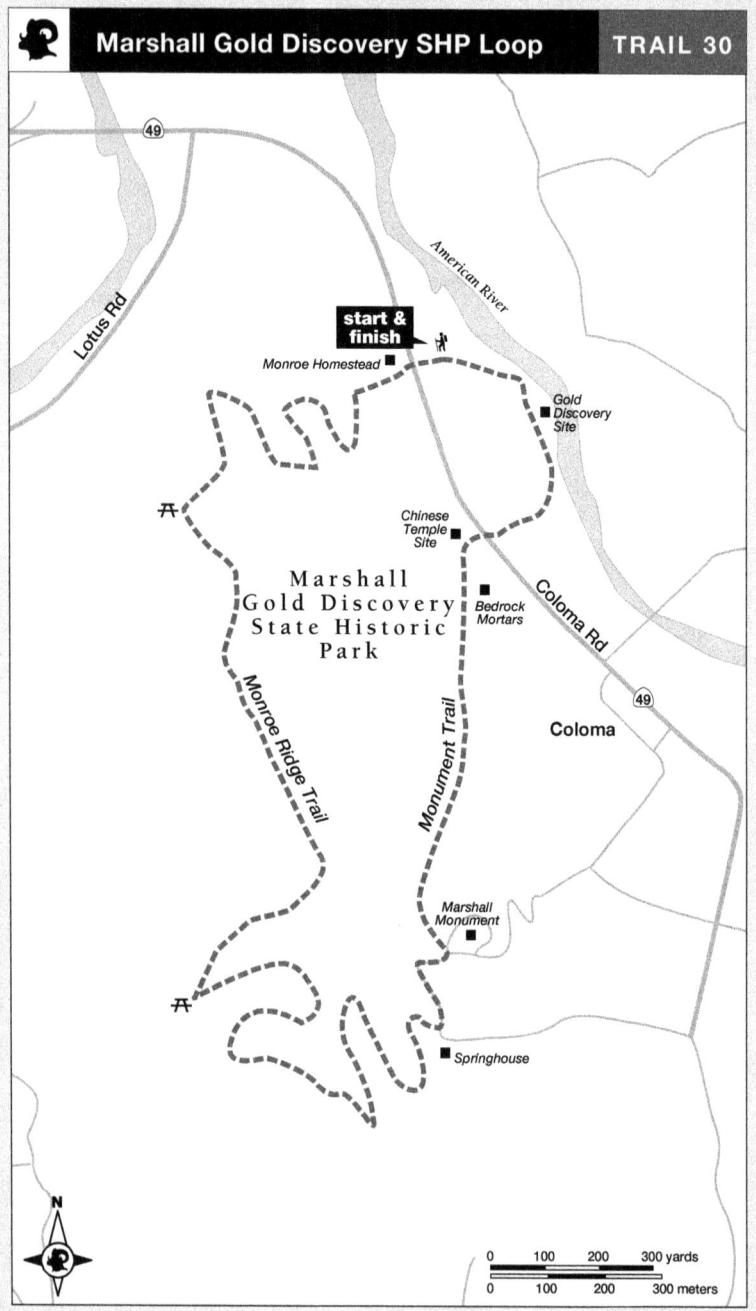

TRAIL 30 Sierra Foothills

Marshall Gold Discovery State Historic Park Loop

The Monroe Ridge and Monument trails explore some of the less-visited parts of Marshall Gold Discovery State Historic Park. Perhaps the most historic site in California, the park commemorates the place where gold was discovered in California in 1849. This route provides excellent views of the Coloma Valley and the South Fork American River, as well as a varied sampling of the area's rich Gold Rush history.

Best Time

This is a year-round, relatively low-elevation trail (780–1275 feet). It can get hot on summer afternoons, making it a good morning hike.

Finding the Trail

From Sacramento, take Hwy 50 east to Placerville. Take Hwy 49 north from Placerville to Coloma. Drive through Marshall Gold Discovery State Park and turn right into the North Beach parking area. Drive to the south end of the parking area and park. The trail begins across the highway in a meadow near an orchard.

Logistics

This trail is in a State Park, where entrance fees are charged. Purchase a parking permit at the entrance of the North Beach parking area or at the Park visitors center.

TRAIL USE
Hike, Run
LENGTH
3.6 miles, 2–3 hours
VERTICAL FEET
±496
DIFFICULTY
- 1 2 **3** 4 5 +
TRAIL TYPE
Loop
SURFACE TYPE
Dirt

FEATURES
Parking Fee
Fall color
Canyon
River
Wildlife
Historic
Interpretive
Photo Opportunity
Great Views
Steep

FACILITIES
Toilets

Trail Description

The trail passes a large granite rock with several grinding holes, reminding us that history did not start here with the arrival of Europeans and the discovery of gold.

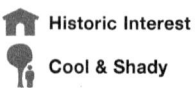
Historic Interest
Cool & Shady

From the south end of the North Beach parking area, ▶1 carefully cross Hwy 49 to the meadow on the other side. A sign says MONROE RIDGE TRAIL—MARSHALL MONUMENT—2.3 MILES. Cross the meadow and pass the Monroe Orchard on your right. Much of what later became the park was purchased from the Monroe Family, early settlers of the **Coloma Valley** who came to the state as slaves. Freed when California entered the union, the Monroe Family were respected local farmers and landowners.

Just as the trail begins to climb, you pass the monument identifying the Monroe Family homesite. The well-shaded trail climbs up through oak woodland with thick understory of native blackberry and non-native vinca. After two switchbacks, the trail negotiates a short wood stairway and bridge that crosses the **Lotus Ditch**, which transports water diverted upstream from the South Fork American River to various farms and properties in the Coloma Valley.

Soon the invading vinca gives way to typical poison oak and other native shrubs of the Sierra foothills. There are occasional glimpses of the South Fork American River through the live oak forest as the trail continues its moderate ascent of **Monroe Ridge** through a series of well-graded switchbacks.

Soon the trail reaches the ridgetop and gently climbs toward the ridge's northern high point. The oak forest gives way to tree-size manzanita bushes punctuated with ponderosa, gray pines, and open grassy swales.

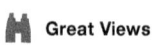
Great Views

Within a little less than 1.0 mile from the trailhead, the trail reaches the high point on the north end of Monroe Ridge. The brush and trees open up, providing great views of most of the park below, as well as of the South Fork American River and hair-raising Troublemaker Rapid to the east. ▶2 A

Marshall Gold Discovery State Historic Park Loop TRAIL 30

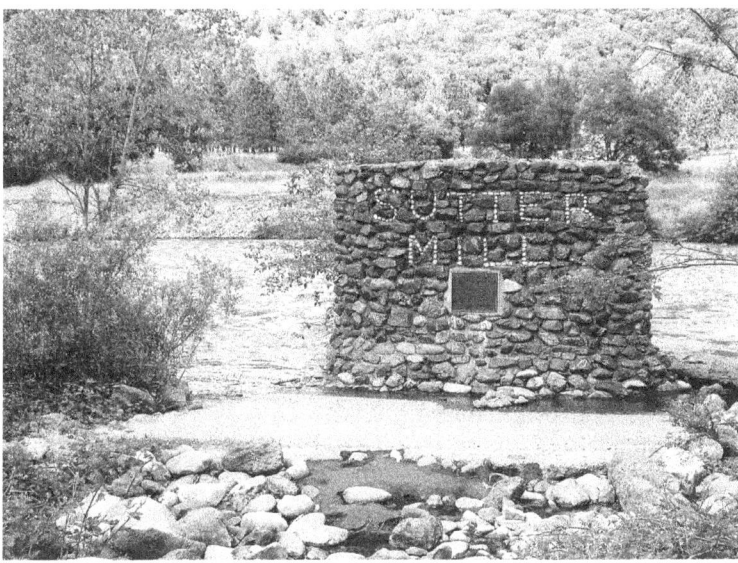

The Marshall Park Loop Trail *takes you past the actual site of John Marshall's discovery of gold in California.*

shaded picnic table provides an excellent rest stop with a view.

From the picnic table, the trail continues south, undulating along the top of Monroe Ridge through broken forest. An observant hiker will spy the white monolith of the **Marshall Monument** to the southeast. Soon thereafter, a short spur trail on the left takes you to an old mine shaft in the ridge. The open pit leading to the shaft is fenced off for public safety. Many foolish hikers rue the day they tried to explore an old Mother Lode mine.

After crossing under a power line, the trail cuts over to the west side of the ridge and then begins to switchback through black oaks, crisscrossing the ridgetop several times as it climbs toward the ridge's ultimate "summit."

About 0.66 mile from the first picnic table, the trail reaches the 1275-foot peak of the ridge,

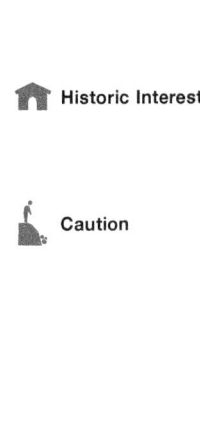

Historic Interest

Caution

Steep

Sierra Foothills 237

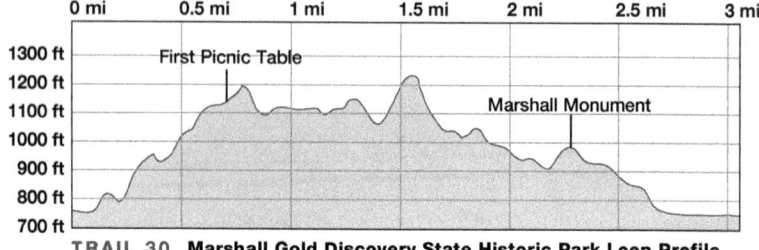

TRAIL 30 Marshall Gold Discovery State Historic Park Loop Profile

Great Views

where a second picnic table ▶3 provides yet another opportunity to rest and observe the west end of the Coloma Valley.

From the second picnic table, the trail crosses over the ridge from west to east one more time and then begins to drop swiftly down toward the Marshall Monument in a series of long switchbacks. The trail reaches an old dirt road providing access to a large spring and springhouse that formerly served the park. After following the dirt road a short ways, the Monroe Ridge Trail ends at the paved road that leads to the Marshall Monument.

Turn left and walk up the paved road for about 100 yards to ▶4 the Monument, which consists of a picnic area, parking lot, and a large mound on which stands a pedestal and statue of John Marshall pointing to the location on the river where he found gold and forever changed California.

Historic Interest

From the foot of the stone stairs that climb the Monument mound, head north past a park residence and look for the sign directing you to the visitors center. Here the wide **Monument Trail**, lined with a split rail fence, drops steeply down toward the center of the park and the river. The trail negotiates another wood bridge and stairway over the Lotus Ditch and soon thereafter reaches a point just above a large grassy picnic area along Hwy 49.

At this point, the trail passes a large granite rock with several grinding holes. Unfortunately, the

Historic Interest

Marshall Gold Discovery State Historic Park Loop | TRAIL **30**

Nisenan and Miwok people who once lived here were largely wiped out by the Gold Rush, which brought greed, conflict, and disease to the valley they called Callumah.

Just past the grinding rock, the trail turns sharply right, follows the picnic area fence line, and goes through a meadow that was once the site of a Chinese Taoist Temple. Chinese workers came to California to labor in the gold mines, only to find discrimination. But a few managed to work their way out of poverty to open a store, bank, and temple in Coloma, which was regarded as the queen of the mining camps.

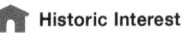
Historic Interest

From the picnic area and temple site, the trail crosses Hwy 49 (be sure to look both ways for traffic) and becomes part of the riverside **Gold Discovery Trail**. Follow the trail across a meadow toward the river and then turn north along the river, past the actual site of **Sutter's Mill** (which is a couple of hundred yards north of the sawmill replica across from the visitors center).

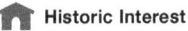
Historic Interest

The trail soon reaches the south end of the North Beach parking area ▶5 and the trailhead.

🚶	**MILESTONES**
▶1	0.00 Start at trailhead (south end of North Beach parking area)
▶2	0.91 North Picnic Table on Monroe Ridge
▶3	1.57 South Picnic Table on Monroe Ridge
▶4	2.58 Marshall Monument
▶5	3.60 Return to trailhead

CHAPTER 4

Sierra Nevada

31. Mount Judah Loop Trail
32. Pacific Crest Trail: Castle Peak Area
33. Salmon Lake Trail to Loch Leven Lakes
34. Grouse Lakes Loop Trail
35. Picayune Valley Trail: Granite Chief Wilderness
36. Lake Margaret Trail: Caples Creek Proposed Wilderness
37. Granite and Hidden Lakes Loop
38. Shealor Lake Trail: Caples Creek Proposed Wilderness
39. Winnemucca–Round Top Lakes Loop: Mokelumne Wilderness
40. Caples Creek–Silver Fork Loop: Caples Creek Proposed Wilderness
41. Horsetail Falls Trail
42. Twin Lakes Trail: Desolation Wilderness
43. Lyons Creek Trail: Desolation Wilderness

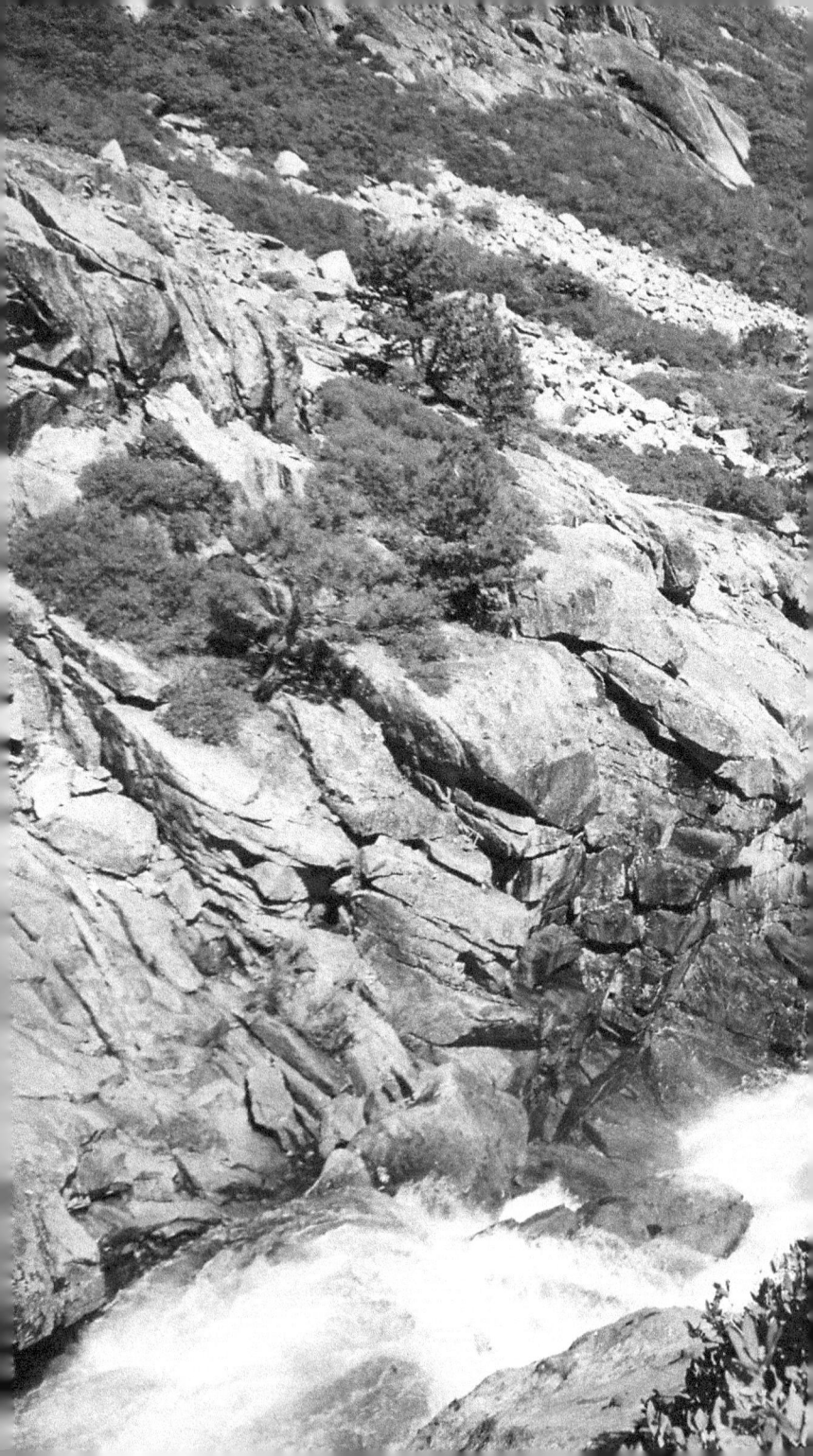

AREA OVERVIEW

Sierra Nevada

John Muir played an early role in drawing public attention to the need to protect the outstanding scenery and recreation opportunities of the Sierra Nevada. Much of his "Range of Light" was set aside in its natural state in parks and federal reserves. All the trails in Chapter 4 are located on National Forest lands, some which have been designated as Wilderness to preserve their undeveloped character. The trails explore mid-elevation forests cut by streams and rivers, and rocky highlands dotted with alpine lakes. Many of these trails are buried in snow for much of the winter and spring, but provide a welcome respite to the summer heat that dominates the lower elevations.

Maps and Permits

All of the trails featured in this chapter are located on federally managed public lands in the Tahoe and Eldorado National Forests. The Forest Service publishes recreation maps depicting the road and trail systems for each forest, as well as campgrounds and other developed facilities. The Forest Service also publishes detailed topographic maps for each Wilderness Area featured in this chapter. For viewing topography and physical features on the non-wilderness trails, USGS 7.5-minute quad maps are best. The Forest Service maps are available at most outdoor–recreation equipment stores or can be ordered from the agency via the Internet or by regular mail. Details are found in the appendix.

Trailhead parking and the use of National Forest trails are generally free. However, the trails that enter Wilderness require a permit. Some of the Wilderness trails featured in this chapter have quotas that limit the number of visitors in order to preserve the Wilderness experience. Details on where to acquire wilderness permits are found in the appendix.

Overleaf and opposite: *Pyramid Creek just below Horsetail Falls (Trail 41)*

AREA MAP

The Sierra Nevada

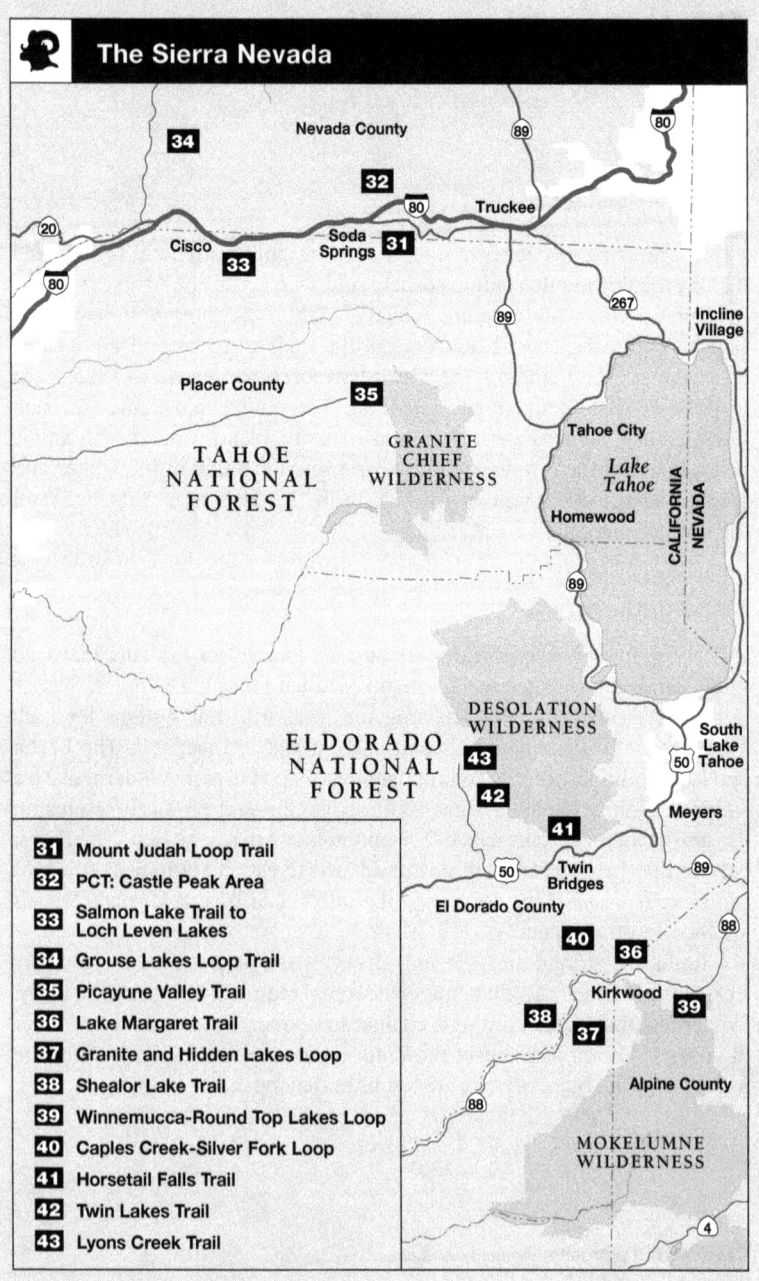

31. Mount Judah Loop Trail
32. PCT: Castle Peak Area
33. Salmon Lake Trail to Loch Leven Lakes
34. Grouse Lakes Loop Trail
35. Picayune Valley Trail
36. Lake Margaret Trail
37. Granite and Hidden Lakes Loop
38. Shealor Lake Trail
39. Winnemucca-Round Top Lakes Loop
40. Caples Creek-Silver Fork Loop
41. Horsetail Falls Trail
42. Twin Lakes Trail
43. Lyons Creek Trail

TRAIL FEATURE TABLE

Sierra Nevada

TRAIL	Difficulty	Length	Type	USES & ACCESS	TERRAIN	FLORA & FAUNA	OTHER
31	4	4.6	Loop	Hiking, Dogs	Meadow, Canyon	Wildflowers, Birds	Historic, Views, Photo
32	4	6.72	Point-to-Point	Hiking, Dogs	River, Waterfall, Canyon	Wildflowers, Fall Colors	Geologic, Views, Steep, Camping
33	3	5.0	Point-to-Point	Hiking, Dogs	Lake		Views, Photo
34	5	10.1	Loop	Hiking, Horses, Biking, Dogs	River, Waterfall, Lake, Wetland, Canyon, Mountain	Wildflowers	Views, Camping
35	4	8.66	Point-to-Point	Hiking, Horses, Permit, Dogs	River, Waterfall, Wetland, Canyon	Wildflowers, Fall Colors	Views, Camping, Photo
36	3	4.7	Point-to-Point	Hiking, Dogs	River, Lake, Wetland	Wildflowers, Birds	Views, Photo
37	4	7.0	Loop	Hiking, Dogs	River, Lake, Wetland		Views, Camping, Photo
38	2	3.2	Point-to-Point	Hiking, Running, Child Friendly, Dogs	Lake, Canyon	Wildflowers	Geologic, Views, Camping, Photo
39	4	4.74	Loop	Hiking, Permit, Dogs	River, Waterfall, Meadow, Canyon	Wildflowers, Fall Colors	Historic, Views, Steep
40	5	8.6	Loop	Hiking, Horses, Running, Biking, Dogs	River, Waterfall, Wetland, Canyon	Wildflowers, Fall Colors, Birds, Wildlife	Views, Steep, Camping
41	2	3.0	Loop	Hiking, Running, Biking, Child Friendly, Fee, Dogs	River, Waterfall, Canyon		Geologic, Views, Photo
42	4	5.0	Point-to-Point	Hiking, Permit, Dogs	River, Waterfall, Lake, Meadow	Wildflowers	Views, Steep, Camping
43	5	10.0	Point-to-Point	Hiking, Permit, Dogs	River, Waterfall, Lake, Wetland	Wildflowers	Views, Steep, Camping, Photo

USES & ACCESS
- Hiking
- Horses
- Running
- Biking
- Child Friendly
- Handicap Access
- $ Fee
- Permit Required
- Dogs Allowed

TYPE
- Loop
- Out & Back
- Point-to-Point
- V Variable

DIFFICULTY
- 1 2 3 4 5 +
less   more

TERRAIN
- River or Stream
- Waterfall
- Lake
- Wetland
- Meadow
- Canyon
- Mountain

FLORA & FAUNA
- Wildflowers
- Fall Colors
- Birds
- Wildlife

FEATURES
- Historic Interest
- Geologic Interest
- Great Views
- Steep
- Secluded
- Camping
- Photo Opportunity

TRAIL SUMMARIES

Sierra Nevada

TRAIL 31
Hike
4.6 miles, Loop
Difficulty: 1 2 3 **4** 5

Mount Judah Loop Trail 253
Following one of the more scenic segments of the Pacific Crest Trail (PCT) south from Donner Pass, this loop trail provides commanding views of the high peaks along the Sierra crest north of Lake Tahoe. It also offers an astounding alpine wildflower display during the midsummer season and an opportunity to easily "bag" a Sierra peak. Along the way, you can get a rough idea of what early pioneers suffered as they hauled their wagons over the mountain range and of the historic effort of the railroad workers who forged a route across the crest.

TRAIL 32
Hike
6.7 miles, Out & Back
Difficulty: 1 2 3 **4** 5

Pacific Crest Trail:
Castle Peak Area.................... 259
A favorite of Sacramentans desiring a taste of the high country, this popular hike offers incredible alpine vistas and a great summer wildflower display. It also provides access to the proposed Castle Peak Wilderness, a long-time protection priority for conservationists. Along the way, you get an introduction to the Sierra's diverse glacial and volcanic geology and may be tempted to bag 9103-foot Castle Peak.

Salmon Lake Trail
to Loch Leven Lakes 265
The hike to Loch Leven Lakes is probably the most beloved of the high mountain trails visited by Sacramentans. This easy day hike or short backpack trip not only visits the three Loch Leven Lakes, it also offers a short side trip to lovely Salmon Lake. Along the way, you get spectacular views of the rugged North Fork American River canyon and surrounding peaks.

TRAIL 33

Hike
5.0 miles, Out & Back
Difficulty: 1 2 **3** 4 5

Grouse Lakes Loop Trail 273
The Grouse Lakes area is truly Sacramento's nearby "land-o-the-lakes." This long but rewarding loop hike will bring you within view of more than fifteen lakes of all sizes, and to the shores of seven of the lakes. The extensive trail system provides many options to explore this beautiful area by foot, bike, or horse. Whether you are looking to swim, stalk wily trout, or watch a sunset over an alpine lake, this is the place to be.

TRAIL 34

Hike, Bike, Horse
10 miles, Loop
Difficulty: 1 2 3 4 **5**

Picayune Valley Trail:
Granite Chief Wilderness 281
The grand scenery and solitude provided by this trail are worth the drive. Sharp peaks, granite ridges, and sheer cliffs dominate the glacially scoured Picayune Valley. Old-growth forests, lush meadows, and colorful aspens dot the valley floor, and the trail leads to a scenic cascade and an even more spectacular waterfall. This trail packs a lot of outstanding Sierra landscape into a relatively small area and a short hike.

TRAIL 35

Hike, Horse
8.7 miles, Out & Back
Difficulty: 1 2 3 **4** 5

TRAIL 36

Hike
4.7 miles, Out & Back
Difficulty: 1 2 **3** 4 5

Lake Margaret Trail:
Caples Creek Proposed Wilderness 287

Lake Margaret is tucked away in a heavily forested glaciated valley pocked with ponds and small lakes and studded with granite rock formations. Although a short hike from Hwy 88, this subalpine jewel provides surprising seclusion. Lake Margaret offers a great opportunity to set up a base camp and explore a virtually trail-less portion of the Caples Creek Proposed Wilderness.

TRAIL 37

Hike
7.0 miles, Loop
Difficulty: 1 2 3 **4** 5

Granite and Hidden Lakes Loop 293

This hike showcases two lakes—Granite and Hidden—that offer good destinations for a day hike or an easy overnight backpack trip. You can make it a loop hike and add some additional miles and a third and larger lake—Silver—to the tour. Campgrounds and three resorts around Silver Lake offer excellent base-camp opportunities to explore this scenic area adjacent to the Mokelumne Wilderness.

TRAIL 38

Hike, Run
3.2 miles, Out & Back
Difficulty: 1 **2** 3 4 5

Shealor Lake Trail:
Caples Creek Proposed Wilderness 301

The Shealor Lake Trail is easily accessible from Hwy 88 and it's a relatively easy walk for less-experienced hikers and families with children (age 10 or older). The trail provides wildly contrasting alpine scenery, including dark volcanic peaks and lighter-colored granite canyons. Pretty Shealor Lake is a great destination for a picnic, swim, or to simply lie on a warm granite rock and look at the clouds.

Winnemucca–Round Top Lakes Loop: Mokelumne Wilderness............ 307

This signature hike is beloved by Sacramentans for its spectacular alpine vistas, magnificent wildflowers, sparkling lakes, and outstanding fall color. The dark volcanic ridges and peaks provide a brooding backdrop to Winnemucca and Round Top lakes, two of the prettiest lakes in the northern Sierra. The volcanic soils also support an unusually rich wildflower display.

TRAIL 39
Hike
4.7 miles, Loop
Difficulty: 1 2 3 **4** 5

Caples Creek–Silver Fork Loop: Caples Creek Proposed Wilderness 313

This loop trail in the Caples Creek Proposed Wilderness provides access to scenic glaciated topography, old-growth forests, rugged river canyons, and sparkling cascades. The area's extensive trail system accesses many streamside and meadow campsites and provides plenty of opportunities for seclusion. It's a nice destination for a long day hike or an even better two- to three-day backpack trip.

TRAIL 40
Hike, Run, Bike, Horse
8.6 miles, Loop
Difficulty: 1 2 3 4 **5**

Horsetail Falls Trail.................. 321

When Sacramentans want to visit a lovely Sierra waterfall, all they have to do is drive up Hwy 50 and hike 1.5 miles to visit spectacular Horsetail Falls. Easily one of the top ten waterfalls in California, Horsetail competes with the falls of Yosemite Valley when it comes to scenic grandeur. Even if you don't make it all the way to the base of the falls, the cascades on lower Pyramid Creek make a good destination for a fine family outing.

TRAIL 41
Hike, Run, Bike
3.0 miles, Loop
Difficulty: 1 **2** 3 4 5

TRAIL 42

Hike
5.0 miles, Out & Back
Difficulty: 1 2 3 **4** 5

**Twin Lakes Trail:
Desolation Wilderness**............. 327

The relatively short but steep hike to Twin Lakes in the Desolation Wilderness is a classic alpine hike in the northern Sierra. The glaciated granite, sparse forest cover, cascading streams, and alpine lakes provide a true High Sierra feel minus about 2000 feet in elevation. The destination—Lower Twin Lake—provides a rewarding, if chilling swim.

TRAIL 43

Hike
10 miles, Out & Back
Difficulty: 1 2 3 4 **5**

**Lyons Creek Trail:
Desolation Wilderness**............. 333

Although many people focus on the ultimate destinations of this trail—Sylvia and Lyons lakes in the Desolation Wilderness—its real attractions are the beautiful waterfalls and wildflowers along the way. The trailside cascades and flower-spangled meadows make the Lyons Creek Trail one of the more beautiful routes into the Desolation Wilderness. It makes for a scenic, if long, day hike, or an ideal backpack trip.

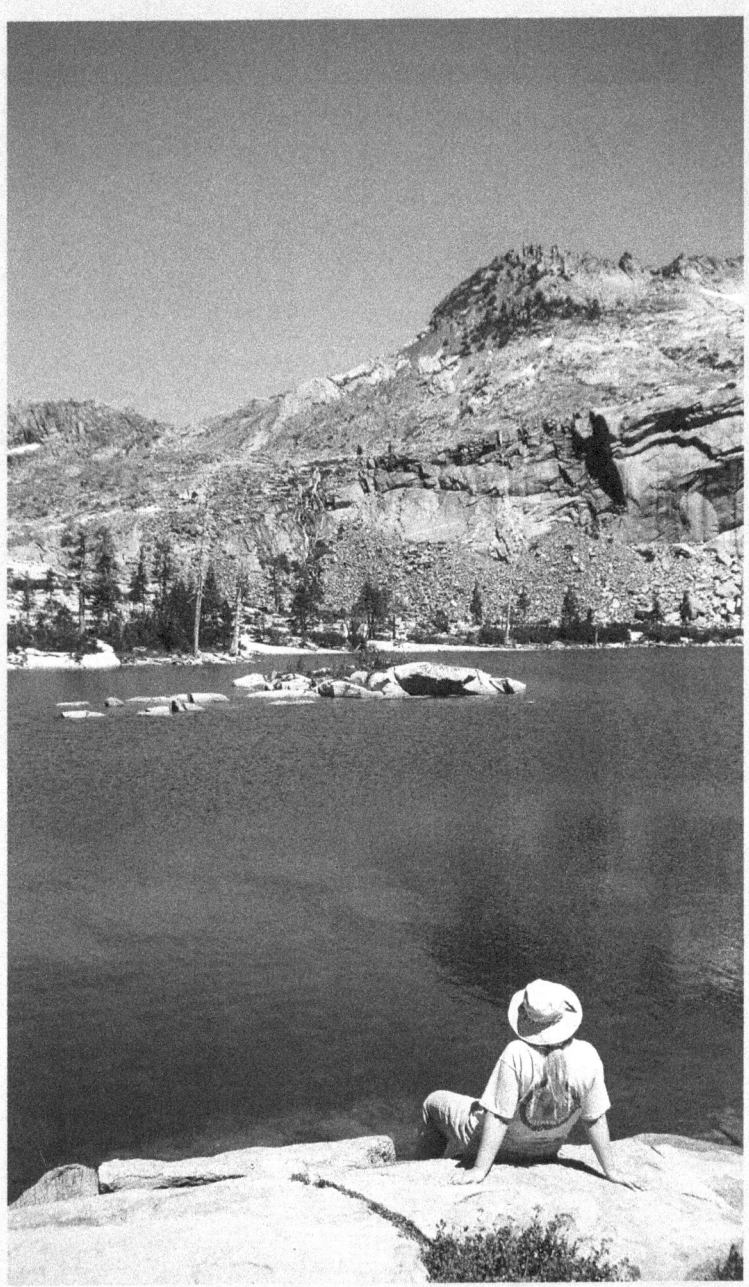

The reward at the end of steep Twin Lakes Trail *is beautiful lower Twin Lake.*

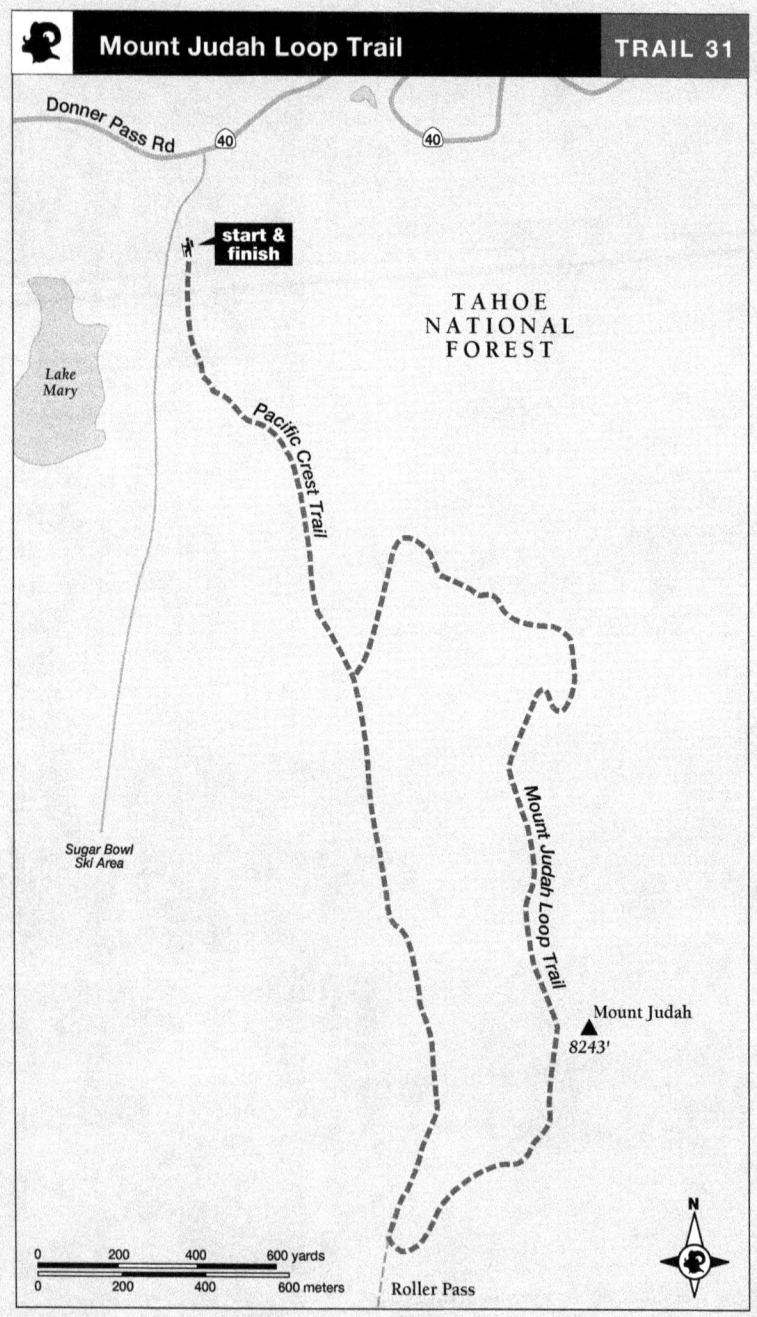

TRAIL 31 Sierra Nevada

Mount Judah Loop Trail

Following one of the more scenic segments of the Pacific Crest Trail (PCT) south from Donner Pass, this loop trail provides commanding views of the high peaks along the Sierra crest north of Lake Tahoe. It also offers an astounding alpine wildflower display during the mid-summer season and an opportunity to easily bag a Sierra peak. Along the way, you can get a rough idea of what early pioneers suffered as they hauled their wagons over the mountain range and of the historic effort of the railroad workers who forged a route across the crest. Unfortunately, this loop trail is something less than a wilderness experience due to both its popularity and its proximity to the nearby highway and adjacent ski areas, but the views and wildflowers more than make up for its lack of seclusion.

Best Time

The optimal visiting time is from mid-July to October. Some snow may linger in forested areas and along north-facing slopes through late July and early August.

Finding the Trail

From Sacramento, take Interstate 80 east 93 miles to the Soda Springs exit. Turn right on old Hwy 40 and drive 3.0 miles east to Donner Pass. Just past Donner Ski Ranch (on your left), turn right into the paved parking area and follow the narrow road 100 yards to the PCT trailhead. Depending on how early in the day it is, you can either park in the paved area

TRAIL USE
Hike
LENGTH
4.6 miles, 2–4 hours
VERTICAL FEET
±1155
DIFFICULTY
- 1 2 3 **4** 5 +
TRAIL TYPE
Loop
SURFACE TYPE
Dirt
Rock

FEATURES
Dogs Allowed
Meadow
Mountain
Wildflowers
Birds
Historic
Great Views
Photo Opportunity
Steep

FACILITIES
None

The trail crosses an open ski run, spangled in midsummer with paintbrush, arrowleaf groundsel, mule ears, corn lily, and pennyroyal.

marked PCT PARKING or park closer to the trailhead along the narrow road.

Logistics

Mountain bikes are prohibited on the PCT section of the loop. There is little or no water available along this trail, so bring plenty to drink.

Trail Description

From the trailhead, follow ▶1 the **Pacific Crest Trail** (PCT) south through a small grove of fir and lodgepole pines. Beyond the trailhead kiosk, the trail begins a steep but short climb, switchbacking five or six times up a talus and boulder slope. The tread on this section of the loop is rough, with large stones and a few rock steps. Almost immediately, you enjoy views of nearby **Lake Mary** directly below, with Summit Valley and the shallow wetland of former Lake Van Norden to the west. Toward the south, you will see the peaks that define the south rim of Summit Valley, including Mount Lincoln, Mount Disney, and the Crows Nest—all festooned with the runs and lifts of the Sugar Bowl ski area.

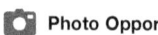
Photo Opportunity

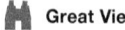
Great Views

Soon the trail moderates with a predominantly packed-dirt tread as it begins to traverse southward along the west slope of **Mount Judah**. The trail makes its way through a sparse grove of Jeffrey pines, negotiates two switchbacks to gain additional elevation, and enters a more verdant fir forest. After two more switchbacks, the trail crosses an open ski run.

Nearly a mile from the trailhead, your route reaches ▶2 the first loop junction, which leads upward to your left. Continue straight and to the south on the PCT, crossing a jeep trail, leaving the open ski run, snaking under a ski lift, and then continuing a gentle climb through the fir forest.

Mount Judah Loop Trail | TRAIL 31

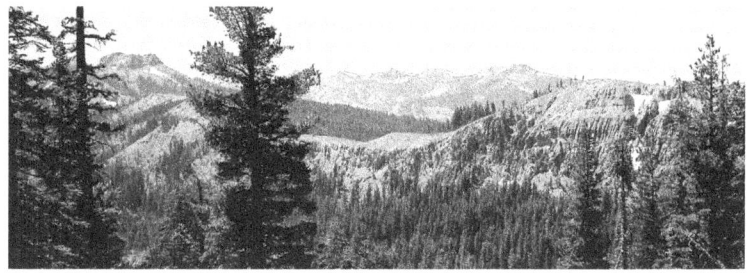

Looking south along the Sierra Crest *from the Pacific Crest Trail at historic Roller Pass*

Boulders from the ridge above appear to be a jumble of small rocks mixed in concrete. Known as breccia, these rocks provide a clue that you will soon be leaving the Sierra's granite pluton behind to discover a more recent volcanic overlay. The PCT passes a ski-lift station down the slope on your right, and continues to climb gently through red firs and small meadows providing splashes of wildflower color, including purple gentian and penstemon.

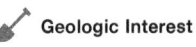 Geologic Interest

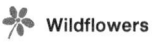 Wildflowers

About 1.8 miles from the trailhead, the PCT reaches the second loop junction, ▶3 which heads up the slope on your left. From this junction, it is worth continuing straight on the PCT about 300 yards farther south to visit **Roller Pass**. This is the saddle between **Coldstream Valley** to the east and Summit Valley to the west. It was once one of two passes used by the pioneers to cross the Sierra. Even though it was less steep and rocky than Donner Pass, directly to the north, Roller Pass was still steep enough to require the use of logs as rollers under the wagons, which were pulled up to the saddle with rope and tackle.

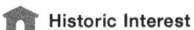 Historic Interest

After marveling at the effort it must have take to cross the mountain range in wagons, retrace your steps north back to the second junction and take your leave of the PCT by turning right on the **Mount Judah Loop Trail**. The trail heads upslope in a northeasterly direction toward Mount Judah. The ascent soon steepens, and the predominantly

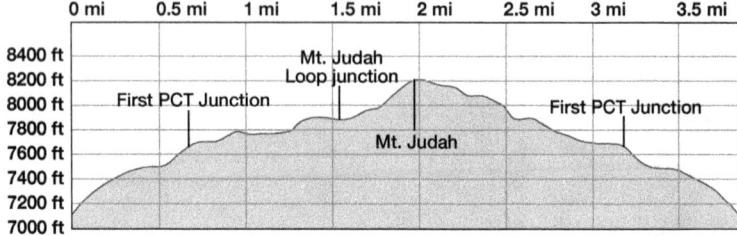

TRAIL 31   Mount Judah Loop Trail Profile

Great Views

fir forest begins to give way to higher altitude-loving hemlocks. The trail then switchbacks across the nose of the ridge and breaks out above tree line. Here is the first unobstructed view south of a scenic phalanx of peaks along the Sierra crest, including nearby Mount Lincoln (capped with a ski lift), Anderson Peak, Tinker Knob, Lyon Peak, Needle Peak, and 9083-foot-high Granite Chief. The trail continues its climb past outcrops of breccia lava flow and open talus slopes covered with mule ears, phlox, and other flowers that tax rudimentary botanical skills.

Summit

About 2.3 miles from the trailhead, ▶4 you reach the 8243-foot-high summit of **Mount Judah**. The mountain was named after Theodore Judah, the architect and promoter of the Central Pacific Railroad. It was his chosen route that led the railroad over (and under) Donner Pass. Ironically, he died before the first rail was laid down, but the adjacent peak now bears his name.

Great Views

From the top of Mount Judah, the view expands to the east to include Donner Lake, the town of Truckee, and the ski-run-scarred slopes of Lookout Mountain, and northward to the brooding chocolate brown battlements of Castle Peak. If you are lucky, you may see a goshawk swoop by. Sit on a boulder, eat lunch, and enjoy the view.

From its high point, the trail leads directly north down to a saddle between Mount Judah's north summit and its slightly lower south summit.

Mount Judah Loop Trail — TRAIL 31

A short trail leads up to the south summit, but the loop trail drops down from the saddle and begins to traverse northward along the eastern slope of the mountain. Your route quickly drops below the tree line, entering a mixed forest of hemlock and fir. The wildflower display continues, with phlox, forget-me-nots, and other colorful flowers lining the trail. Snow patches may linger on this section of the trail well into late July and even early August. A couple of switchbacks drop the trail down to a saddle between Mount Judah's south summit and **Donner Peak** just to the north. For those tempted to bag another peak, it looks like a short and easy scramble nearly to the top of Donner Peak, but the peak's perpendicular summit blocks require class 3 rock-climbing skills.

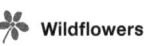
Wildflowers

At the saddle, the loop trail merges with an old jeep route that climbs up from Summit Valley and heads down into Coldstream Canyon. ▶5 Turn left onto the jeep trail and head southwest back toward the PCT. The trail drops down below a seeping slope that supports a veritable garden of lupine, paintbrush, wandering daisy, cow's parsnip, horse mint, and groundsel. Shortly, the loop trail leaves the jeep route by turning right and dropping down to the first junction with the PCT (Milestone 2). ▶6 Turn right at this junction and ▶7 retrace your steps along the PCT to the trailhead.

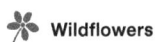
Wildflowers

🚶 MILESTONES

▶1	0.0	Start at PCT trailhead
▶2	0.9	First loop junction, continue straight on PCT
▶3	1.8	Leave PCT, turn left on second loop junction
▶4	2.3	Top of Mount Judah
▶5	3.1	Turn left on old jeep route
▶6	3.7	Turn right onto PCT
▶7	4.6	Return to trailhead parking area

PCT: Castle Peak Area

TRAIL 32

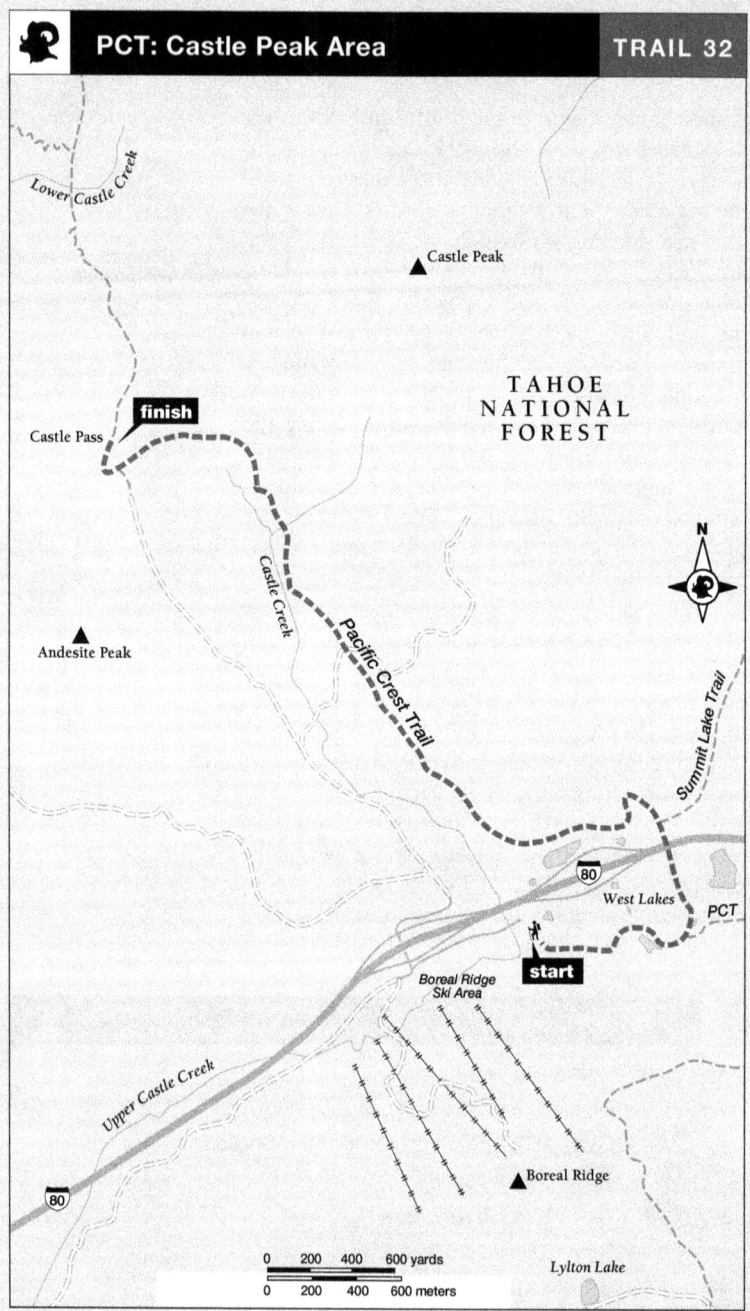

TRAIL 32 Sierra Nevada

Pacific Crest Trail: Castle Peak Area

A favorite of Sacramentans desiring a taste of the high country, this popular hike offers incredible alpine vistas and a great summer wildflower display. It also provides access to the proposed Castle Peak Wilderness, a long-time protection priority for conservationists. Along the way, you get an introduction to the Sierra's diverse glacial and volcanic geology, walk through culverts under Interstate 80, and may be tempted to "bag" 9103-foot Castle Peak. Despite climbing 700 feet, this is a well-graded and moderate section of the Pacific Crest Trail. This area is also a popular winter destination for cross-country skiers and snowshoers.

TRAIL USE
Hike
LENGTH
6.72 miles, 3–5 hours
VERTICAL FEET
±700
DIFFICULTY
- 1 2 3 **4** 5 +
TRAIL TYPE
Out & Back
SURFACE TYPE
Dirt

FEATURES
Dogs Allowed
Meadow
Mountain
Stream
Wildflowers
Fall Color
Camping
Geology
Interpretive
Great Views
Steep

FACILITIES
Restrooms
Picnic Tables
Seasonal Water

Best Time

Depending upon the snow pack, this trail is accessible from July through October. Late July through August is the best time to enjoy alpine wildflowers.

Finding the Trail

From Sacramento, drive 96 miles east on Interstate 80 to the Castle Peak–Boreal exit. Take the exit and continue east 0.4 mile on the frontage road past the Boreal ski area to the Boreal–Pacific Crest Trail parking area and PCT trailhead.

Logistics

This is an introductory day hike to the beautiful Castle Peak area. Those who want a more challenging trip can proceed from Castle Pass to climb

Castle Peak and its namesake volcanic ramparts are visible as you work your way past glaciated granite bedrock.

another 1.5 miles and 1200 feet to reach Castle Peak. Or they can continue a bit over a mile or so on the PCT to visit Round Valley and the Sierra Club's Peter Grubb Hut. There are suitable camping spots in upper Castle Valley and Round Valley.

Trail Description

From the parking area, ▶1 go east on the connector trail to the Pacific Crest Trail (PCT) through lodgepole pines and white firs, over a bridge spanning a seasonal creek.

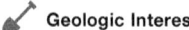 Meadow

A short distance from the trailhead is the first of two junctions for the **Glacier Meadow Interpretive Loop Trail**, which circles north through the forest, connects with the CalTrans rest stop on I-80, and then circles back to your trail. There are a number of interpretive signs along the loop concerning the role of glaciers in Sierra Nevada geography. You may want to take this loop at the beginning of your hike, which will add about a bit less than 0.33 mile to your overall trip. If you don't, ▶2 veer right to continue on the PCT connector trail and you will come shortly to the second junction with the Glacier Meadow Loop. ▶3 Veer right again, and continue east on the PCT connector trail past a large pond on the right

Geologic Interest

The connector trail meets the **Pacific Crest Trail** proper at the edge of a brushy meadow. ▶4 Turn left and walk north along the meadow's edge, which follows the foot of a low ridge that just might be the remains of glacial moraine. Soon, traffic noise heralds the first of two large culverts that allow the PCT to pass under I-80.

Climbing up a seasonally flowing gully from the trail underpass, you come to a signed four-way junction. The trail to the right leads to Summit Lake. The trail to the left goes to the CalTrans rest area on the north side of the freeway. ▶5 Proceed straight on the

Pacific Crest Trail | TRAIL 32

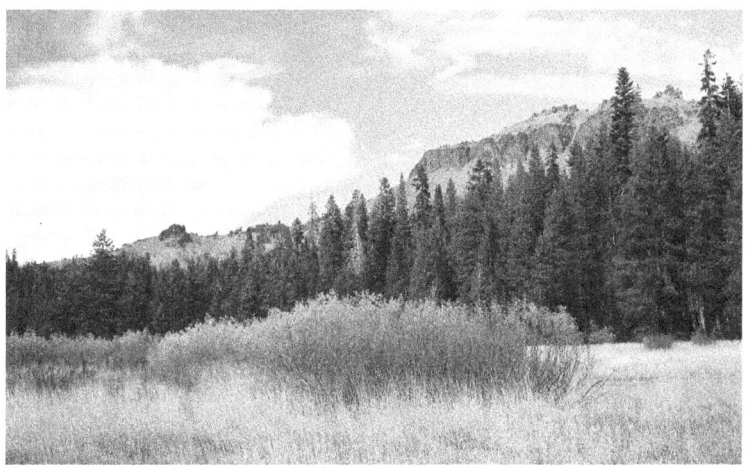

Castle Valley meadows *are dominated by the ramparts of Castle Peak.*

PCT as it bends westward over the moraine that you paralleled on the other side of the freeway. The trail climbs over the moraine through fir forest punctuated by occasional clumps of aspens. Soon, you will see a small pond and the CalTrans rest stop on your left. A use-trail veers left to the rest stop, but the PCT continues straight west and then bends northwest as it gently climbs over the low ridge forming the eastern boundary of **Castle Valley**.

The trail descends nearly to the bank of upper **Castle Creek** and then proceeds northwestward through forest above the valley's open meadow. Views of the scenic meadow and its sinuous creek may to tempt you to utilize a couple of use-trails that lead down through the trees to the left to access the valley floor, which may be seasonally spangled with wildflowers. Excellent campsites are found at the meadow's edge in the upper portion of Castle Valley.

More than 2.0 miles from the trailhead, the PCT crosses an old jeep trail climbing up from Castle Valley. ▶6 Continue straight as the PCT begins

Stream

Great Views

Camping

Sierra Nevada 261

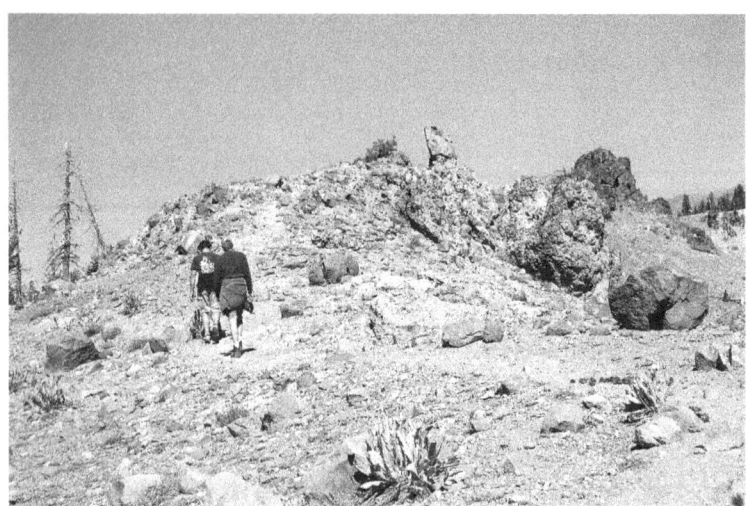

A spur trail leads from the Pacific Crest Trail at Castle Pass to the top of Castle Peak.

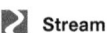
Stream

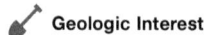
Geologic Interest

a steeper but still well-graded ascent. Soon, the trail crosses one flowing stream and several seeps that feed into Castle Creek. The trail continues to climb moderately through thick forest and bends westward. The geology along the trail changes from traditional Sierra granitics to andesitic volcanics. Views from the trail are dominated by Castle Peak's dark ramparts, upslope to the right.

About 3.75 miles from the trailhead, the PCT connects with the end of the **Castle Pass truck road**, used by less-active folk to drive up from

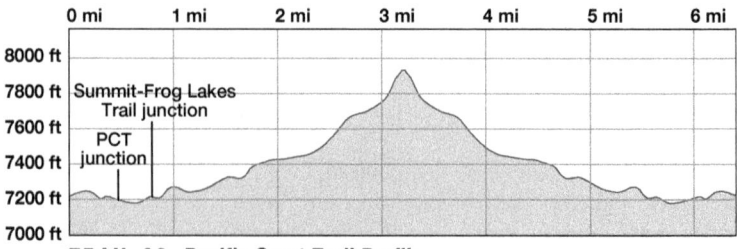

TRAIL 32 **Pacific Crest Trail Profile**

Pacific Crest Trail | TRAIL **32**

Castle Valley. ▶7 Turn right, and a short ascent brings you nearly above the tree line at ▶8 lovely Castle Pass. Above and to your right is the ridge and the spur trail leading 1.5 miles to the top of Castle Peak. Andesite Peak can be seen to your left. The view north of the pass is of scenic Round Valley. Far on the northern horizon, on a clear day, you may be able to see Mount Lassen. Sit down on a volcanic rock, eat your lunch, and enjoy the view.

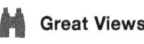 **Great Views**

▶9 Retrace your steps to the trailhead.

MILESTONES

▶1	0.00	Boreal/PCT trailhead.
▶2	0.20	First Glacier Meadow Loop junction, veer right to stay on the PCT
▶3	0.30	Second Glacier Meadow Loop junction, veer right to stay on the PCT
▶4	0.58	Pacific Crest Trail junction, turn left to go north
▶5	1.00	Four-way trail junction, go straight to follow PCT
▶6	2.20	Cross jeep trail, continue straight on PCT
▶7	3.32	Junction with Castle Pass truck road, turn right to follow PCT
▶8	3.36	Castle Pass
▶9	6.72	Retrace steps back to Boreal/PCT trailhead

Salmon Lake Trail – Loch Leven Lakes TRAIL 33

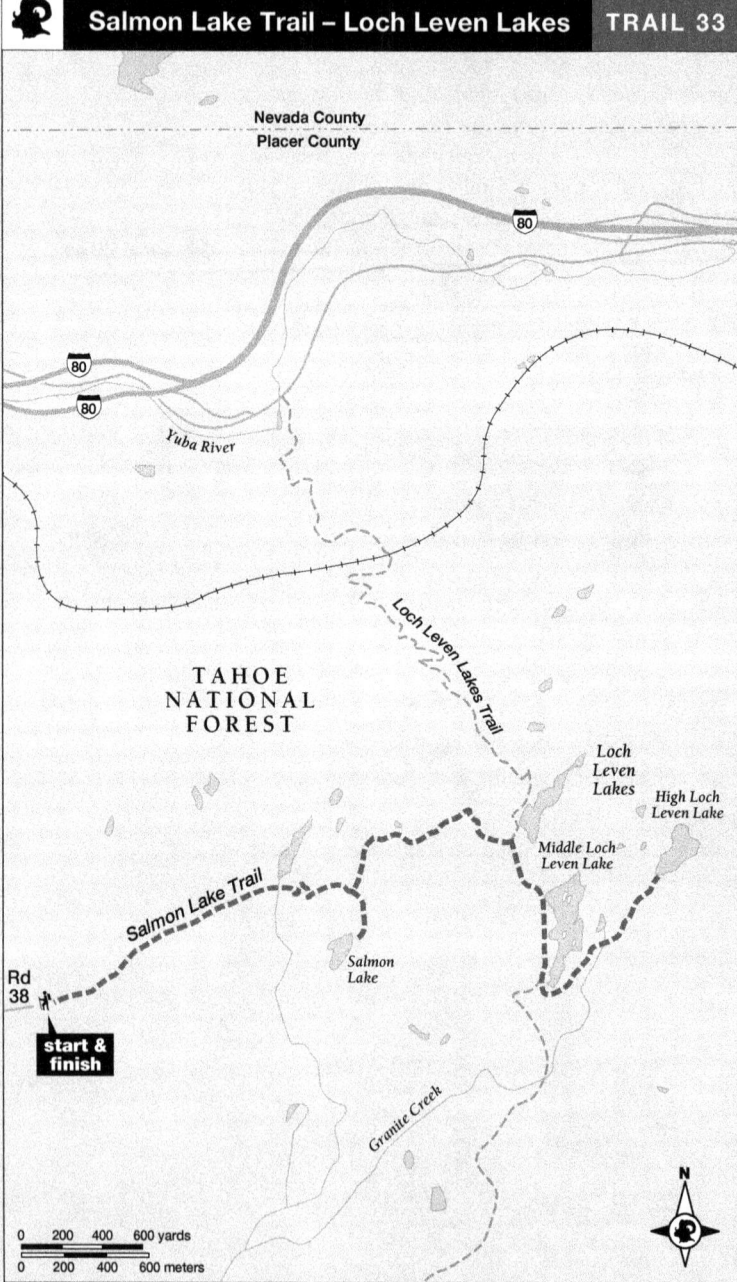

TRAIL 33 Sierra Nevada

Salmon Lake Trail to Loch Leven Lakes

The hike to Loch Leven Lakes is probably the most beloved of the high mountain trails visited by Sacramentans. This easy day trip is a quick drive up I-80 from the state's capital and offers outstanding alpine scenery. The only drawback is that the traditional route to Loch Leven lakes requires you to slog up a 1000-foot-high ridge across railroad tracks, all the while accompanied by the sound of I-80 traffic and trains. But the "back" way into Loch Leven Lakes, via the Salmon Lake Trail, avoids most of the climb, all of the noise, and visits more lakes. All that is required is some patience driving on a relatively well-maintained dirt road. What's not to like?

TRAIL USE
Hike
LENGTH
5.0 miles, 3–4 hours
VERTICAL FEET
±275
DIFFICULTY
- 1 2 **3** 4 5 +
TRAIL TYPE
Out & Back
SURFACE TYPE
Dirt
Rock

Best Time

The lakes are between 6700 and 7000 feet in elevation and therefore are typically snowed in until late June or July, depending on the previous winter's snowfall. The hiking season lasts through October. The one drawback to using the Salmon Lake Trail is that although one can slog through snow if climbing up to Loch Leven Lakes using the traditional route, it's best to wait until the snow is fully melted before driving the seldom-plowed back road to the Salmon Lake Trailhead.

FEATURES
Dogs Allowed
Lakes
Camping
Great Views
Photo Opportunity

FACILITIES
None

Finding the Trail

Drive east on Interstate 80 about 73 miles to the Yuba Gap exit. Turn right on Yuba Gap Road, drive 0.2 mile, and turn right on Long Valley Road (a sign says LAKE VALLEY RESERVOIR, LODGEPOLE

A large granite rock jutting out into High Loch Leven Lake makes an excellent lunch spot.

CAMPGROUND—1.8, SILVER TIP PICNIC AREA—2.0). Drive 1.3 miles and turn left on Road 19 (also known as Mears Meadow Road). Drive 4.0 miles (past the right turn to the Silver Tip Picnic Area) and turn left on Road 38 (a sign says HUYSINK LAKE—1.0, SALMON LAKE TRAIL—2.0). Drive 2.0 miles past Huysink Lake to the Salmon Lake Trailhead. Look for the trailhead sign on the left of the road. Just past the trailhead, there are parking areas to the right and left of the road. You leave pavement once you turn on Road 19. The surface is rocky but negotiable by highway vehicles (good tires are recommended).

Logistics

If your hiking group has another car, you can leave a car at the traditional Loch Leven Lakes trailhead near the Big Bend visitors center, hike in on the Salmon Lake Trail, and hike down to the Big Bend Trailhead. To find this trailhead, take the Big Bend exit off Interstate 80. Turn right and drive approximately 0.3 mile to the Loch Leven Lakes Trailhead parking area on the left side of the road. The trail starts across the road from the parking area. Camping is permitted at Salmon Lake and all the Loch Leven Lakes, but this is a heavily used area so don't expect to have it all to yourself. Please take care to camp more than 100 feet from the lakes and all other water sources.

Trail Description

From the trailhead at about 6600 feet in elevation, ▶1 the **Salmon Lakes Trail** makes its way northeastward through a small willow thicket and edges around a meadow. It then begins a moderate 200-foot climb up a ridge through an old-growth red fir forest. When it tops the ridge, the environment becomes drier and the forest diversifies with Jeffrey

Salmon Lake Trail to Loch Leven Lakes | TRAIL 33

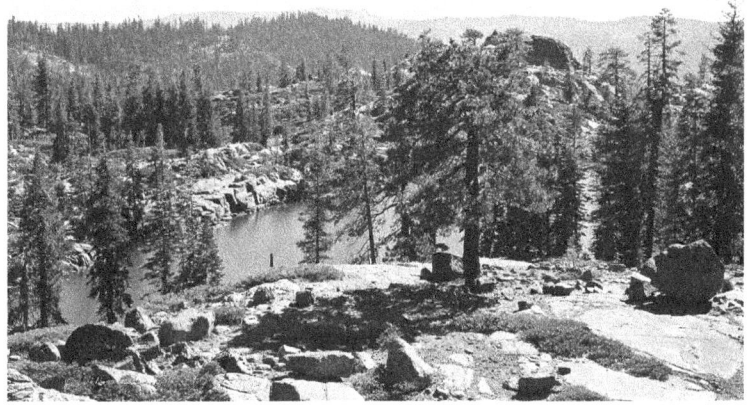

Salmon Lake *as viewed from its namesake trail on the way to lower Loch Leven Lake*

pines and lodgepole pines. The trail drops down from the ridge and into rolling country broken by granite outcrops and an open forest with an understory of ceanothus, pinemat manzanita, and lush fern gardens.

The trail crosses the outlet of a finger-shaped shallow lake on your left. Lily pads suggest that this may be excellent habitat for the elusive and endangered mountain yellow-legged frog. Then the trail drops down into a shallow gully, and the formerly dirt tread of the trail becomes rocky. It then climbs a couple of short switchbacks out of the gully and over a low ridge. Here it leaves the forest for an open expanse of glaciated granite slabs with a scattering of glacial erratics (large boulders left by the glacier). The open area provides expansive views south to the North Fork American River canyon. To the southeast is the granite knob of Cherry Point, and beyond is the dark and rugged façade of Snow Mountain. Walk about 100 feet south off the trail

 Lake

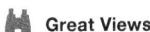 Great Views

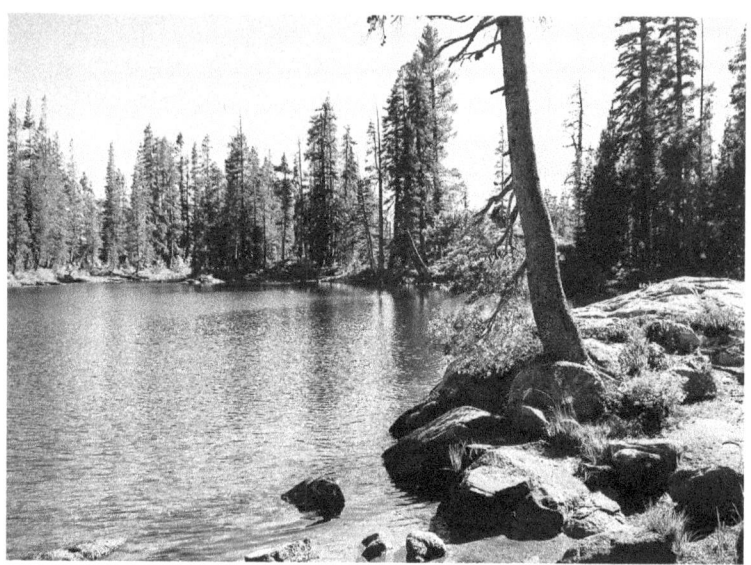

Lower Loch Leven Lake

and you will also get a good view of Salmon Lake just below the ridge.

Return to the trail, which continues east as it drops down over granite shelves and through copses of fir and lodgepole to the **Salmon Lake Spur Trail**. A sign indicates that Salmon Lake is 0.25 mile to the right and **Loch Leven Lake** is 1.0 mile to the left. ▶2 Turn right to make your way 0.3 mile (according to the topo map program) to ▶3 **Salmon Lake**.

The spur trail climbs briefly to a saddle between two large granite outcrops and then drops gently down through a draw. It then proceeds through a stand of lodgepole pines to Salmon Lake at about 6700 feet in elevation. You may find catfish gliding languidly through the shallows of small but pretty Salmon Lake, which has several large flat rocks suitable for sunning. There is an open flat area east of the lodgepole pines suitable for camping. Once surfeited with Salmon Lake, retrace your steps to the

 Lake

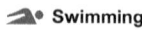 **Swimming**

Camping

Salmon Lake Trail to Loch Leven Lakes TRAIL 33

Salmon Lake Trail junction and ▶4 veer right toward **Loch Leven Lakes**.

The trail continues northeast along and over a series of spur ridges that break off from the Yuba/American divide just to the north. It briefly parallels a low ridge on your right and then makes its way over rolling ground until climbing 100 feet over another low ridge heralded by large granite slabs. The usual ducks and lines of rocks mark your route over the slabs as the trail climbs moderately upward and then drops down to enter a fir forest with a scattering of giant Jeffrey pines.

Traversing the south-facing slope of a ridge, the trail makes its way through firs and Jeffreys and across a small stringer meadow. It easily climbs 100 feet again to top the ridge. As the trail begins to drop downward, you get glimpses of **Lower Loch Leven Lake** through the trees. After two short switchbacks downward, the Salmon Lake Trail meets its junction with the Loch Leven Lakes Trail on the shores of Lower Loch Leven Lake.

 Lake

Lower Loch Leven Lake offers good swimming and is popular for fishing. There are a handful of illegal (closer than 100 feet from the water) campsites to the north and west of the lake. The lower lake is the one that everyone visits (since it's 2.7 miles from the Loch Leven Lakes Trailhead near Big Bend and only 1.7 miles from the Salmon Lake Trailhead), so if you are looking for a bit more solitude or just need to stretch your legs a bit farther, ▶5 turn right on the **Loch Leven Lakes Trail** and head south.

Swimming

A sign says MIDDLE LOCH LEVEN LAKE 0.25, CHERRY POINT TRAIL—0.5, HIGH LOCH LEVEN LAKE—1.0. As you make your way south of the lower lake, you pass a legal campsite with a fire ring. The trail drops down a short and steep rocky draw, levels out, and then climbs gently over a rise to drop down to scenic **Middle Loch Leven Lake**. The middle lake's numerous rocky coves and three small wooded

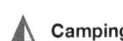 Camping

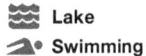 Lake
Swimming

Sierra Nevada   269

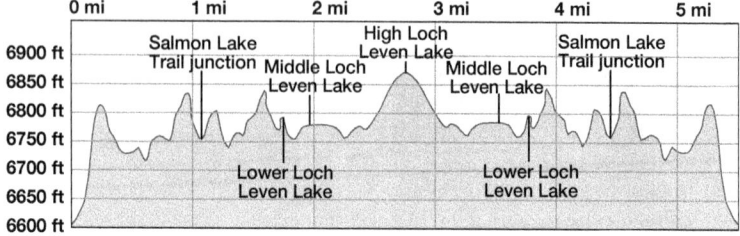

TRAIL 33 Salmon Lake Trail to Loch Leven Lakes Profile

islands, all backdropped by a low granite ridge, make it the prettiest of the Loch Leven chain.

The trail proceeds past an illegal campsite and then parallels the west side of the middle lake, past a flat area just beyond the regulation 100-foot limit. The trail continues south. Every time you think you've left Middle Loch Leven Lake behind, the trail reaches yet another cove of the lake—and it gets prettier as you go south. At the very southern end of the middle lake, the Loch Leven Lakes Trail reaches a junction with the **Cherry Point Trail**, which heads off to the right. ▶6 Veer left to continue on the Loch Leven Lakes Trail to the third lake in the chain.

The trail circles the south end of the middle lake and crosses an open granite bench dominated by a view of Snow Mountain. The trail may be indistinct as it crosses the open granite slabs, depending on the status of ducks and rock lines, but it tends east/northeast across the usually dry and shallow outlet of the middle lake and into a rocky and wooded draw. The trail then veers to the north and proceeds up the draw on its west side, crosses through a stand of lodgepole pines on the right, and then continues up the draw on its east side.

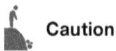 Caution

The trail climbs out of the draw and continues steeply uphill through two short switchbacks over high granite shelves requiring care in foot placement. This is by far the roughest section of the entire

Salmon Lake Trail to Loch Leven Lakes | TRAIL 33

trail. The climb lessens as it enters a stand of firs. To the left, you glimpse a small, unnamed lake through the trees. A little farther up the trail, Middle Loch Leven Lake reappears about 100 feet below and to your left, at the foot of the granite ridge you are ascending.

Gently climbing north/northeast through stands of firs and lodgepoles, the trail crosses the now ubiquitous granite slabs and then reaches the top of a low rise, which creates the south shore of ▶7 **High Loch Leven Lake**. Suitable campsites are found along the southeast side of the lake. If you are up for a short cross-country scramble across broken granite and through low chaparral, a rocky **butte** north of the lake promises an outstanding view of the entire Loch Leven Lakes chain.

Retrace your steps to ▶8 the Salmon Lake Trailhead.

≋ Lake
▲ Camping
≈ Swimming
🔭 Great Views

MILESTONES

▶1	0.00	Salmon Lake Trailhead
▶2	0.60	Junction with Salmon Lake Spur Trail, turn right
▶3	0.90	Salmon Lake, then retrace steps to Salmon Lake Trail
▶4	1.20	Veer right to continue on Salmon Lake Trail
▶5	1.80	Junction with Loch Leven Lakes Trail, turn right
▶6	2.30	Junction with Cherry Point Trail, turn left
▶7	2.80	High Loch Leven Lake
▶8	5.00	Retrace steps to Salmon Lake Trailhead

Grouse Lakes Loop Trail

TRAIL 34

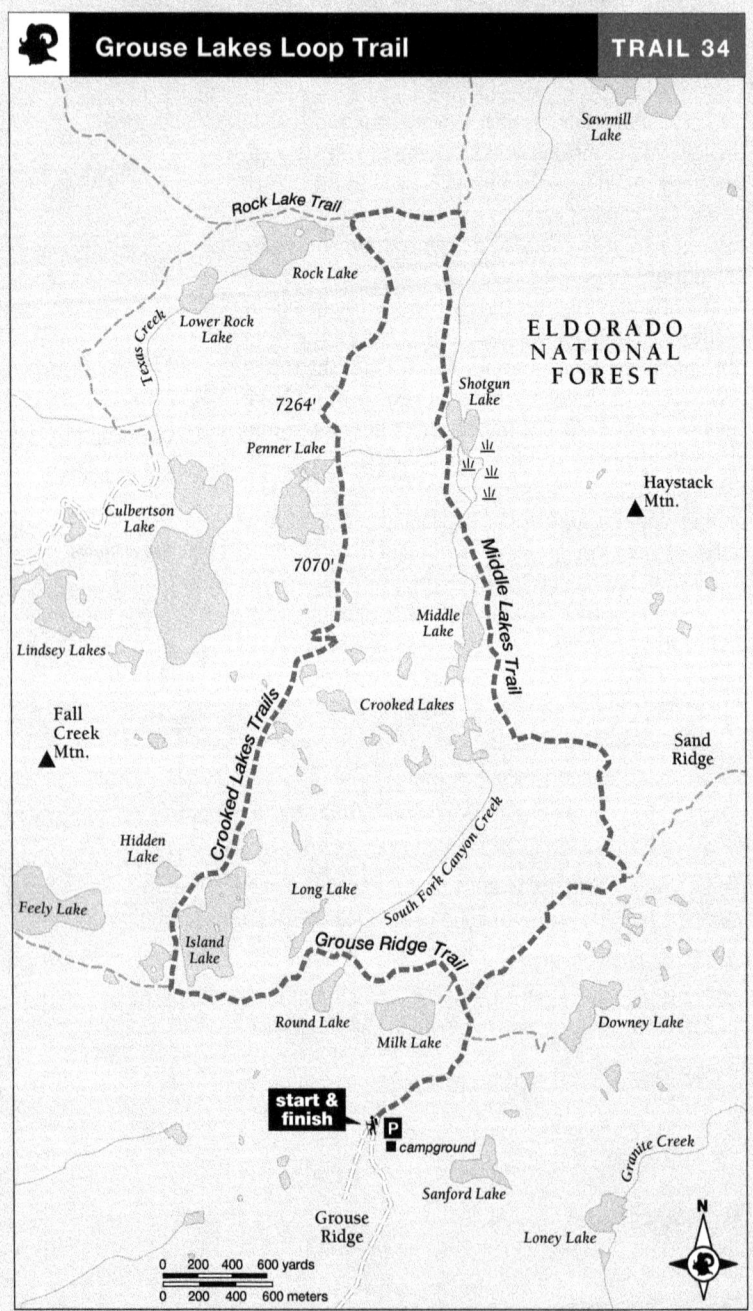

TRAIL 34 Sierra Nevada

Grouse Lakes Loop Trail

The Grouse Lakes area is truly Sacramento's "land-o-the-lakes." This long but rewarding loop hike will bring you within view of more than fifteen lakes of all sizes, and to the shores of seven of the lakes. Whether you are to swim, stalk wily trout, or watch a sunset over an alpine lake, this is the place to be. Despite its long history of public use, much of the area is privately owned, so please respect property rights. The old network of jeep roads that formerly connected the lakes has been closed to motor vehicle use, creating a wonderful area to explore by foot, bike, or horse.

TRAIL USE
Hike, Bike, Horse
LENGTH
10.1 miles, 6–7 hours
VERTICAL FEET
±1125
DIFFICULTY
- 1 2 3 4 **5** +
TRAIL TYPE
Loop
SURFACE TYPE
Dirt
Rock

Best Time

At 7500 feet, the trailhead and its access road can be snowed in well into late June or early July some years. The typical hiking season is July–October.

Finding the Trail

From Sacramento, take Interstate 80 east past Auburn, Colfax, and Dutch Flat. Take the Hwy 20 exit, turn right and go under the freeway and drive 5.5 miles west on Hwy 20. Turn right on Bowman Road. Drive north on Bowman Road. Turn right on Grouse Ridge Road. Drive east and north on Grouse Ridge Road as it slowly climbs Grouse Ridge. About 0.2 mile past the Grouse Ridge Campground, the road makes a sharp left curve to head up to the Grouse Ridge Lookout. Turn right at the curve and park at the Grouse Ridge Trailhead parking area.

FEATURES
Dogs Allowed
Lakes
Mountain
Canyon
Meadow
Stream
Waterfall
Wildflowers
Camping
Great Views

FACILITIES
Vault Toilets

Logistics

The northern cove of Penner Lake becomes a separate lake in the low-water months of fall.

The scenic Grouse Ridge Campground makes an excellent base camp for day hikes to explore the Grouse Lakes area. If the Grouse Ridge Road and trailhead is still snowed in, you might want to continue north on Bowman Road, past the Grouse Ridge Road turnoff, to the Carr–Lindsey Lakes Road. Turn right on Carr–Lindsey Lakes Road and drive northeast to the Carr Lake turnoff. Turn right and proceed to the parking area on the northern end of Carr Lake. From there, you can walk along the road, past the closed Carr Lake Campground to Trail 13E13, which takes you past Feeley Lake to the junction with Trail 12E11, with Island Lake just beyond. The Carr Lake Road and trailhead are about 1000 feet lower in elevation than the Grouse Ridge Trailhead, so they can be accessible a few weeks earlier than Grouse Ridge.

Trail Description

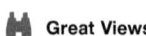 **Great Views**

From the parking area, ▶1 enjoy the view of the **Grouse Lakes basin**, with lakes peeking through the forests or standing exposed in barren, rocky areas. Rugged Fall Creek Mountain to the northwest, Bowman Mountain beyond, Old English Mountain to the north, and rounded Haystack Mountain to the northeast define the basin's perimeter. A sign at the trailhead says MIDDLE LAKE—2.0, SAWMILL LAKE—5.0, GLACIER LAKE—5.0.

The **Grouse Ridge Trail** drops down the trailhead on the ridge and follows an old jeep route. Almost immediately, you come to an unsigned trail junction on the right that leads to the Grouse Ridge Campground. Continue left as the trail drops past an old truck carcass and then enters scattered lodgepole pines and red fir. Looking off the ridge to your right, you have good view of pretty-as-a-picture

Grouse Lakes Loop Trail | TRAIL **34**

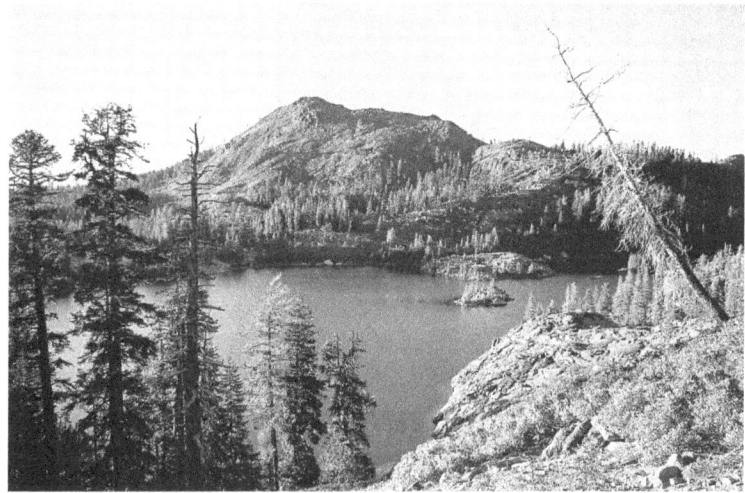

Fall Creek Mountain and Island Lake *comprise just one of the spectacular views from the Grouse Lake Loop Trail.*

Sanford Lake. To your left, you see **Milk Lake**, one of the first lakes to visit on the loop hike.

After about 0.5 mile, you come to another unsigned trail junction that leads over the low ridge on your right to **Downey Lake**. Continue straight on the Grouse Ridge Trail.

Shortly after the Downey Lake trail junction, you reach a junction with Trail 13E13 (Sand Ridge Trail). ▶2 Turn left to proceed to Milk Lake. The trail continues downward but now in a westerly direction through firs. It then levels out on well-packed dirt tread and within less than 0.5 mile, comes to the Milk Lake Spur Trail on the left. It is well worth the short walk over the low ridge down to scenic Milk Lake, which is a great day destination for less ambitious hikers.

From the Milk Lake junction, continue west on Trail 13E13 as it continues in a downward trend and crosses the outlet stream from **Round Lake**. This is actually the **South Fork Canyon Creek**, which you

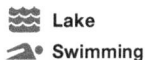

Lake
Swimming

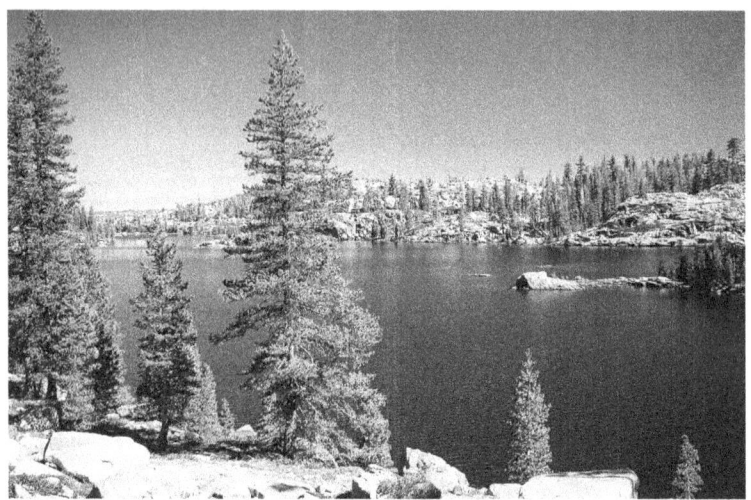

The many coves and rocks of Island Lake *invite swimming.*

will visit later on in the loop. A short spur trail also leads to Round Lake. After crossing the South Fork Canyon Creek, the trail begins climbing a ridge that separates Milk, Round, and Long lakes from **Island Lake**. As the trail tops this glaciated ridge, you will see below you Island Lake with its inviting coves and islands.

The trail passes Island Lake to the south and comes to the junction with Trail 12E11 (Crooked lakes Trail). A sign says PENNER LAKE—2.0. ▶3 Turn right on this trail and hike north past a shallow unnamed lake on your left, to the west shore of Island Lake. A favorite swimming destination for many, Island Lake is big on scenery but short on solitude. There is a suitable campsite on the granite slabs overlooking the western shore of Island Lake but camping here should be avoided since this is private land.

Continue north on the trail through lodgepoles, firs, and bracken ferns, and you soon come to the first of many ponds and small lakes that make up

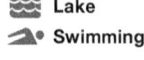
Lake
Swimming

the **Crooked Lakes** chain. As the trail tops a small rock outcrop, you get a view of most of the chain, with Sand Ridge in the background and the brooding fastness of the Black Buttes beyond. The trail proceeds in a northwesterly direction past another small lake (which makes a perfect playpen for an otter) and then ascends a nondescript ridge. A couple of switchbacks through manzanita and Jeffrey pines lead to a bench as the trail traverses past modest peak 7073 on your right. A little farther north and you'll come to the colorful rocky basin that holds scenic **Penner Lake**.

The trail drops down to the east side of the lake, but you may not be able to resist the urge to explore the rocky shelves overlooking the lake's south end. Penner Lake is set in a saddle between two unnamed peaks (7070 to the south and peak 7264 to the north). The dark metamorphic rocks that dominate most of the Grouse Lakes basin changes to pinkish red-and-white rocks around Penner Lake, adding to the lake's spectacular scenery. There are suitable if exposed campsites on the lake's east shore promontory, on the rock benches south of the lake, and some less suitable campsites that may not be beyond the 100-foot no-camping limit. Both potential camping areas are on public land. As the trail continues north, you reach the northern cove of Penner Lake.

 Lake

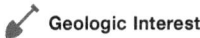 Geologic Interest

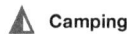 Camping

The trail crosses Penner Lake's outlet stream and then begins to climb peak 7264. A sign says CROOKED LAKES TRAIL. After a short 200-foot climb, the trail reaches a saddle and then drops down toward **Rock Lake**. Although now closed to motor vehicles, this section of trail retains its jeep route roots and drops steeply downward until it levels out in the flats north of Rock Lake, which can be seen through the trees.

The trail reaches the junction with Trail 12E12 (Rock Lake Trail). A sign says SAWMILL LAKE—1.5,

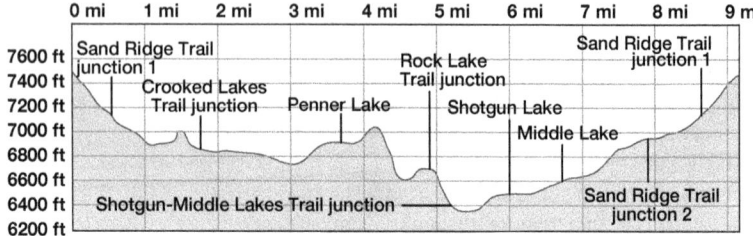

TRAIL 34 Grouse Lake Loop Trail Profile

PENNER LAKE—1.0, LINDSEY LAKE—3.0. ▶4 Turn right, in the direction indicated for **Sawmill Lake**. The trail heads east and drops down a thickly forested slope.

After losing nearly 400 feet in elevation, your pathway reaches the junction with Trail 13E28 (Shotgun/Middle Lakes Trail). At about 6375 feet in elevation, you are at the lowest point in the loop, and it will be all uphill from this point. There are several signs at the junction, but the one pertinent to your itinerary says MIDDLE LAKE—2.0, GROUSE RIDGE—4.0. ▶5 Turn right and head south.

Trail 13E28 climbs gently southward through forest that thins out as the trail approaches the rocky gorge of the South Fork Canyon Creek. The trail parallels this dark rocky gorge for nearly 0.5 mile. Early season hikers are treated to views of its many cascades, but this portion of the South Fork is all but dry come fall. After re-entering the forest, the trail comes to large but shallow **Shotgun Lake**. Much of the lake's southern shore is a large meadow with buggy but otherwise ideal campsites—but these too are on private land.

Following the now more-placid South Fork as it meanders it way through a series of stringer meadows, the trail pushes southward through more lodgepoles and firs. Your route crosses the shallow South Fork and continues south while climbing gently. A solid stand of lodgepoles blocks the view of

Stream

Waterfall

Meadow

Grouse Lakes Loop Trail | TRAIL **34**

shallow **Middle Lake**, but its presence is announced by a simple trailside sign. From here the trail begins climbing in earnest, 400 feet up to the base of **Sand Ridge**.

The trail comes to the junction with Trail 13E13 (Sand Ridge Trail). A sign says CARR LAKE—3, GROUSE RIDGE—2. ▶6 Turn right and proceed in a southwesterly direction as the trail begins climbing up toward the foot of **Grouse Ridge**.

Another 250-foot elevation gain over about 0.8 mile brings you to the junction with the Grouse Ridge Trail, ▶7 and to the right, the trail that leads to Milk, Round, and Island Lakes. Proceed straight to climb the 300 feet up the ridge ▶8 back to the trailhead.

MILESTONES

- ▶1 0.00   Grouse Ridge Trailhead, proceed downhill
- ▶2 0.51   Junction with Trail 13E13 (Sand Ridge Trail), turn left
- ▶3 1.80   Junction with Trail 12E11 (Crooked Lakes Trail), turn right
- ▶4 5.60   Junction with Trail 12E12 (Rock Lake Trail), turn right
- ▶5 6.00   Junction with Trail 13E28 (Shotgun/Middle Lakes Trail), turn right.
- ▶6 8.70   Junction with Trail 13E13 (Island Lake/Sand Ridge Trail), turn right
- ▶7 9.50   Junction with Grouse Ridge Trail, go straight
- ▶8 10.01 Return to Grouse Ridge Trailhead

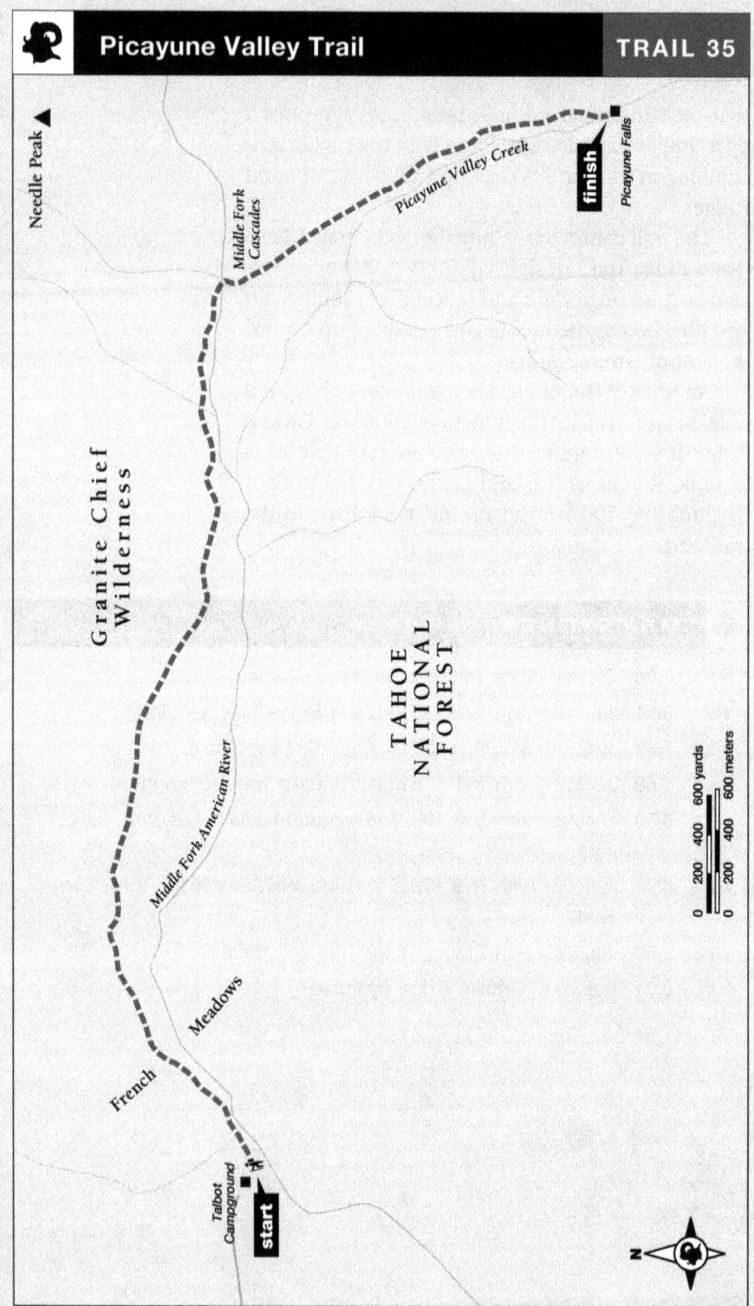

TRAIL 35 Sierra Nevada

Picayune Valley Trail: Granite Chief Wilderness

The grand scenery and solitude found along this trail are worth the drive. Sharp peaks, granite ridges, and sheer cliffs dominate the glacially scoured Picayune Valley. Old-growth forests, lush meadows, and aspens dot the valley floor, and the trail leads to a scenic cascade and an even more spectacular waterfall. This trail packs a lot of outstanding Sierra landscape into a relatively short hike.

Best Time

The best time is June to October. In heavy snow years, access roads and trail may still be blocked until July.

Finding the Trail

From Sacramento, drive 36 miles east on Interstate 80 to Auburn. Take the Foresthill Road–Secret Ravine exit, turn right on Foresthill Road, and proceed through the stoplight and across the Foresthill Bridge. Drive 18 miles northeast on Foresthill Road, through the town of Foresthill. Just before reaching the town center, turn right on Mosquito Ridge Road (Forest Road 96), and proceed 32 long, winding miles to French Meadows Reservoir. Continue another 7.0 miles east on Forest Road 96 to the Talbot Campground and the Picayune Valley Trailhead.

TRAIL USE
Hike, Horse
LENGTH
8.66 miles, 4–6 hours
VERTICAL FEET
±800
DIFFICULTY
- 1 2 3 **4** 5 +
TRAIL TYPE
Out & Back
SURFACE TYPE
Dirt

FEATURES
Dogs Allowed
Wilderness permit required
River
Stream
Waterfall
Canyon
Meadows
Wildflowers
Fall color
Camping
Great Views
Photo Opportunity

FACILITIES
Vault Toilet

Ranging from 8000 to 9000 feet in altitude, Lyon, Needle, Granite Chief, and Mildred peaks ring the upper end of Picayune Valley, exposing precipitous granite facades that slope downward to the broad valley floor.

River

Waterfall

Logistics

It takes three hours to get to the trailhead. You may want to camp overnight at the Talbot Campground or one of the many campgrounds along the road in order to provide a full day for hiking. Better yet, backpack into the Picayune Valley and use it as a base camp to explore the Granite Chief Wilderness.

Trail Description

From the day-use parking area at the **Talbot Campground**, ▶1 proceed east across the stream. The trail follows a former road for about a mile through an open U-shaped valley, dotted with groves of Jeffrey pines and black oaks, and fields of ceanothus and manzanita. As the road/trail climbs easily eastward, the forest begins to close in and large old-growth Jeffries appear along its length. Soon the former road ends, the trail turns to single track, and its rate of climb increases.

About 1.3 miles from the trailhead, the trail reaches the **Granite Chief Wilderness** boundary, ▶2 which is marked by a sign. Your route continues to climb moderately, crossing several small tributaries to the **Middle Fork American River**, which is hidden in the forest and rolling terrain of the broad valley visible to the south. The trail continues its way along the foot of the valley's north slope, providing expansive views southward across the valley of rocky and rugged Mildred Ridge. The trail steepens as it climbs upward toward the sharp prominence of **Needle Peak**, and the sound of flowing water announces your proximity to the Middle Fork American River.

The trail drops down to the **Middle Fork** and crosses it just downstream of a scenic cascade. Caution should be used in crossing during the early season when snowmelt increases the flow. After crossing the river, follow a spur trail upstream to

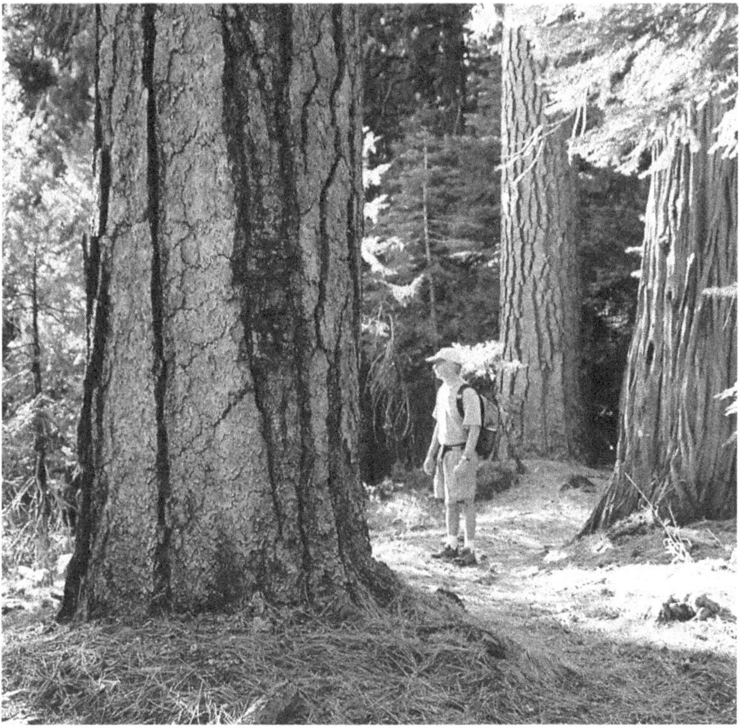

Picayune Valley Trail | TRAIL **35**

Old growth Jeffrey pines and cedar *shade parts of the Picayune Valley Trail.*

better view the cascade. Just beyond the crossing, the **Picayune Valley Trail** climbs the Middle Fork's south bank and ▶3 turns southward. A few small open areas offer potential campsites.

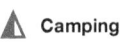 Camping

The trail breaks out of the forest and crosses an open granite knob dotted with Jeffrey pines and clumps of manzanita. The knob provides an outstanding view south of the 200-foot-high rock escarpment that delineates the boundary between lower and upper **Picayune Valley**.

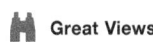 Great Views

As the trail heads south, it crosses spring-fed streams and wet meadows ringed with willows, aspens, and cottonwoods, broken by rocky areas supporting groves of pines and cedars. The trail

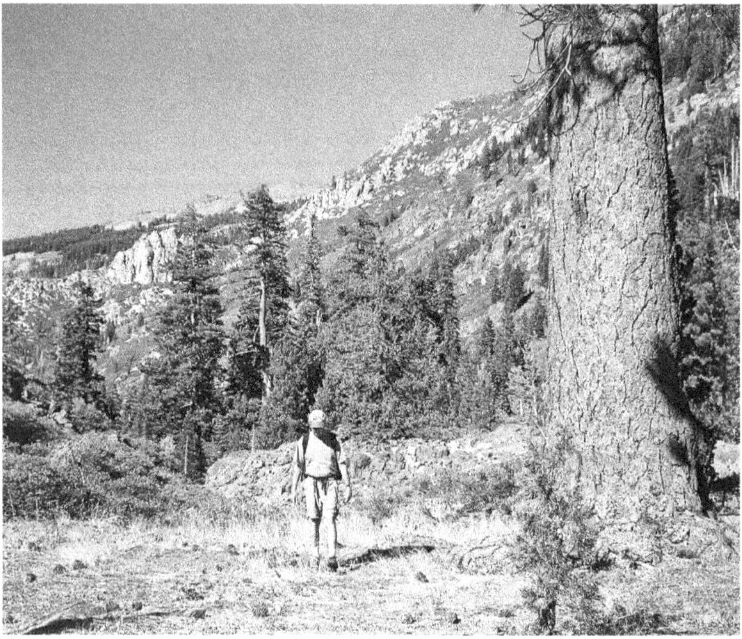

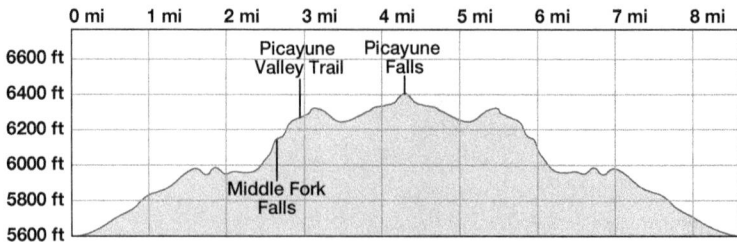

Granite buttresses *surround the wide glaciated valley of the Picayune.*

⚠ Camping

parallels Picayune Valley Creek as it heads toward the rocky escarpment. There are several potential campsites along this stretch of the trail.

At the foot of the escarpment, the trail begins to climb upward. A large open area guarded by a giant Jeffrey pine appears on the right. ▶4 A spur trail breaks off to the right, you follow it across this

TRAIL 35 Picayune Valley Trail Profile

Picayune Valley Trail | TRAIL 35

open expanse and then drop down toward Picayune Valley Creek. At the bottom of the rocky creek, turn left and follow the spur trail upstream to ▶5 scenic **Picayune Falls**.

Sit down and have lunch while enjoying the falls and the surrounding alpine scenery. Campsites are available in the large open area near the trail. Campers also have the option to continue up the escarpment to explore upper Picayune Valley.

▶6 Retrace your steps to the trailhead.

Waterfall

Camping

MILESTONES

- ▶1 0.00 Talbot Campground Trailhead, head east
- ▶2 1.33 Granite Chief Wilderness boundary, continue east
- ▶3 2.50 Middle Fork American River crossing, head south
- ▶4 4.30 Turn right on use-trail at bottom of escarpment
- ▶5 4.33 Picayune Valley Falls
- ▶6 8.66 Retrace steps to trailhead

Lake Margaret Trail

TRAIL 36

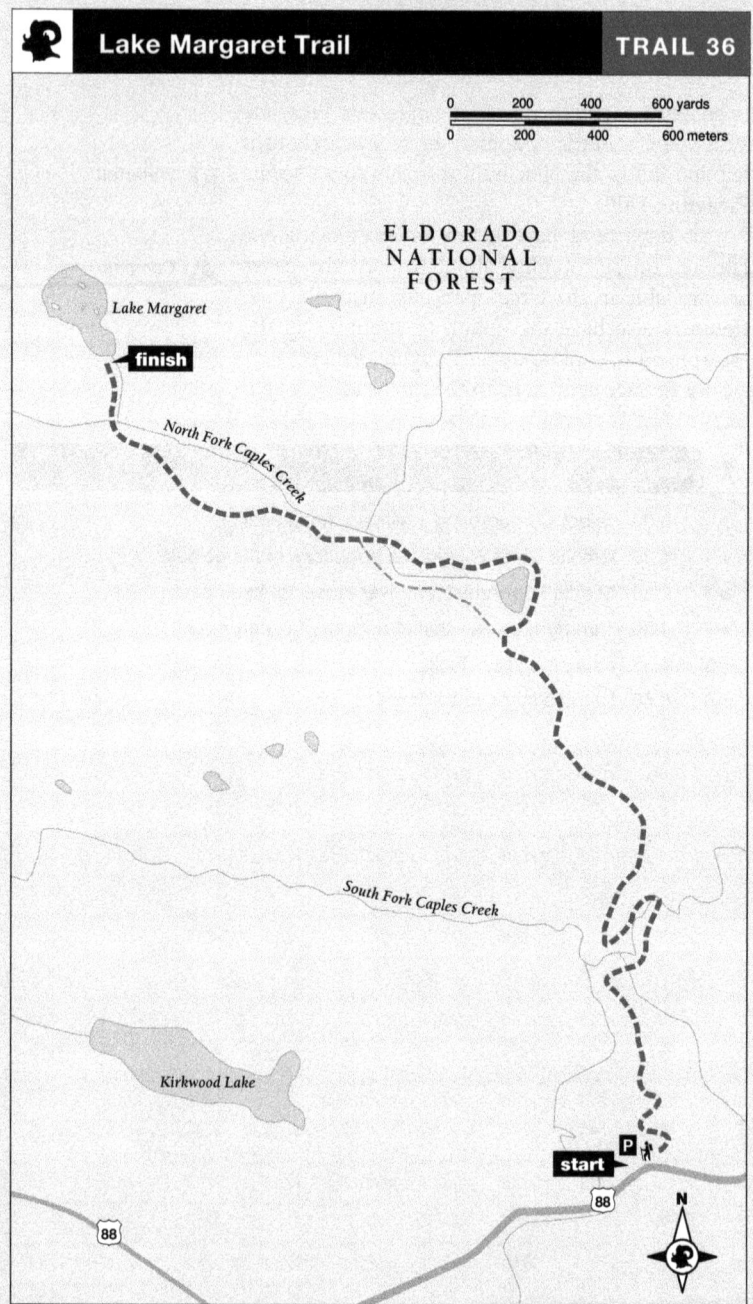

TRAIL 36 Sierra Nevada

Lake Margaret Trail: Caples Creek Proposed Wilderness

Lake Margaret is tucked away in a heavily forested glaciated valley pocked with ponds and small lakes and studded with granite rock formations. Although a short hike from Hwy 88, this subalpine jewel offers surprising seclusion. The up-and-down topography of the country also requires a bit more effort than implied by the short trail length depicted on the maps. Surrounded by granite ramparts, Lake Margaret offers a great opportunity to base camp and explore a virtually untracked portion of the Caples Creek Proposed Wilderness.

Best Time

This trail lies at just under 8000 feet in elevation, so the snow pack doesn't clear from it until late June or early July. The hiking season can stretch into October.

Finding the Trail

From Sacramento, drive 58.5 miles on Hwy 50 past Placerville to Pollock Pines. Take the Sly Park exit, turn right, and follow Sly Park Road 4.6 miles to the intersection with Old Mormon Emigrant Trail Road; turn left. Drive past Sly Park reservoir and continue approximately 25 miles to the junction of Old Mormon Emigrant Trail and Hwy 88. Turn left and drive east approximately 12.8 miles on Hwy 88. Look for a sign indicating the Lake Margaret Trailhead. Turn left into the trailhead parking lot.

TRAIL USE
Hike
LENGTH
4.7 miles, 3–4 hours
VERTICAL FEET
±250
DIFFICULTY
- 1 2 **3** 4 5 +
TRAIL TYPE
Out & Back
SURFACE TYPE
Dirt

FEATURES
Dogs Allowed
Stream
Lake
Meadow
Wildflowers
Birds
Camping
Great Views

FACILITIES
None

The South Fork Caples Creek meadow offers good spring wildflower display and excellent opportunities for birdwatching.

Logistics

Due to its proximity to Hwy 88 and Lake Tahoe, this trail can be busy on summer weekends. The two stream crossings required by this hike can be challenging when spring snowmelt or upstream reservoir releases in the fall swell the normally placid flow of Caples Creek.

Trail Description

From the trailhead parking area, at 7725 feet in elevation, ▶1 hikers get a good overview of the heavily forested glaciated valley that encompasses, hidden **Lake Margaret**, numerous unnamed pothole lakes and ponds, and the two forks of **Caples Creek**. The trailhead sign says LAKE MARGARET—2.5 MILES, although one topo map program has figured it to be 2.35 miles instead. Head north and down a rocky slope shaded by Jeffrey and lodgepole pines. After descending over a couple of granite benches, the trail reaches the edge of a large meadow incised by the meandering bends of the **South Fork Caples Creek**. The open, grassy meadow and its winding creek beckon anglers and picnickers alike, and also provides good views to the south of the Thimble and other volcanic peaks that separate Caples Lake and Silver Lake.

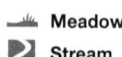 Meadow
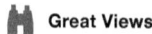 Stream

Great Views

Stream

The trail bends east briefly, skirts the edge of the meadow, and within slightly less than 0.5 mile from the trailhead, reaches the South Fork ford, which may or may not have a log crossing. ▶2 If the log has been washed out, you can ford the stream here, which should be easy enough during the summer months, but could be tricky during high water caused by snowmelt or upstream reservoir releases (typical during the late fall after the Labor Day holiday). You may have better luck finding other log crossings farther upstream, where the creek banks are closer together. After crossing, the trail follows

Lake Margaret Trail | TRAIL 36

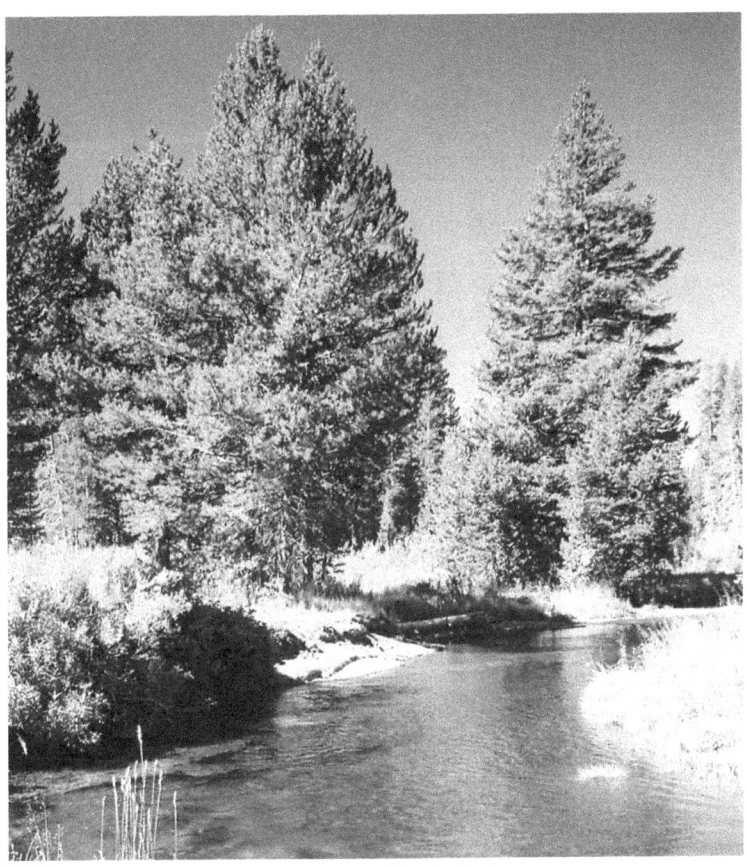

Hiking to Lake Margaret *requires a crossing of Caples Creek.*

the creek westward briefly and then comes to an unsigned trail junction. The left branch is a fishing trail. Turn right to continue on the trail to Lake Margaret.

The trail continues north, climbing 125 feet in elevation up a rocky draw. The path can get sketchy as it crosses large granite slabs, so look for ducks marking the route. The trail soon tops a ridge among a profusion of lodgepole pines and then heads downhill again as it makes its way over

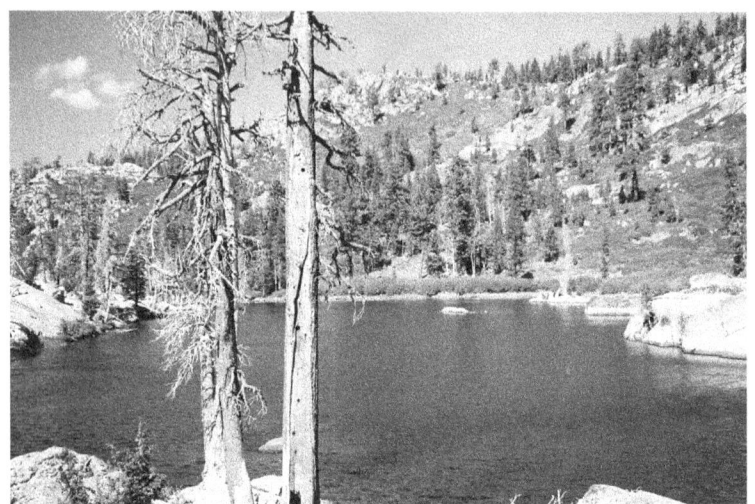

A relatively short hike brings you to secluded Lake Margaret.

the glacier-scoured, uneven terrain. As its proceeds downhill, the trail passes a forest-shrouded shallow pond (which may be dry by September). Both the Eldorado National Forest and Mokelumne Wilderness maps show the trail passing this pond to the west, but the trail actually curves around the east side of the pond. Then it drops down a rocky gully, requiring some scrambling.

The trail soon crosses a seasonal tributary, and just beyond that reaches the **North Fork Caples Creek**. There it turns west and follows the south

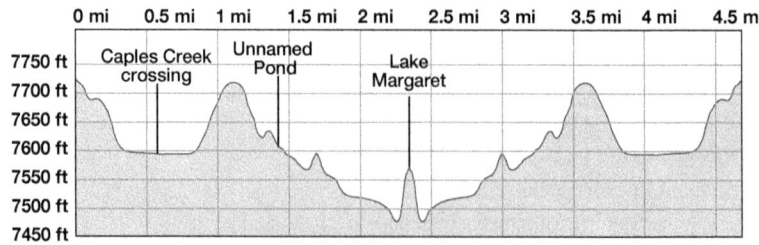

TRAIL 36 Lake Margaret Trail Profile

Lake Margaret Trail TRAIL 36

side of the creek for about 0.5 mile. The trail makes its way through a small aspen grove and willow thicket, which provide seasonal color and relief from the dark forest and boulders. The trail reaches the North Fork ford approximately 1.12 miles from the first ford on the South Fork. ▶3 The North Fork has less flow than the reservoir-enhanced South Fork and can be easily forded, except during the height of spring snowmelt.

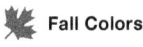 Fall Colors

After crossing the North Fork, the trail proceeds northeast a short distance up a draw and over yet another glaciated rocky bench. It then drops into the granite pothole that provides the scenic setting for ▶4 Lake Margaret. Legal campsites beyond the regulation 100-foot no-camping area of the lakeshore are limited, but they can be found on the granite bench south of the lake. Although quite cold, the lake offers excellent sunning rocks and plenty of bouldering opportunities for those who like to clamber around on rocks. It also makes a great base camp to explore the trackless and heavily forested granite jumbles that make up the nearly trail-less upper Caples watershed.

Lake
Camping
Swimming

When you are done exploring Lake Margaret and its environs, ▶5 retrace your steps to the return to the trailhead.

🚶 MILESTONES

- ▶1   0.0   Start at trailhead on Hwy 88
- ▶2   0.45   Cross South Fork Caples Creek
- ▶3   2.25   Cross North Fork Caples Creek
- ▶4   2.35   Lake Margaret
- ▶5   4.70   Retrace steps to trailhead

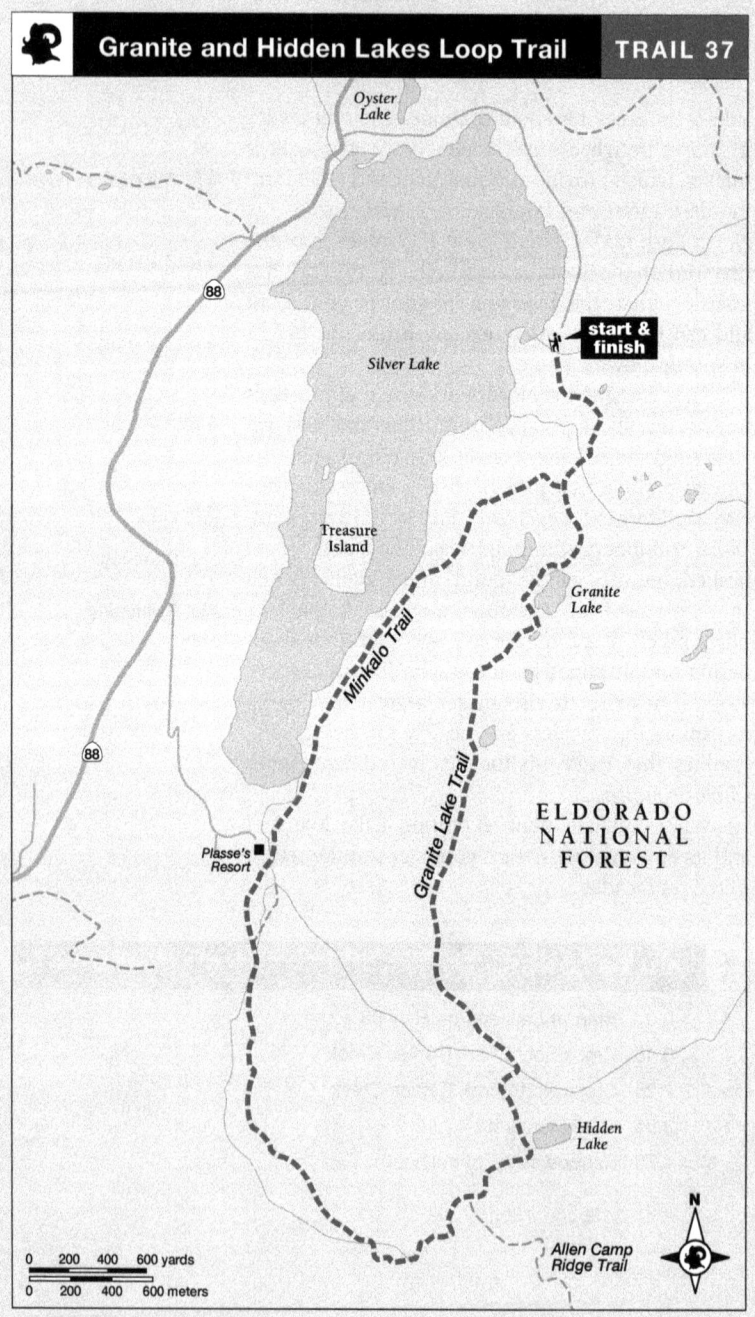

TRAIL 37 Sierra Nevada

Granite and Hidden Lakes Loop

This hike showcases two scenic lakes—Granite and Hidden—that offer good destinations for a day hike or an easy overnight backpack trip. Or make it a loop hike and add a third and larger lake—Silver—to the tour, as well as some additional miles. Campgrounds and three resorts around Silver Lake offer excellent base-camp opportunities to explore this trail and other routes to the adjacent Mokelumne Wilderness.

Best Time

This is a fairly high-elevation trail. The hiking season is generally June through October.

Finding the Trail

From Sacramento, drive 58.5 miles on Hwy 50 past Placerville to Pollock Pines. Take the Sly Park exit, turn right and follow Sly Park Road 4.6 miles to the intersection with Old Mormon Emigrant Trail Road and turn left. Drive past Sly Park reservoir and continue approximately 25 miles to the junction of Old Mormon Emigrant Trail and Hwy 88. Turn left on Hwy 88 and drive 5.3 miles east past the Plasse and Kay's resorts turnoffs, over the Silver Lake dam, to the Kit Carson Lodge road, and turn right. At this point, you will be driving on a largely unsigned road network serving cabins on the north and northeastern shores of Silver Lake. The directions may seem confusing, but you can't go wrong if you continue to follow your way east and south around the lake. On the Kit Carson Lodge road, drive 0.3 mile and

TRAIL USE
Hike
LENGTH
7.0 miles, 4–6 hours
VERTICAL FEET
±700
DIFFICULTY
- 1 2 3 **4** 5 -
TRAIL TYPE
Loop
SURFACE TYPE
Dirt

FEATURES
Dogs Allowed
Meadow
Stream
Lake
Camping
Great Views
Photo Opportunity

FACILITIES
None

> The volcanic soils along the Allen Camp Trail retain more moisture than the granitics, adding lushness to the vegetation not found along the drier Granite Lake Trail.

turn left at the **Y**. Drive another 0.5 mile and turn left at the **Y** at Kit Carson Lodge sign. Drive another 0.2 mile, and turn right at the **Y**. Drive another 0.1 mile and turn right at the **Y**. Continue 0.3 mile over a large, granite bedrock area dotted with a few cabins, to the Minkalo Trail sign on the left. There are a handful of parking spaces by the trailhead sign and several more about 100 feet up the road.

Logistics

This is a popular trail, so trailhead parking fills up fast on summer weekends. Various signs along this route offer a confusing and sometimes conflicting variety of trail names. Officially, the Minkalo Trail (17E72) leads from the trailhead south along the east shore of Silver Lake to Plasse's Resort. The Granite Lake Trail (17E23) splits off from the Minkalo Trail and makes its way past Granite and Hidden Lakes to the Allen Camp Trail (17E19). The Allen Camp Trail drops down to Plasse's Resort. If you can find your way through the resort's maze-like campground, you will reach the southern terminus of the Minkalo Trail and can make your way back to the trailhead.

Trail Description

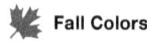
Fall Colors

The **Minkalo Trail** ▶1 sign says GRANITE LAKE—1.0, PLASSE'S—3.0. The trail climbs through a broken forest of fir and lodgepole as it circles behind a granite bluff on your right. A small copse of aspen provides fall color. The tread varies between decomposed granite, bedrock, and loose rock as it continues south past a shallow pond and meadow and over a footbridge spanning a seasonal stream. As the trail climbs up a slope studded with large granite outcrops and lodgepole pines, good views are provided of the dark volcanic massif of Thunder Mountain

Granite and Hidden Lakes Loop | TRAIL **37**

to the northeast and deep blue **Silver Lake** to the northwest.

Less than 0.5 mile from the trailhead, you come to the junction of the Minkalo Trail and the **Granite Lake Trail**. A sign points left to the GRANITE LAKE TRAIL. The Minkalo Trail goes right to skirt the east shore of Silver Lake on its way to Plasse's Resort. This will be your return route if you choose to make this a loop trip. ▶2 Turn left on the Granite Lake Trail to make your way to its namesake as the trail climbs gently through lodgepole and fir trees past a small pond frequented by Canada geese. Lake

After an easy 300-foot climb from the trailhead, the Granite Lake Trail soon reaches a large bedrock bench that leads to pretty **Granite Lake**. ▶3 The lake at first seems rather small, but the initial view is just the northern cove of the lake. Continue south on the trail and the lake soon reveals a size even Goldilocks would like (just right!). Several flat bedrock slabs surrounding the lake and its shallow water (which warms nicely in later summer months) provide perfect swimming conditions. Campers may be tempted by some lakeside flat areas, but look for other sites to the south and west of the lake, which are beyond the required 100-foot no-camping limit. Some folks may prefer to spend the day at Granite Lake, but they should expect lots of visitors because of its proximity to the trailhead. **Hidden Lake** is worth the continued hike and climb.

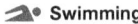 Swimming

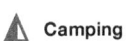 Camping

The trail circles around the south end of Granite Lake and continues south past another small pond and through an area of large granite boulders and bedrock dotted with stands of lodgepole pines. On a nearly flat grade, the trail enters a red-fir forest broken by stringer meadows ringed by the ubiquitous lodgepoles. After climbing and descending a gentle rise, the trail continues on a nearly flat grade through broken forest.

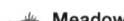 Meadow

Sierra Nevada

Lake

Camping

Great Views

Great Views
Photo Opportunity

About 1.75 miles from Granite Lake, the trail crosses a seasonal stream and then abruptly climbs 200 feet up to Hidden Lake. Hidden Lake is set in a forested bowl dominated by the granite buttresses of **Squaw Ridge**, which forms the eastern boundary of the **Mokelumne Wilderness**. The dark surrounding forest gives Hidden Lake a more gem-like quality, and the overall setting is more intimate than the open expanse around Granite Lake. Appropriate campsites are available west and south of the lake.

At this point, you have to decide whether you want to turn around and retrace your steps to the trailhead or climb the 400 feet up to the **Allen Camp Trail** and then drop down to Plasse's Resort. From there, you can follow the Minkalo Trail along Silver Lake's east shore to its junction with the Granite Lake Trail. On the plus side is a stunning view you'll have from a knob near the junction of the Granite Lake and Allen Camp trails, as well as a dramatic change in geology and vegetation. The down side includes motorcycle use of the Allen Camp Trail and some route confusion traversing Plasse's Resort. Read on and decide.

As the trail reaches the west end of Hidden Lake, a sign says PLASSE'S—3.0 and points the way southwestward. The trail turns a sharp right ▶4 and almost immediately begins a moderate climb through red firs and past a medium-sized meadow. It then abandons its well-engineered grade altogether and simply zigzags steeply uphill past another meadow. Thankfully, this steep pitch is short.

The trail's uphill climb moderates and the forest opens to the right. A spur trail to the right leads 100 feet to a granite knob that provides a stunning view of Silver Lake, Thunder Mountain, and the Crystal Range in the distance. A separate trail leads away from the knob and reconnects with the Granite Lake Trail where it meets the Allen Camp Trail at a four-way junction (the Granite Lake Trail, the Allen

Granite and Hidden Lakes Loop | TRAIL 37

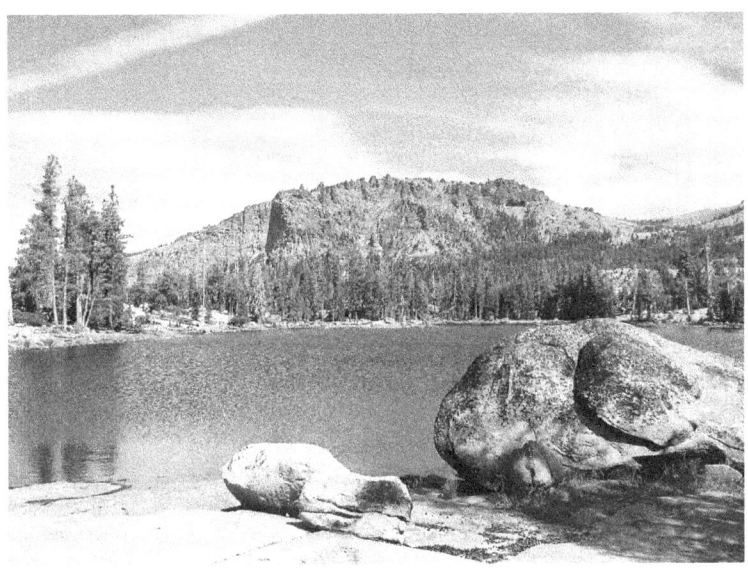

Thunder Mountain *dominates the skyline above Granite Lake.*

Camp Trail in two different directions, and the scenic knob spur trail). At this four-way trail junction, you are 3.35 miles and 700 feet from where you started.

To the left, the Allen Camp Trail leads up to the top of Squaw Ridge; to the right, it leads down to Plasse's Resort. A sign says PLASSE'S RESORT—2.0. Unfortunately, this scenic trail, which follows a stream and a series of deep green meadows ringed by old-growth firs, is open to motorcycle use. So the trail itself has been pounded into thick dust and widened unnecessarily in several sections. Nevertheless, the scenery is worth the walk.

▶5 Turn right on the Allen Camp Trail. Almost immediately you will notice a change in geology. The ever-present granite has been replaced with volcanic breccia.

Geologic Interest

The Allen Camp Trail quickly drops down, off the nearly 8000-foot-high ridgetop to cross a

Sierra Nevada 297

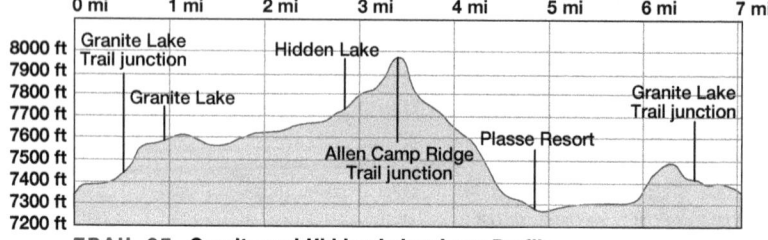

TRAIL 37 Granite and Hidden Lakes Loop Profile

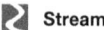

Stream

Lake

headwaters meadow feeding a small stream flowing down to Plasse's Resort. Above you, three large, purplish-gray breccia outcrops dominate the little headwater. The trail drops farther and then switchbacks across the stream. It continues to make its way steeply downhill as it parallels the stream and its lush meadow system along the forest edge.

Soon, the downhill trek moderates and you will see some buildings on your right through the trees. This is the **Stockton Municipal Camp**. The trail soon reaches a Y junction. ▶6 Turn right, walk past a large corral on your left, and enter the Plasse's Resort's sprawling campground and road network. There is no ideal way to make your way through the resort complex—simply follow the campground roads and alphabetically lettered campsites north toward Silver Lake. You will glimpse the main resort buildings on your left. Eventually, you will reach the last road, which parallels Silver Lake's east shore. Turn right and follow this road north. Just beyond Campsite M10, the road crosses a seasonal creek. A home-made sign incorrectly labeled GRANITE LAKE TRAIL nevertheless correctly directs you to a trail leading off ▶7 to your left and east.

Continuing northeast on the trail, you will reach an official Forest Service sign that says MINKALO TRAIL 17E72 and CAMP MINKALO—2.5 MILES. Now that you are beyond the campground and have confirmed that you are indeed on the right trail, proceed northeast through a lodgepole forest with openings that offer occasional glimpse of Silver Lake on your left.

The trail reaches a large meadow. A use-trail splits off to the left and goes through the meadow, but the Minkalo Trail begins climbing steeply up a ridge on your right. This route is also misnamed with another home-made sign saying GRANITE LAKE TRAIL, PLASSE'S STABLES. But rest assured that you are still on the Minkalo Trail. Perhaps because of heavy equestrian use, the tread of the steeply climbing trail degenerates into loose rock and dirt, but after a short 200-foot climb, it reaches an open granite bench that provides good views of Silver Lake and Thunder Mountain. Shortly thereafter, the Minkalo Trail reconnects with the Granite Lake Trail. ▶8 Turn left and ▶9 retrace your steps to the trailhead.

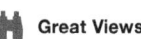 **Great Views**

MILESTONES

- ▶1 0.00 Minkalo Trailhead
- ▶2 0.45 Granite Lake Trail junction, turn left
- ▶3 0.81 Granite Lake, continue straight
- ▶4 2.84 Hidden Lake, turn right
- ▶5 3.35 Allen Camp Ridge Trail junction, turn right
- ▶6 4.52 Y junction at Plasse Resort, turn right, follow campground road
- ▶7 5.10 End of Plasse Campground, cross stream, turn left on trail
- ▶8 6.54 Granite Lake Trail junction, turn left
- ▶9 7.00 Retrace steps to Minkalo Trailhead

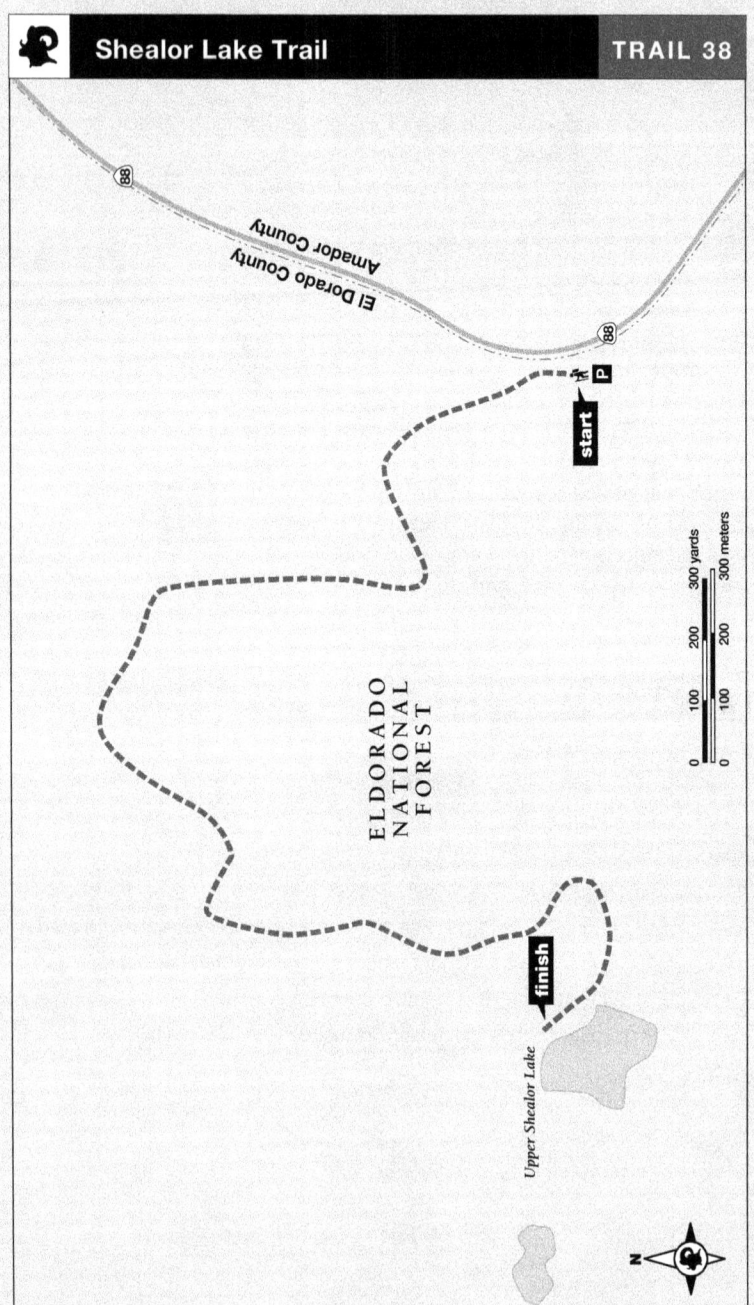

TRAIL 38 Sierra Nevada

Shealor Lake Trail: Caples Creek Proposed Wilderness

The Shealor Lake Trail is easily accessible from Hwy 88 and it's a relatively easy walk for less-experienced hikers and families with children (age 10 or older). The trail provides wildly contrasting alpine scenery, including the dark volcanic peaks in the nearby Mokelumne Wilderness and lighter-colored granite canyons of the Caples Creek Proposed Wilderness. Pretty Shealor Lake is a great destination for a picnic, or a swim, or to simply lie on a warm granite rock and look at the clouds. If you desire a bit more of a challenge, you can make your way cross-country from upper Shealor Lake down to lower Shealor Lake.

Best Time

Topping out at nearly 7600 feet, this is a fairly high-altitude hike. The snow pack usually doesn't abate in this area until late June. The optimum season is July through October. Wildflowers add to the scenery during the high-mountain summer.

Finding the Trail

From Sacramento, drive 58.5 miles on Hwy 50 past Placerville to Pollock Pines. Take the Sly Park exit, turn right, and follow Sly Park Road 4.6 miles to the intersection with Old Mormon Emigrant Trail Road, then turn left. Drive past Sly Park reservoir and continue approximately 25 miles to the junction of Old Mormon Emigrant Trail and Hwy 88. Turn left and drive east approximately 6.0 miles on Hwy 88. Look for a sign indicating the Shealor Lake Trailhead. Turn left into the parking lot.

TRAIL USE
Hike, Run
LENGTH
3.2 miles, 2–3 hours
VERTICAL FEET
±450
DIFFICULTY
- 1 **2** 3 4 5 +
TRAIL TYPE
Out & Back
SURFACE TYPE
Dirt
Rock

FEATURES
Child Friendly
Dogs Allowed
Lake
Canyon
Geology
Wildflowers
Great Views
Photo Opportunity
Camping

FACILITIES
None

The warm rocks surrounding Shealor Lake provide an excellent lunch and nap spot, and the lake itself is a picture-perfect, if chilling, swimming experience.

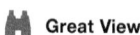 **Great Views**

Logistics

Perhaps because of its short length and ease, this trail is surprisingly less popular than many others along Hwy 88. Nevertheless, the trailhead parking lot can be full and the trail crowded on summer weekends. As usual, weekdays or post–Labor Day weekends are the best times to avoid crowds.

Trail Description

From the parking lot, at 7450 feet, ▶1 proceed due north on the **Shealor Lake Trail** through a grove of red fir and lodgepole pines. The trail soon crosses an ephemeral stream and breaks out of the forest to work its way over a series of granite slabs and benches, climbing easily up toward a visible saddle between two round knobs on the ridge. To the northeast, you see Silver Lake and Thunder Mountain, but better views are available ahead.

About 0.72 mile from the trailhead parking lot, you reach the high point of the trail, ▶2 a saddle just under 7600 feet in altitude. The eastward view from the saddle includes beautiful Silver Lake, as well as the dark volcanic ramparts of Thunder Mountain, Thimble Peak, and several other 9000-plus-foot high peaks that delineate the western boundary of the Mokelumne Wilderness. To the west is the Tragedy Creek drainage and the other drainages that make up the proposed **Caples Creek Wilderness**.

Contrasting sharply with the brown volcanic formations to the east, Tragedy Creek canyon is dominated by white granite cliffs and outcrops. As you stand in the saddle facing west, **upper Shealor Lake** is at your feet, tucked away in the very beginnings of the Tragedy Creek watershed. Tragedy Creek is named after an 1848 incident during which three Mormon scouts were allegedly killed by Indians.

Shealor Lake Trail | TRAIL 38

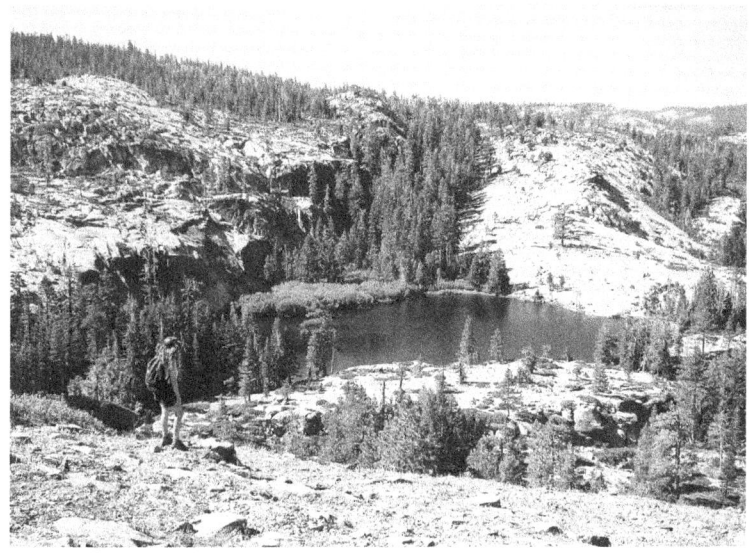

Shealor Lake *is a short but scenic hike from Highway 88.*

From the saddle, proceed down through an open rocky slope punctuated by pine-mat manzanita and an occasional Jeffrey pine. The trail descends in three long switchbacks. Trail sections over bare granite get sketchy but are usually marked with ducks—but you can't really wander astray because upper Shealor Lake remains in sight below you, providing a good beacon. At the farthest northern point of the trail switchback, you can also catch a glimpse of **lower Shealor Lake**, farther down in the Tragedy Creek drainage.

Nearly a mile from the saddle, the trail reaches the relatively flat bottom of Tragedy Creek Canyon, winds its way through a small grove of red fir, and onto the bare granite slabs surrounding the east shore of ▶3 upper Shealor Lake.

 Canyon

 Lake

Those looking to extend their outing and add more of challenge to this easy hike can make their way cross-country about 0.7 mile down to lower

Sierra Nevada 303

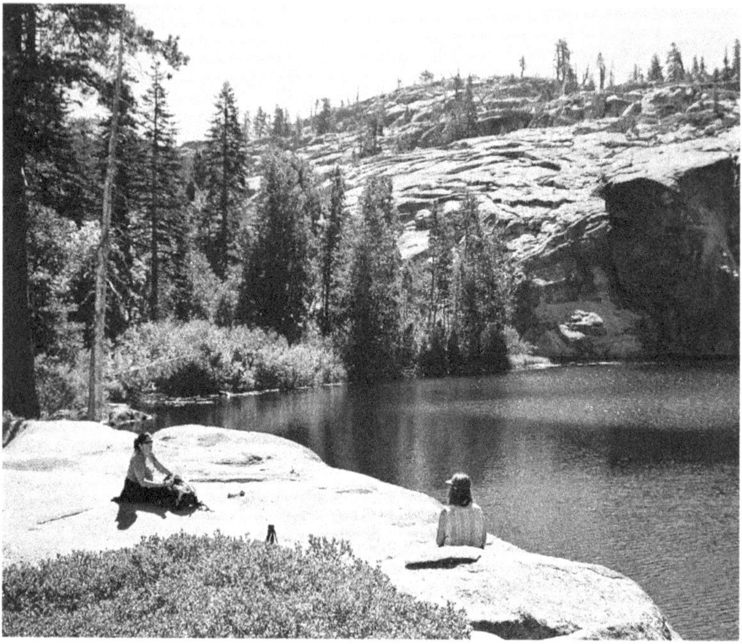

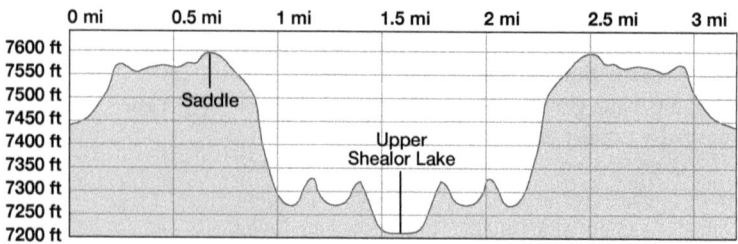

Shealor Lake *makes a great lunch spot.*

Shealor Lake, at 6700 feet. Follow the east side of the outlet stream from upper Shealor and approach lower Shealor from the east to avoid cliffs just south of the lower lake. Cross-country hikers should be familiar with trail-less travel, be able to read a map, and possess and know how to use a compass.

TRAIL 38 Shealor Lake Trail Profile

Shealor Lake Trail | TRAIL 38

If the short amble to the upper lake was your intended outing, ▶4 simply retrace your steps to parking lot when you are ready to bid the upper lake adieu.

MILESTONES

- ▶1   0.00   Start at trailhead on Hwy 88
- ▶2   0.72   Saddle
- ▶3   1.60   Shealor Lake
- ▶4   3.20   Retrace steps to trailhead parking lot

Winnemucca – Round Top Lakes Loop — TRAIL 39

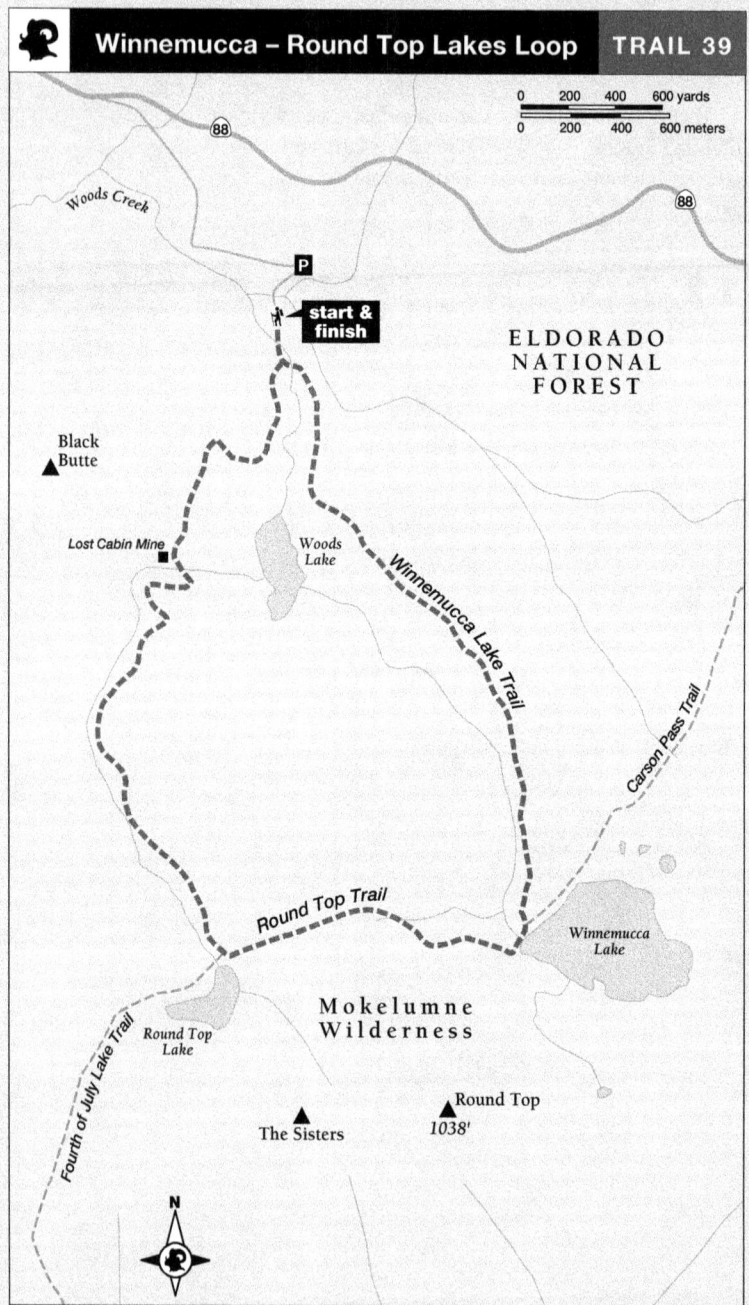

TRAIL 39 Sierra Nevada

Winnemucca–Round Top Lakes Loop: Mokelumne Wilderness

This signature hike is beloved by Sacramentans for its spectacular alpine vistas, magnificent wildflowers, sparkling lakes, and outstanding fall color. The dark volcanic ridges and peaks provide a brooding backdrop to Winnemucca and Round Top Lakes, two of the prettiest lakes in the northern Sierra. The volcanic soils also support an unusually rich wildflower display. As a consequence, be prepared to share this incredible hike with many people during the optimum summer months, and please limit your visit to Winnemucca and Round Top Lakes to day use only, to protect the fragile alpine habitat.

Best Time

The thick Sierra snowpack above 8000 feet limits access to this trail until mid-July. Optimum wildflower-viewing months are July and August. Heather and other ground-covering shrubs offer their own autumnal display of color in September and October.

Finding the Trail

From Sacramento, drive 58.5 miles on Hwy 50 past Placerville to Pollock Pines. Take the Sly Park exit, turn right, and follow Sly Park Road 4.6 miles to the intersection with Old Mormon Emigrant Trail Road, then turn left. Drive past Sly Park reservoir and continue approximately 25 miles to the junction of Old Mormon Emigrant Trail and Hwy 88. Turn left and drive 16.15 miles east on Hwy 800, past Silver and Caples Lakes to the turnoff to Woods Lake. Turn

TRAIL USE
Hike
LENGTH
4.74 miles, 3–5 hours
VERTICAL FEET
±1200
DIFFICULTY
+ 1 2 3 **4** 5 +
TRAIL TYPE
Loop
SURFACE TYPE
Dirt

FEATURES
Dogs Allowed
Wilderness permit
Mountain
Lake
Stream
Fall color
Meadow
Wildflowers
Historic
Great Views
Steep

FACILITIES
Vault Toilets

> Take a quick dip in Winnemucca Lake if you dare, but the water in this alpine gem is always cold.

right (if you reach Carson Pass on Hwy 88, you have gone about 1.85 miles too far). Follow the road approximately 0.95 mile to the trailhead parking lot, just before the road crosses Woods Creek.

Logistics

If you are looking for a wilderness experience, avoid this trail on summer weekends and holidays. Although you miss most of the wildflowers, you can also avoid the crowds altogether by hiking this trail after Labor Day and into October. Woods Lake campground near the trailhead offers a great base camp from which to explore this area.

Trail Description

From the trailhead parking lot, ▶1 continue down the road and over the bridge crossing **Woods Creek**. Go past the sign on the right marking your return route from **Round Top Lake**. Within a short distance, a sign on the left side of the road indicates the start of the **Winnemucca Lake Trail**.

Shortly after leaving the road, the trail ▶2 crosses **Woods Creek** over a sturdy footbridge and makes its way through a forest of lodgepole and white pine.

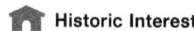 Historic Interest

In about 0.25 mile, the trail passes an arrastra, a circular stone-lined pit once used to crush mining ore. Soon thereafter, the trail enters an open slope with limited shade provided by scattered white pines and hemlocks.

After about 1.3 miles, the trail reaches a trailside sign delineating ▶3 the boundary of the 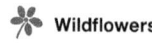 Wildflowers **Mokelumne Wilderness**. The wildflower display begins in earnest here, taking advantage of the open grassy slopes, which are well watered by a small stream on your right fed by Winnemucca Lake. At this point, the trail gradient steepens as it makes its way upward toward the lake.

Winnemucca–Round Top Lakes Loop | TRAIL 39

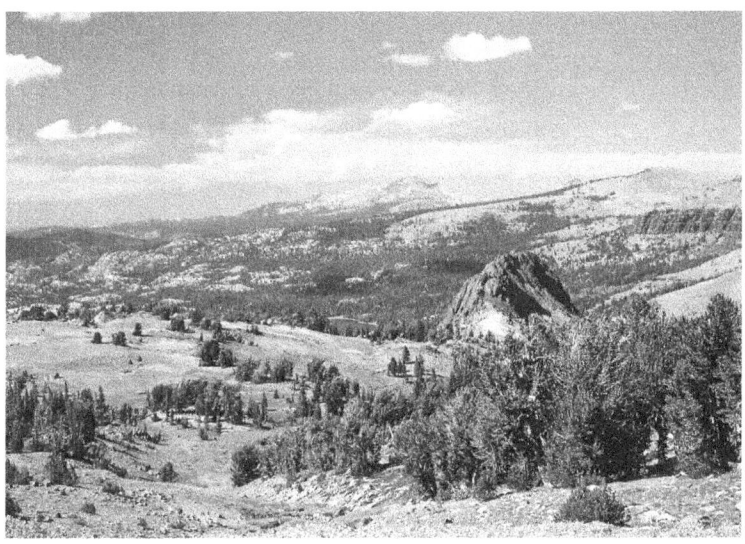

The view south from Round Top Lake, *with Black Butte and the east end of Caples Lake in the center, Little Round Top Peak to the right, and the Crystal Range in the distance*

Less than 0.5 mile after crossing into the Mokelumne Wilderness, the trail enters a shallow bowl that contains **Winnemucca Lake**. Shortly before reaching the lake, you come to a trail intersection with the **Carson Pass Trail** on your left and the **Round Top Lake Trail** on your right. ▶4 Go right and proceed 50 feet up the trail to Winnemucca Lake. The turquoise-colored lake (great for a quick dip) is dominated by sheer volcanic cliffs rising to the top of 10,381-foot-high Round Top Peak.

 Lake

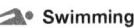 Swimming

After admiring the view, proceed on the Round Top Lake Trail, cross the stream flowing out of Winnemucca Lake, and begin ascending a ridge directly to the west of the lake. Less than 0.5 mile from Winnemucca Lake, you reach a 9400-foot-high saddle, providing great views of nearby Elephants Back peak on the Sierra crest to the northeast, Red Lake Peak across Hwy 88 to the north, and Freel Peak overlooking Lake Tahoe on the far

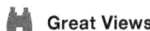 Great Views

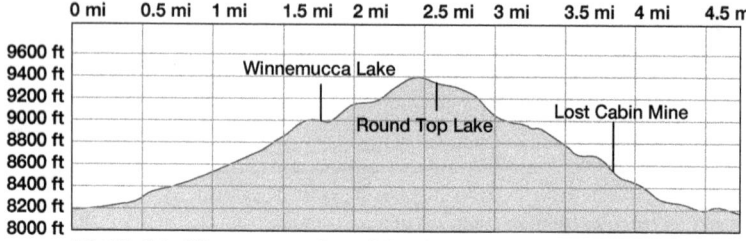

TRAIL 39 Winnemucca–Round Top Lakes Loop Profile

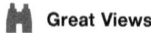

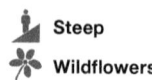

northeastern horizon. After crossing the saddle, the trail drops a short way down to Round Top Lake.

At a bit more than halfway on your loop, ▶5 Round Top Lake provides an ideal lunch spot. Just before reaching the lake, the Round Top Lake Trail intersects with the Fourth of July Lake Trail. Proceed straight on the Fourth of July Lake Trail about 50 feet to Round Top Lake. From here, more energetic hikers can follow the trail over a pass southwest of the lake and drop down to visit **Fourth of July Lake** or even proceed up the slope from the lake to bag Round Top Peak.

Round Top Lake itself is beautifully framed to the south by The Sisters, a series of volcanic crags directly west of Round Top Peak. The view to the south of the lake is of a broad glaciated slope rolling down to Black Butte and Caples Lake beyond. A nearly constant cold wind makes the lake a challenge for even the hardiest of swimmers.

Once fully satisfied with lakeside scenery, retrace your steps to the trail junction and go left (south) on the Round Top Lake Trail. The trail descends steeply as it parallels the lake's outlet stream. Seasonal wildflowers remain abundant as the route winds its way through a series of small flats dominated by dwarf willows lining the stream. Soon, the trail drops steeply through a hemlock forest until it reaches the remains of a stone structure on your right, the first of several reminders of the ▶6 **Lost Cabin Mine**.

Winnemucca–Round Top Lakes Loop | TRAIL 39

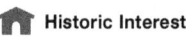 Historic Interest

Strung out along the trail, a rusted Model T pickup, a mining pit, a closed tunnel, and couple of not-so-lost cabins herald the mine proper. Please appreciate this bit of the Sierra's hard-rock mining heritage but leave it untouched. At this point, the trail heads to the right and then switchbacks to the left and passes below the mine cabins. It soon connects with the jeep road that services the mine, which drops down toward the Woods Lake Campground. Just before reaching the campground, the trail leaves the jeep road and proceeds left through a forest of lodgepole and white fir to reconnect with the paved **Woods Lake Road**. Turn left on the road and walk less than 0.1 mile to ▶7 the trailhead parking lot.

MILESTONES

- ▶1 0.00 Start at trailhead
- ▶2 0.15 Footbridge over Woods Creek
- ▶3 1.35 Mokelumne Wilderness boundary
- ▶4 1.73 Winnemucca Lake, turn right at trail junction
- ▶5 2.60 Round Top Lake, turn right to visit, then retrace steps to trail to continue
- ▶6 3.96 Lost Cabin Mine
- ▶7 4.74 Trailhead parking lot

Caples Creek - Silver Fork Loop   TRAIL 40

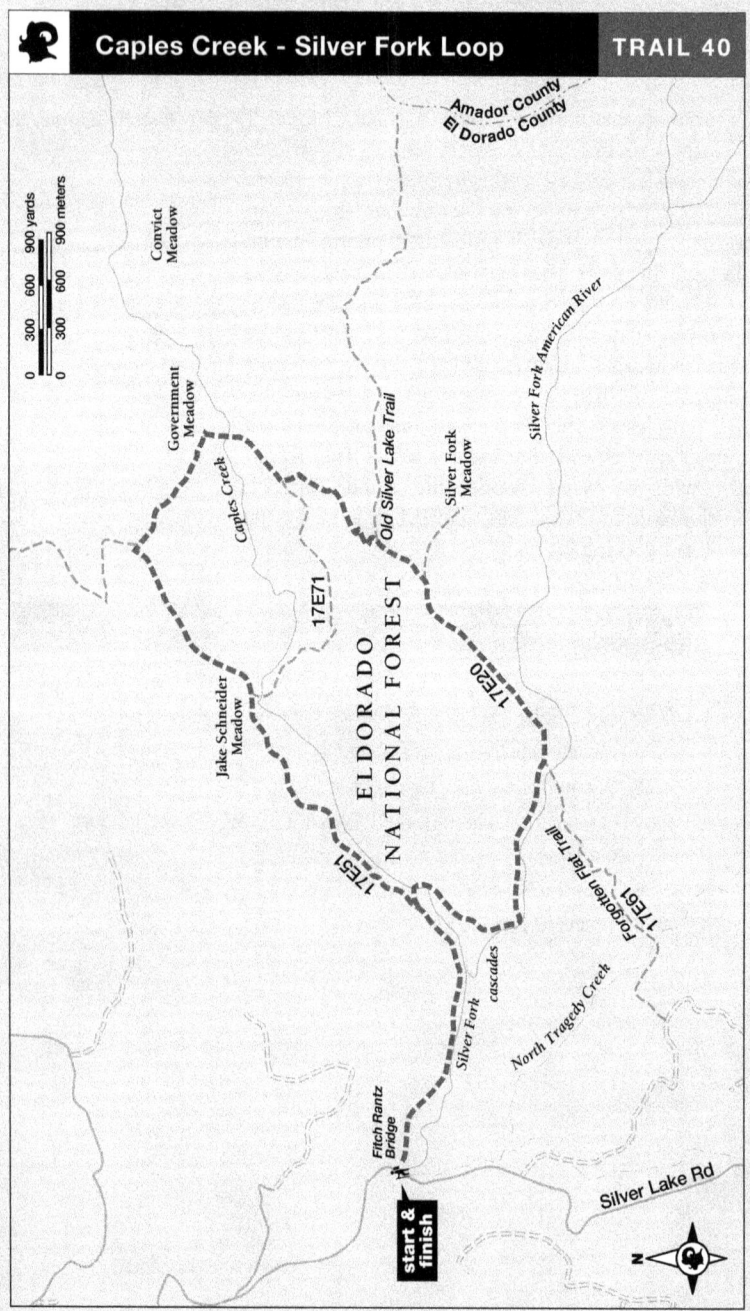

TRAIL 40 Sierra Nevada

Caples Creek–Silver Fork Loop: Caples Creek Proposed Wilderness

The proposed Caples Creek Wilderness is relatively small in comparison to the Mokelumne Wilderness to the south and the Desolation Wilderness to the north, but its glaciated topography, rugged river canyons, old-growth forests, and extensive trail system provide plenty of opportunities for true wilderness solitude. The trail system is easily accessible from multiple trailheads off Hwy 50 and Hwy 88. This hike is accessed from Hwy 50 and features a loop that makes a good long day hike or two- to three-day backpack trip. There are many streamside and meadow campsites to choose from, providing a great opportunity to base camp and explore. Anglers can fish for trout in both Caples Creek and the Silver Fork, and all visitors will enjoy the sparkling cascades of both streams.

Best Time

Elevations range from 5600 feet at the trailhead to 6800 feet, making the lower portion of the area available as early as May or June, but the higher elevations may still have snow through July. The best hiking season is June through October.

Finding the Trail

From Sacramento, drive 75 miles east on Hwy 50 to the small town of Kyburz. Turn right on Silver Lake Road and proceed 8.4 miles. Just before the road curves right and crosses the Silver Fork over a bridge, there is a road on the left with a TRAILHEAD sign. Turn left and park at the trailhead.

TRAIL USE
Hike, Run, Bike, Horse
LENGTH
8.6 miles, 5–6 hours
VERTICAL FEET
±1200
DIFFICULTY
- 1 2 3 4 **5** +
TRAIL TYPE
Loop
SURFACE TYPE
Dirt

FEATURES
Dogs Allowed
River
Stream
Waterfalls
Canyon
Meadow
Wildflowers
Fall Color
Birds
Wildlife
Camping
Great Views
Secluded
Steep

FACILITIES
None

The wildflower display in Jake Schneider Meadow can be spectacular.

Logistics

Some of the trails in this area are open to motorized use, but the area is not heavily used by vehicles. Creek crossings may be dangerous during spring runoff.

Trail Description

From the trailhead, ▶1 proceed up the old jeep road (now closed to four-wheeled vehicles) marked on the Forest Service map as Trail 17E51. The former road climbs through firs and cedars and soon becomes a foot trail. As you continue up the trail, the sound of water lets you know that you are getting closer to the **Silver Fork American River** on your right. A bit over 0.75 mile, the trail provides a view of the confluence between the Silver Fork and **Caples Creek**. While you enjoy the view of this cataract tumbling its way through smooth water-worn granite, contemplate the fact that at one time, this beautiful site was threatened by a proposed hydroelectric dam (now foreclosed by the Forest Service's Wilderness recommendation for the area). At this point, your southeast-trending trail will make a right turn and proceed northeast.

  River

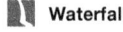 Waterfall

Approximately 1.2 miles from the trailhead, you come to a small meadow and the first of many trail junctions. A sign says GOVERNMENT MEADOW—2.0 MILES and HWY 88—5.0 MILES. Your route, Trail 17E51, continues straight ahead in a northeast direction, toward Government Meadow. Take a good look at ▶2 Trail 17E20 coming in from your right, because 6.2 miles from now you will be walking down that trail to close the loop. Continue on Trail 17E51 through a forest of firs and cedars broken by an occasional meadow speckled with seasonally appropriate wildflowers. The trail parallels Caples Creek for more than a mile, providing plenty of

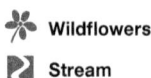 Wildflowers
  Stream

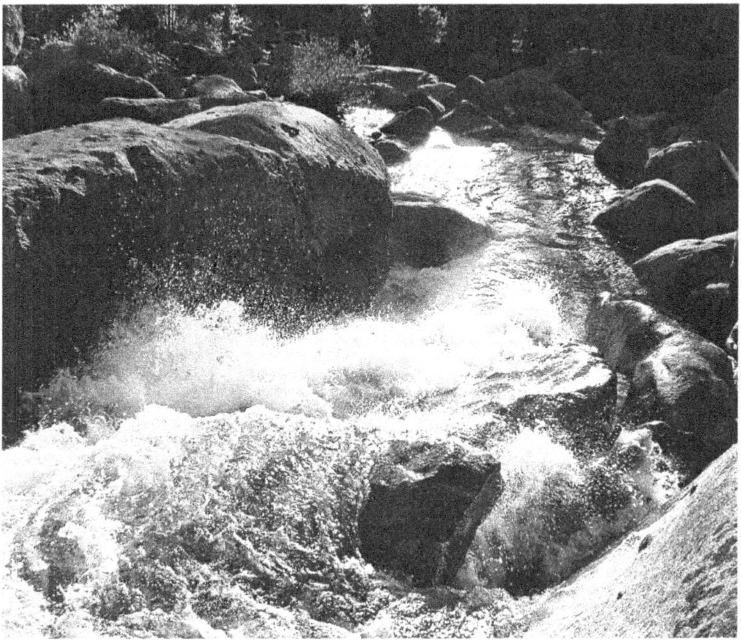

Caples Creek–Silver Fork Loop | TRAIL 40

The Silver Fork American River *tumbles over numerous cascades.*

opportunity to explore the stream, swim its pools, and stalk its wild trout.

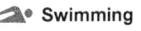 Swimming

After 1.11 miles, the trail breaks out of the forest into **Jake Schneider Meadow**, the largest meadow on your route. The tread can get sketchy later in the summer due to the high grass, but look for and head to a signpost in the middle of the meadow. This is the junction with Trail 17E71. The sign directs hikers straight ahead to the HAY MEADOW TRAIL and to the right, SILVER FORK ROAD—5.0 MILES. Decent campsites may be found if you turn right on this trail and proceed 100 yards toward the creek. ▶3 But your route continues straight, northeast on the Hay Meadow Trail 17E51, leaving Jake Schneider Meadow and Caples Creek behind. Almost immediately beyond Jake Schneider Meadow, the trail begins its first

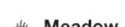 Meadow

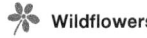 Wildflowers

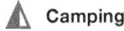 Camping

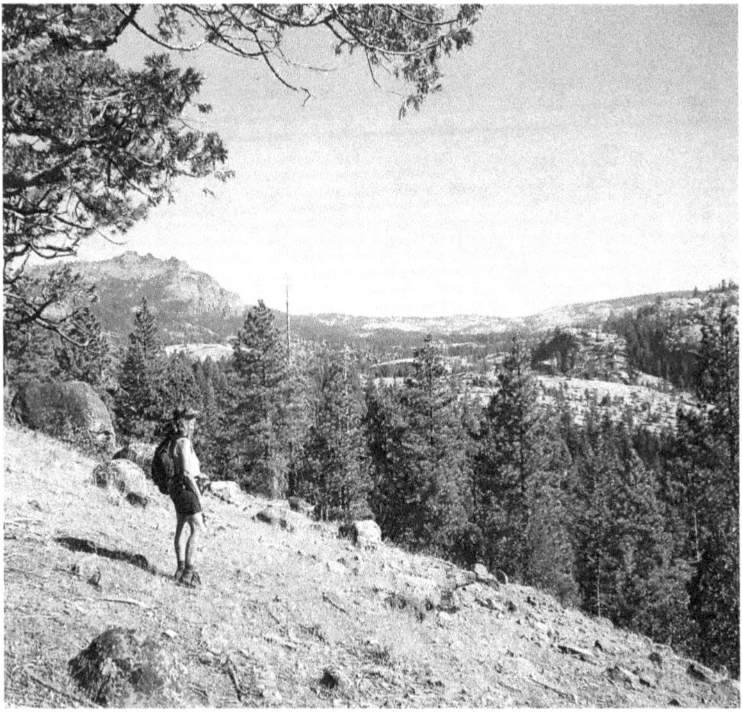

View of the upper Silver Fork Canyon and Thunder Mountain *from the Caples–Silver Fork Loop Trail*

major climb, up a draw with granitic ramparts on each side, shaded by an occasional Jeffrey pine.

In slightly more than 0.75 mile, the trail climbs 350 feet to the junction with Trail 17E20. A sign indicates that the Hay Flat Road is 3.0 miles straight ahead, ▶4 but your path is to the right on Trail 17E20, with the sign promising that **Government Meadow** is only 0.5 mile and the Silver Fork Road 3.0 miles. This trail proceeds 0.5 mile through fir and lodgepole forest southeast to Government Meadow, a stringer meadow carved by a seasonal creek. Another 0.5 mile down this trail brings you to Caples Creek. There is a good campsite on the north

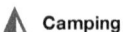
Camping

Caples Creek–Silver Fork Loop TRAIL 40

bank. The ford across the creek is shallow and easy most of the hiking season, but could be challenging during spring snowmelt.

After fording Caples Creek, the trail heads southwest and begins to climb 180 feet in elevation through a thick fir forest. Within another 0.5 mile, it reaches a seasonal pond. Unheralded by any signpost, there is a barely discernable junction with Trail 17E71 at this point. But your route continues straight to the southwest on Trail 17E20. After leaving the pond and unmarked trail junction, the trail begins to climb the steep south slope of Caples Creek canyon in earnest. Through a couple of steep pitches and switchbacks, the trail gains 400 feet in elevation over the next mile. As you climb, expansive views of the glacier-carved canyon provide a good excuse to pause and catch your breath.

Topping out in a forested flat, you reach the high point of the trail (6800 feet) and the junction with the **Old Silver Lake Trail** to your left. ▶5 A sign notes that this trail leads to Hwy 88 in about 2.0 miles, but your path continues straight forward on Trail 17E20 in a southwesterly direction, with the sign's promise that the Silver Fork is only 2.0 miles ahead. Within 0.25 mile of passing the Old Silver Lake Trail junction, the trail comes to the edge of the wide and scenic **Silver Fork** canyon. Go left about 100 yards off the trail to acquire a clear view of this U-shaped, glacier-carved canyon, which is dominated by a granite dome in the foreground and the dark volcanic bluffs above Silver Lake on the horizon. After enjoying the view, proceed back to the trail as it descends more than 400 feet into the Silver Fork canyon. After reaching the broad-bottomed Silver Fork canyon, the trail continues southeast for about 1.0 mile, eventually coming close to and paralleling the sparkling Silver Fork.

The trail and the canyon turn to the northwest and within 0.5 mile reach the junction with Trail

Stream

Steep

Canyon

Great Views

Stream

Sierra Nevada 317

River

Camping

Waterfall

17E63, which crosses the Silver Fork and heads south to Forgotten Flat. ▶6 From this junction, continue straight on Trail 17E20 as it follows the Silver Fork downstream. A sign optimistically promises that Caples Creek is only 1.0 mile and the trailhead only 2.0 miles away, but both are underestimates. The trail continues along the bank of the Silver Fork as it winds lazily through a series of deep pools (just begging to be fly-fished) overhung by large firs, cedars, and lodgepole pines. Potential campsites abound in the next 0.5 mile, but avoid using those that are less than 100 feet from the Silver Fork.

About 1.0 mile beyond the Forgotten Flat Trail junction, the Silver Fork canyon abruptly steepens as the Silver Fork begins to drop through a spectacular series of unnamed cataracts on its way to its confluence with Caples Creek. Above these falls, the trail clings to the steep slope, literally held in place by old-growth sugar pine, Douglas fir, and ponderosa. Some true giants flank the trail, permanently misted by the tumbling water nearby.

To avoid the cliff face that creates the Silver Fork cataracts, the trail turns northeast and traverses into the Caples Creek canyon. About a 0.5 mile past the Silver Fork cataracts, Trail 17E20 reaches the canyon floor and then crosses a footbridge spanning Caples Creek. Just beyond the footbridge, you return to the junction with Trail 17E51 in a small

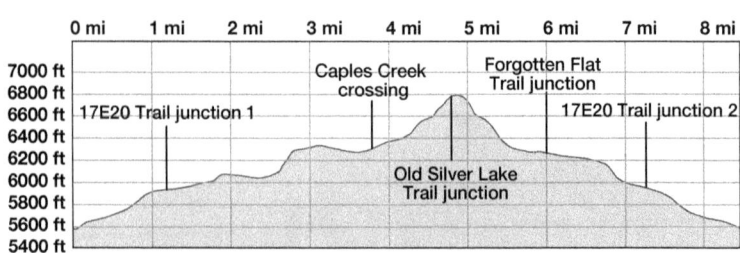

TRAIL 40 Caples Creek–Silver Fork Loop Profile

Caples Creek–Silver Fork Loop | TRAIL 40

meadow. You have just completed the Caples Creek/Silver Fork loop.

Turn left at the Trail 17E20/17E51 junction ▶7 and ▶8 proceed 1.2 miles back to the Silver Fork Road trailhead.

MILESTONES

- ▶1 0.00 Start at trailhead off Silver Fork Road
- ▶2 1.20 Junction with Trail 17E20, continue straight
- ▶3 2.31 Jake Schneider Meadow and Junction with Trail 17E71, continue straight
- ▶4 3.11 Junction with Trail 17E20, turn right
- ▶5 4.90 Junction with Old Silver Lake Trail, continue straight
- ▶6 6.18 Junction with Forgotten Flat Trail 17E63, continue straight
- ▶7 7.41 Junction with Trail 17E51, turn left
- ▶8 8.61 Return to trailhead

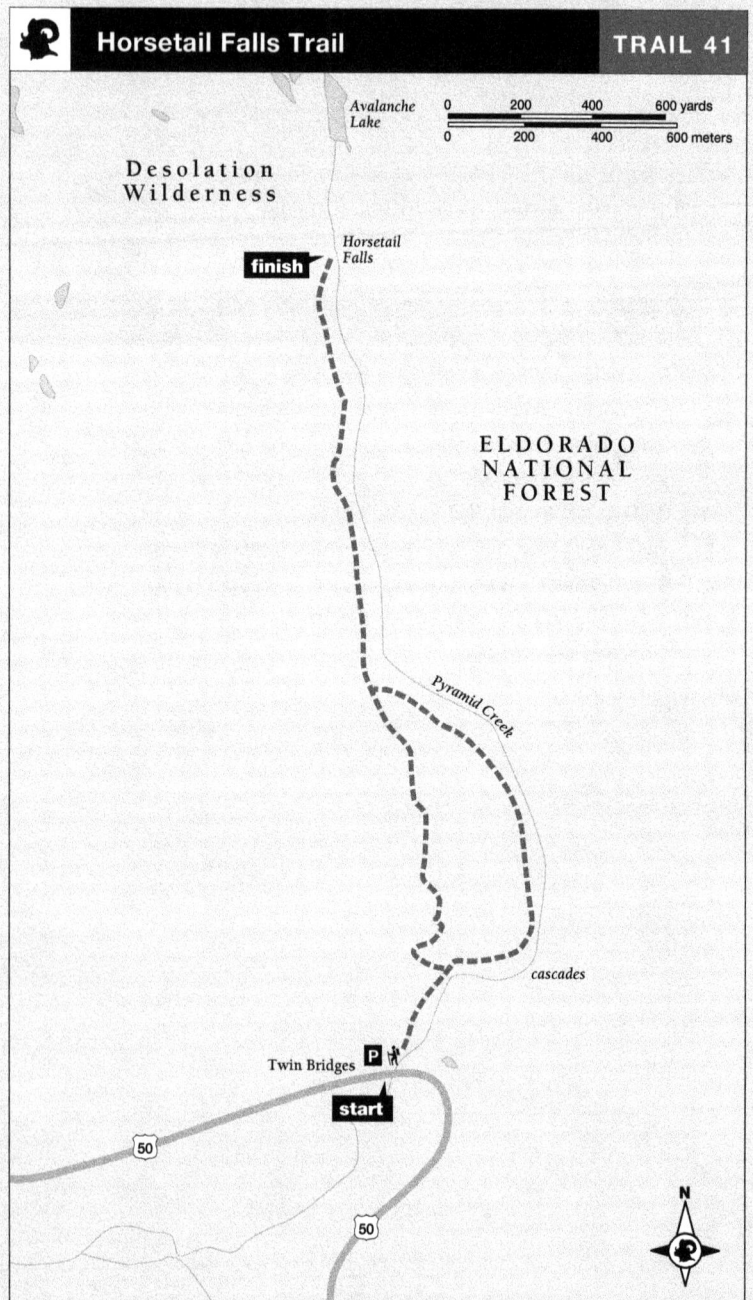

TRAIL 41 Sierra Nevada

Horsetail Falls Trail

Sacramentans desiring to view one of the most scenic waterfalls in the Sierra Nevada need only drive a short distance up Hwy 50 and hike 1.5 miles to visit spectacular Horsetail Falls. Easily one of the top 10 waterfalls in California, Horsetail competes with the falls of Yosemite Valley when it comes to scenic grandeur. Unfortunately, it also competes with Yosemite Valley in terms of crowds and parking fees. But its proximity to Sacramento and its easy access are hard to beat. Even if you don't make it all the way to the base of the falls, the cascades on lower Pyramid Creek make for a fine family outing.

Best Time

Horsetail Falls is at its booming best in June. Earlier hikers may hit snow. But the falls remain spectacular even during lower summer and fall flows. The typical hiking season is June-October.

Finding the Trail

From Sacramento, drive east 86 miles on Hwy 50. Just before the highway climbs out of the South Fork American River Canyon to ascend Echo Summit, turn left into the Twin Bridges/Horsetail Falls Trailhead parking area.

Logistics

There is a $3 fee for the use of the Twin Bridges/Horsetail Falls Trailhead parking area. Despite the implications of various maps and trail guides, the

---

TRAIL USE
Hike, Run, Bike
LENGTH
3.0 miles, 2–3 hours
VERTICAL FEET
±560
DIFFICULTY
- 1 **2** 3 4 5 +
TRAIL TYPE
Loop
SURFACE TYPE
Dirt
Rock

FEATURES
Dogs Allowed
Child Friendly
Parking fee
Stream
Waterfall
Canyon
Great Views
Photo Opportunities
Geology

FACILITIES
Toilets
Water

Horsetail Falls is the big kahuna of all Pyramid Creek drops.

Horsetail Falls Trail virtually disappears at Horsetail Falls. Several deaths have occurred from people climbing too close to the falls and slipping on permanently wet rock. It's best to appreciate the falls from a distance and from no closer than its base.

Trail Description

From the trailhead, ▶1 your route begins a moderate climb through cedars and firs, with a rich understory of bracken ferns. The trail alternates between decomposed granite, dirt, and granite bedrock. Some bedrock sections of the trail may be difficult to follow depending on the status of the ubiquitous "ducks" and stones lining the pathway edge. The trail follows **Pyramid Creek** through a wide canyon so newly scoured (at least in geologic terms) by a glacier that the creek has not had the time to create its own streambed. As a result, it often sheets over bedrock slabs and breaks into multiple channels as it searches for the quickest path downhill.

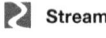 Stream

Within 0.25 mile, you reach the junction with the lower **Pyramid Creek Loop Trail**. ▶2 Since this provides an opportunity to see some creek cascades that are worth visiting, turn right at the sign that helpfully points your way to the CASCADE VISTA and follow the loop as it continues to climb alongside the creek. The trail crosses a large open bedrock area. To follow the trail, look for diamond-shaped plates hammered in the occasional tree and also ducks along the way. You can't go wrong if you stick pretty close to the creek on your right.

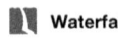 Waterfall

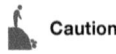 Caution

The trail comes to the first of a series of nearly continuous cascades that sheet over granite bedrock. These initial cascades can be easily reached with young children in tow, although great care should be taken to keep children well back from the cascades because they could easily be swept away in high flows. Above the granite bench to your left

Horsetail Falls Trail   TRAIL 41

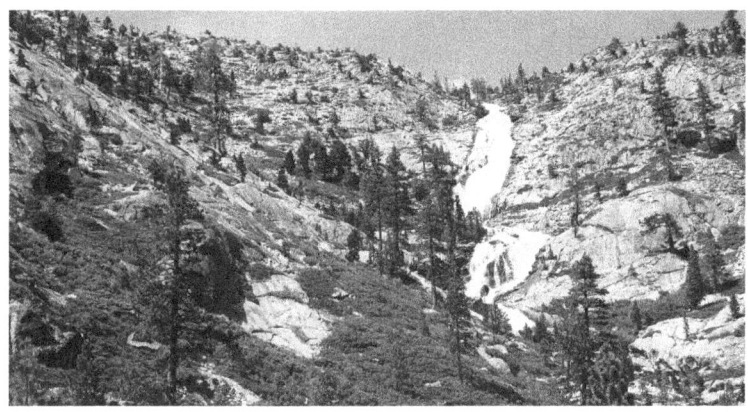

Horsetail Falls *tumbles into the wide glaciated valley drained by Pyramid Creek.*

(which your trail soon ascends), you can enjoy your first unobstructed view north of **Horsetail Falls**. Now turn around and take in the equally stunning view to the southwest of Lover's Leap and the upper American River canyon.

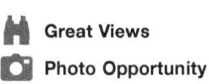

Great Views

Photo Opportunity

Following more of a route than a trail, continue northward parallel to Pyramid Creek, climbing steadily across a broad expanse of smooth granite bedrock. Footprints in frequent sandy sections of the trail, as well as infrequent ducks and diamond plates nailed in trees confirm that you are headed in the right direction. The trail climbs steadily upward and tops the granite bench or rock step. Perhaps for the first time, you may clearly see that you are standing in a broad valley scraped down to bedrock by a mighty force of nature. The U-shaped valley, landscape-sized rock steps, large boulders (known as "erratics") sitting on the land like forgotten toys left by a careless toddler, and the striations and polish of the bedrock underfoot are all classic symptoms of an area formerly covered by glacier, perhaps as recently as 14,000 years ago. In fact, geology professors use the Pyramid Creek area as an outdoor classroom to teach about classic Sierra Nevada glaciology.

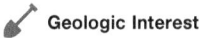

Geologic Interest

Sierra Nevada   323

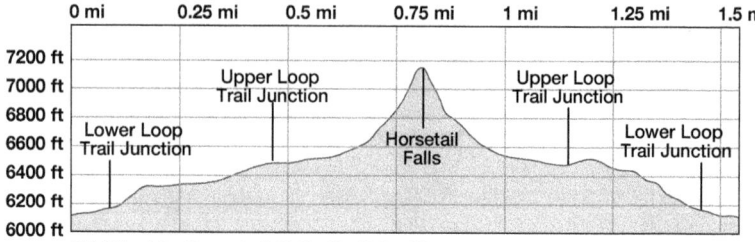

TRAIL 41 Horsetail Falls Trail Profile

Pots of newly created soil in the granite bedrock support small stands of lodgepole pines, firs, and an occasional giant Jeffrey pine. The trail becomes more distinct as it continues to climb and reaches the unsigned upper junction with the **Horsetail Falls Trail**. ▶3 Turn right, and within 100 yards, the trail reaches the boundary of the **Desolation Wilderness**. Fill out the required wilderness permit and place it in the box provided. Large granite slabs on the right offer a mixture of shady and sunny spots adjacent to the some of the mini-cascades and pools that characterize this section of Pyramid Creek. Another 150 yards up the trail, there is a deeper pool suitable for a quick (if bitingly cold) dip.

The trail continues climbing on rough, rocky tread and then enters a stand of Jeffrey pine, cedar, and fir, as well as the first quaking aspen on this route. The trail soon becomes indistinct but generally follows the base of the western canyon slope and the valley. During high flows, much of the trail is flooded in this section because of the creek's shallow and sometimes nonexistent streambed. Soon, the tread gives out altogether, as your route makes its way over granite jumbles, around flooded tree roots, and then between a large tilted rock slab on the right and the bedrock of the canyon wall rising to the left.

The climb steepens considerably, and the route, marked by occasional ducks, zigzags roughly upward requiring large steps over rocky shelves

- Stream
- Swimming

Horsetail Falls Trail | TRAIL **41**

and boulders. Soon, you come to pool at the base of Horsetail Falls. Find a sunny granite slab, plunk down, lean back to enjoy the spray booming off the rocks above, and have lunch. ▶4 All but the most skilled cross-country hikers should turn back at this point, as the route simply gets steeper, wetter, and more dangerous as it climbs steep and slippery cliffs past the falls.

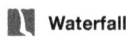 Waterfall

 Caution

Steep

To return, retrace your path to the wilderness boundary. ▶5 About 125 yards south of the boundary, turn right at the base of a large Jeffrey pine marking the upper junction with the Pyramid Creek Loop Trail. Continue downward on the main Pyramid Creek Trail over open bedrock punctuated by glacial erratics and scattered Jeffrey pines. When the trail reaches the lip of the rock bench, it switchbacks downward and then gets indistinct as it crosses more bedrock. Look for ducks that lead you more to the left, toward the base of the cascades you visited on your way up while following the lower Pyramid Creek loop. You will pick up the trail again in the manzanita field at the base of the slope. Ignore bogus routes that lead you to the right. Continue to veer left until you reach the lower junction with the Pyramid Creek Loop Trail. ▶6 Turn right and retrace your steps 0.25 mile back ▶7 to the trailhead parking area.

MILESTONES

- ▶1 0.00 Horsetail Falls Trailhead
- ▶2 0.25 Lower Junction with Pyramid Creek Loop, turn right
- ▶3 0.75 Upper Junction with Pyramid Creek Loop, turn right
- ▶4 1.50 Base of Horsetail Falls, retrace steps
- ▶5 2.25 Upper Pyramid Creek Loop junction, turn right
- ▶6 2.75 Lower Pyramid Creek Loop junction, turn right
- ▶7 3.00 Horsetail Falls Trailhead

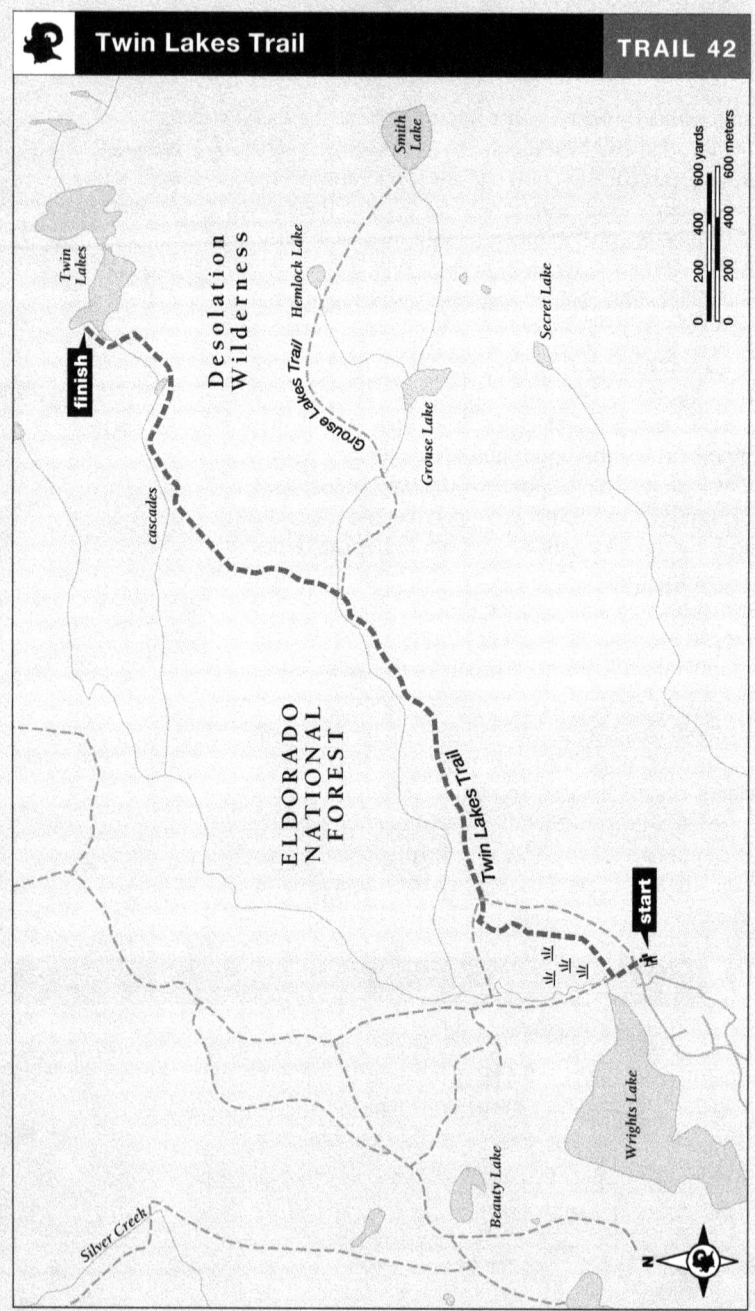

TRAIL 42 Sierra Nevada

Twin Lakes Trail: Desolation Wilderness

The relatively short but steep hike to Twin Lakes in the Desolation Wilderness is a classic alpine hike in the northern Sierra. The glaciated granite, sparse forest cover, cascading streams, and alpine lakes provide a true High Sierra feel, minus about 2000 feet in elevation. The destination—Lower Twin Lake—makes for a rewarding, if chilling, swim.

The trail is accessible from a comfortable base camp at scenic Wrights Lake. There are number of other hiking options from this trailhead and other nearby trails leading to the Desolation Wilderness. Although overnight camping is allowed at Twin Lakes and other nearby lakes, a wilderness permit is required, and the popularity of this trail makes a solitary wilderness experience unlikely.

Best Time

This trail is best visited July through October. The lower section of the trail may be accessible earlier in light-snow years, but even then count on slogging through snow once you get above 7500 feet. The best wildflower display is in July-August.

Finding the Trail

From Sacramento, take Hwy 50 east through Placerville, Pollock Pines, and the upper South Fork American River canyon. Approximately 77 miles from Sacramento and 4.5 miles east of the small community of Kyburz, turn left from Hwy 50 onto Wrights Lake Road (Note: This intersection is easy to miss. If you come to Twin Bridges and the Horsetail

TRAIL USE
Hike
LENGTH
5.0 miles, 3–6 hours
VERTICAL FEET
±1000
DIFFICULTY
- 1 2 3 **4** 5 +
TRAIL TYPE
Out & Back
SURFACE TYPE
Dirt
Rock

FEATURES
Wilderness Permit
Dogs Allowed
Mountain
Lakes
Stream
Waterfall
Wildflowers
Camping
Great Views
Steep

FACILITIES
Toilets
Water

> The peninsula at Lower Twin Lake is an excellent lunch spot, with warm rock slabs for sunning, a few trees for shade, and good access to the lake for swimming.

Falls Trailhead on Hwy 50, you have driven too far east). The paved Wrights Lake Road climbs steeply out of the canyon and is not advisable for large recreational vehicles or vehicles towing trailers. Drive north on Wrights Lake Road approximately 7.6 miles to the Wrights Lake Recreation Area. Just past the kiosk, turn right and cross the outlet creek from Wrights Lake, drive past the campground entrance on your right, and continue 0.8 mile as the narrow road follows the southeast shore of Wrights Lake to the trailhead parking area.

Logistics

Permits are required to enter the Desolation Wilderness. Day hikers may fill out a self-serve trailhead permit. Due to quota restrictions, overnight backpackers need to get a permit from the Forest Service before the trip. Wrights Lake makes an excellent base camp, but its campground sites get reserved early. To obtain an overnight wilderness permit or reserve space at a Wrights Lake campsite, call the Forest Service at (530) 644-6048.

Trail Description

From the trailhead parking area, ▶1 proceed through the gate and about 300 feet down the maintenance road. The road curves to the left, and the trail continues on toward a footbridge crossing Wrights Lake's inlet stream.

Just before the footbridge, ▶2 turn right on the **Twin Lakes Trail** (16E17). The trail skirts a wet meadow to the left and follows the base of a forested slope on the right. Look for columbine and other moisture-loving flowers on this flat segment of trail.

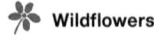
Wildflowers

The Twin Lake Trail meets up with the trail that forms a loop around the meadow system just

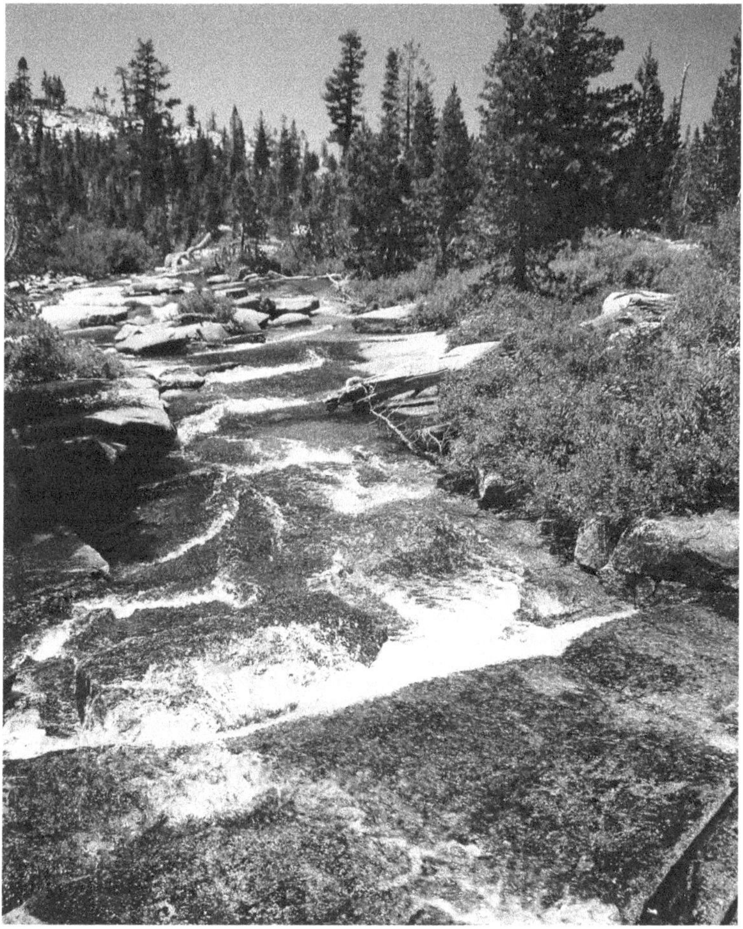

Twin Lakes Trail | TRAIL 42

The outlet creek from Twin Lakes *sluices downhill over a series of granite slabs.*

upstream of Wrights Lake. ▶3 Turn right. Almost immediately, the trail leaves the meadow area behind and begins climbing an open rocky slope covered in brush and dotted with Jeffrey pines. After climbing steeply about 400 feet, the trail approaches and parallels the outlet stream from **Grouse Lake**. The ascent moderates somewhat as the trail enters

 Steep

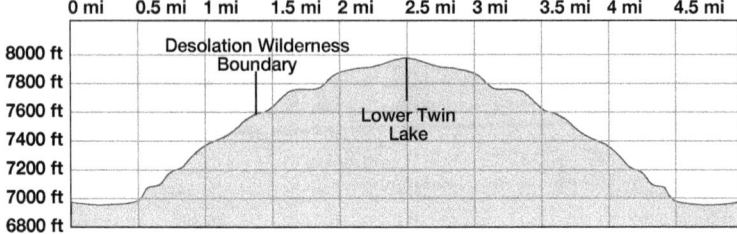
TRAIL 42 Twin Lakes Trail Profile

a lodgepole pine forest and then crosses into the **Desolation Wilderness** (marked by a sign).

The Twin Lakes Trail connects with the **Grouse Lakes Trail**, which heads off to the right. ▶4 Veer left to continue on the Twin Lakes Trail as the trail bends in a more northerly direction. The flatter terrain funnels runoff from the surrounding slopes across the trail, making the route indistinct in some places. Cross the Grouse Lake outlet stream and look for blazes on the trees and for ducks to guide your way as you approach a slope of granite slabs. The trail picks its way up through the slabs as it ascends 120 feet to another forested flat. The trail then bends in a northeasterly direction and nears the outlet stream from **Lower Twin Lake**.

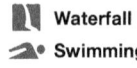
Waterfall
Swimming

Not far to the left of the trail, the stream plunges over a granite shelf into a cool inviting pool, providing an excellent spot to take in the scenery and catch your breath. ▶5 After visiting the waterfall, return to the trail and ascend a slope of granite slabs punctuated by occasional Jeffrey pines.

After climbing another 160 feet, the trail reaches yet another flat area, this one more alpine with its rocky ground covered and grass and few trees. Crossing the flat, the trail reaches ▶6 a pond, from which the outlet creek flows. The trail circles eastward around this shallow tarn, but early season hikers may have to pick their way across large flat rocks to cross the water. Past the pond, a relatively

Twin Lakes Trail   TRAIL 42

short climb over open granite brings you to within view of Lower Twin Lake, set in a scenic bowl of rugged granite slopes dominated by angular Mount Price to the southeast.

At this point, the trail bends north and ▶7 crosses the lake's outlet stream. Early season hikers may have trouble finding suitable stepping stones across the creek due to high flows. Use caution when crossing.

From the crossing, the trail proceeds across ▶8 a short peninsula jutting out into Lower Twin Lake. From here, hikers can explore both Lower and Upper Twin Lakes. Suitable campsites are found in the open area between the lakes. Alternatively, hikers may proceed east from Lower Twin Lake to small **Boomerang Lake** and on to much larger **Island Lake** (about 0.25 mile and 0.5 mile, respectively). Or you can linger at lakeside and soak up the sun before your return trip.

Retrace your steps ▶9 to the trailhead.

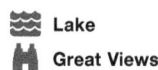

Lake
Great Views

Swimming
Camping

MILESTONES

- ▶1 0.00 Twin Lakes Trailhead, proceed north through gate
- ▶2 0.07 Junction with Twin Lakes Trail, turn right
- ▶3 0.46 Junction Wrights Meadow Loop Trail, turn right
- ▶4 1.36 Junction with Grouse Lake Trail, veer left
- ▶5 1.88 Waterfall, continue straight
- ▶6 2.21 Shallow pond, continue straight
- ▶7 2.41 Lower Twin Lake outlet crossing, continue straight
- ▶8 2.48 Lower Twin Lake peninsula
- ▶9 4.96 Retrace steps to trailhead

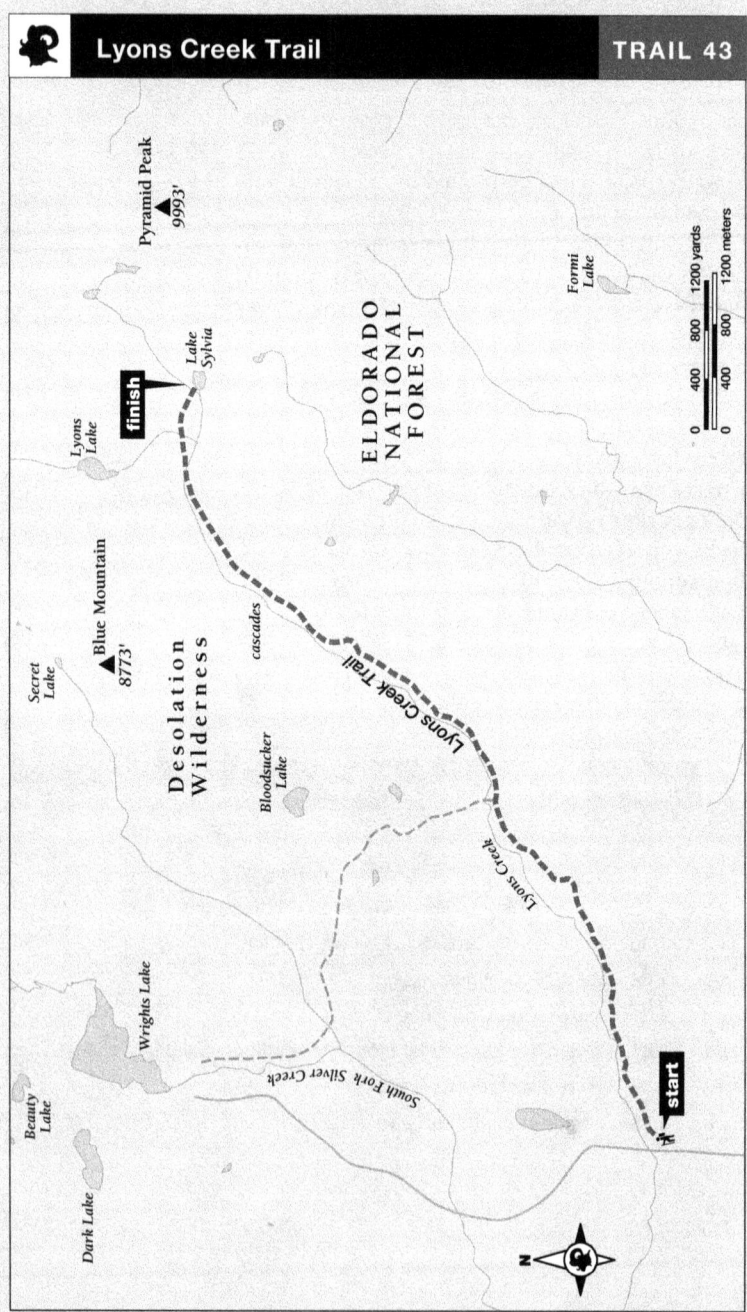

TRAIL 43 Sierra Nevada

Lyons Creek Trail: Desolation Wilderness

Although many people focus on the ultimate destinations of this trail—Sylvia and Lyons lakes in the Desolation Wilderness—its real attractions are the beautiful waterfalls and wildflowers along the way. The trailside cascades and flower-spangled meadows make the Lyons Creek Trail one of the more scenic routes into the Desolation Wilderness. Although it climbs higher than the nearby Twin Lakes Trail, it does so over twice the distance, which makes it a more moderate but diverse route into the Wilderness.

Best Time

This trail climbs from 6600 to over 8000 feet in elevation, so the typical hiking season is June–October. Depending on the snowpack, the lower portion of the trail can be largely snow free as early as June, but the upper portions may not open until mid-July. The best wildflower months are July and August.

Finding the Trail

From Sacramento, take Hwy 50 east through Placerville, Pollock Pines, and along the upper South Fork American River canyon. Approximately 77 miles from Sacramento and 4.5 miles east of the small community of Kyburz, turn left from Hwy 50 onto Wrights Lake Road. (Note: This intersection is easy to miss. If you come to Twin Bridges and the Horsetail Falls Trailhead on Hwy 50, you have driven too far east.) Wrights Lake Road climbs steeply out of the canyon and is not advisable for

TRAIL USE
Hike, Horse
LENGTH
10 miles, 5–7 hours
VERTICAL FEET
±1520
DIFFICULTY
- 1 2 3 4 **5** +
TRAIL TYPE
Out & Back
SURFACE TYPE
Dirt
Rock

FEATURES
Dogs Allowed
Wilderness permit required
Stream
Waterfall
Meadow
Wildflowers
Lakes
Camping
Great Views
Photo Opportunity
Steep

FACILITIES
None

The trail climbs gently up toward the granite fastness of the Desolation Wilderness through a shallow U-shaped valley, scoured by a glacier thousands of years ago.

large recreational vehicles or vehicles towing trailers. Drive north on Wrights Lake Road approximately 3.7 miles to the Lyons Creek Trailhead parking area, on your right.

Logistics

Mountain bikes are allowed on the first 3.0 miles of this trail, until it reaches the Desolation Wilderness boundary. Mountain bikes are prohibited in the Wilderness. Permits are required to enter the Desolation Wilderness. Day hikers may fill out a self-serve trailhead permit. Overnight backpackers need to get a permit from the Forest Service before the trip due to quota restrictions. To obtain an overnight wilderness permit, call the Forest Service at (530) 644-6048.

Trail Description

Fill out the wilderness permit found at the trailhead kiosk. ▶1 From the parking area, proceed east on the **Lyons Creek Trail** past the gate along a closed road for about 0.25 mile. The trail soon turns to single track and begins to climb slowly through firs and lodgepole pines. During mid-summer, the trail will be lined with lupine, giant red paintbrush, wandering daisy, arrowleaf groundsel, mule ears, cows parsnip, and many other types of wildflowers.

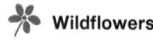
Wildflowers

The trail climbs up toward the **Desolation Wilderness** through a U-shaped valley. Lyons Creek is seldom seen but can usually be heard to your right for much of the trip. Occasional routes used by anglers and swimmers will lead away from the main trail down to **Lyons Creek**. The tread alternates between packed dirt, rocks, gravel, and sand, as it crosses several tributaries (only trickling by July). The trail continues to climb upward, usually gently, sometimes more steeply, but never intensely,

Lyons Creek Trail | TRAIL **43**

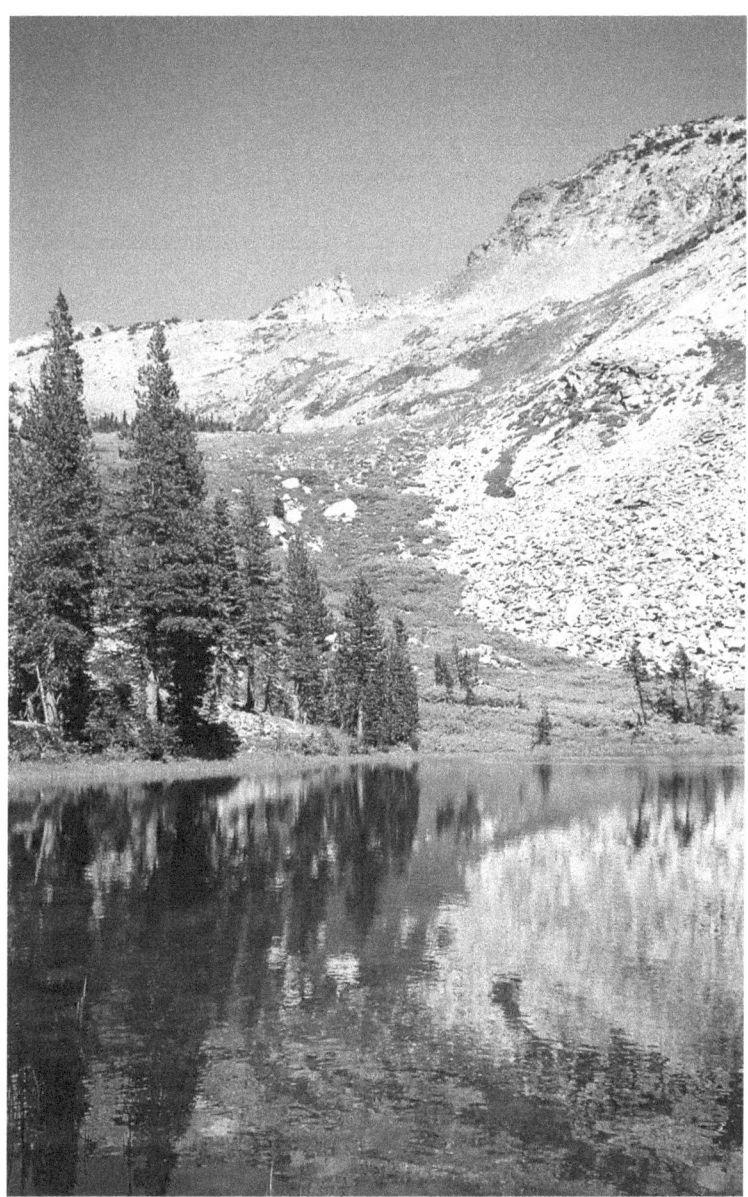

Serene Sylvia Lake *is the perfect destination, at the end of the Lyons Creek Trail.*

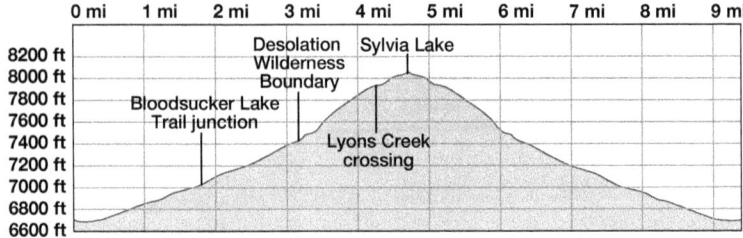

TRAIL 43 Lyons Creek Trail Profile

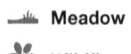 Meadow

🌸 Wildflowers

🅁 Stream

🅽 Waterfall

🏊 Swimming

through small stringer meadows splashed with wildflowers and groves of fir and lodgepole.

In slightly less than 2.0 miles, the trail reaches its junction with the **Bloodsucker Lake Trail**, ▶2 which leads off to the left (north). Continue east on the Lyons Creek Trail. In places, the trail works its way through fern-lined wet meadows and past seeps, which provide a fertile ground for colorful fireweed, columbine, tiger lily, larkspur, penstemon, and corn lily, as you continue your gradual but varying climb upward.

A bit over 3.0 miles from the trailhead, ▶3 the trail crosses into the Desolation Wilderness. The terrain becomes rockier and more open. To your left, Lyons Creek tumbles through some small cascades—but a more dramatic reach of the creek is just ahead. After briefly working its way through a forested area, the trail enters another section of open granite. About 0.66 mile east of the Wilderness boundary, the trail briefly parallels Lyons Creek, which cascades over a series granite ledges and slabs, occasionally forming deep pools perfect for dipping weary feet or swimming for the strong-hearted (the water is cold!). This section of the creek is a destination in its own right.

Refreshed from your dip in Lyons Creek, continue up the trail to the first and largest of three fords crossing Lyons Creek and its tributaries. Care must be taken in early season (particularly during snowmelt), but the crossing can typically be negotiated by boulder hopping after late July.

Beyond the first Lyons Creek crossing the trail enters a red-fir forest and within a few hundred yards, it reaches the Lyons Lake Trail junction, ▶4 which leads northward to your left. To go to Sylvia Lake, continue straight, where you soon cross the outlet creek from Lyons Lake. Again, by mid-season this crossing is usually negotiable via stepping-stones. The trail continues its climb through a largely fir forest, now peppered with shaggy hemlocks.

 Lake

Within 0.25 mile of the Lyons Lake Trail junction, your trail crosses the third and smallest tributary of Lyons Creek, just before climbing over a low ridge to reach ▶5 pretty and placid **Sylvia Lake**. The lake sits in a hemlock-lined basin, which offers several suitable campsites and, judging by the numerous surface strikes, supports a lively trout fishery.

 Lake

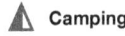 Camping

Retrace your steps to the parking area. ▶6 For those with the extra energy, a side trip to Lyons Lake offers dramatic views of nearby Pyramid Peak, but it will add an additional 1.4 relatively steep miles to your trip. In addition to being farther and higher than Sylvia Lake, Lyons Lake is nearly above tree line at 8400 feet and has few suitable campsites.

MILESTONES

▶1	0.0	Lyons Creek Trailhead
▶2	1.8	Bloodsucker Lake Trail junction, continue straight
▶3	3.1	Desolation Wilderness boundary, continue straight
▶4	4.3	Lyons Lake Trail junction, go straight, toward Sylvia Lake
▶5	5.0	Lake Sylvia
▶6	10.0	Retrace your steps to the trailhead

Appendix 1

Top Rated Trails

Great Valley Trails
Trail 2: River Walk Trail: Cosumnes River Preserve
Trail 10: Jedediah Smith Memorial Trail Loop: American River Parkway
Trail 11: Lake Natoma Loop: Folsom Lake State Recreation Area
Trail 13: Sacramento Waterfront Loop

Coast Range & Sierra Foothills Trails
Trail 15: Blue Ridge Trail: Cache Creek Natural Area
Trail 25: American Canyon Trail: Auburn State Recreation Area
Trail 22: Shingle Falls Trail: Spenceville Wildlife Area
Trail 23: Stevens Trail: North Fork American Wild & Scenic River

Sierra Nevada Trails
Trail 31: Mount Judah Loop Trail
Trail 34: Grouse Lakes Loop Trail
Trail 39: Winnemucca–Round Top Lakes Loop: Mokelumne Wilderness
Trail 40: Caples Creek–Silver Fork Loop: Caples Creek Proposed Wilderness

Appendix 2

Weekend Getaways

If you are looking for a 2–3 day weekend getaway from home, here are some suggested campground, overnight accommodation, and trail combinations.

Great Valley Getaways

Unfortunately, there is a dearth of public campgrounds in the Great Valley region. The best bet is the Sacramento Municipal Utility District's (SMUD) Rancho Seco Recreation Area Campground (RVs and tents). Phone: 24-hour information line at (209) 748-2318, or for reservations call (916) 732-4913. Website: www.smud.org/about/recreation/rancho.

To compensate for its lack of campgrounds, the Sacramento metropolitan area offers a wide variety of overnight accommodations. Check out the Delta King Hotel, in the historic *Delta King* Riverboat moored at the Old Sacramento waterfront. Phone (800) 825-5464. Website: www.deltaking.com.

Another option is the Lake Natoma Inn in Folsom, on the banks of beautiful Lake Natoma. Phone: (800) 808-5253, website: www.lakenatomainn.com.

Nearby Great Valley trails include the Howard Ranch Trail, River Walk Trail in the Cosumnes River Preserve, Sacramento Waterfront Loop in Old Sacramento, the Jedediah Smith Memorial Trail Loop, and the Lake Natoma Loop in the Folsom State Recreation Area.

Coast Range Getaways

Cache Creek Canyon Regional Park includes a nice family campground on the banks of Cache Creek. The park is at 1475 Hwy 16, Rumsey, CA 95679. For reservations, call the Yolo County Parks Department at

(530) 666-8775; reservation email is katherineweiss@yolocounty.com. Website: www.yolocounty.org/prm/cachecreekpark.htm.

For home-style accommodations, check out the Rumsey Canyon Inn. Phone: (530) 796-2400, website: www.rumseycanyoninn.com.

If you're looking for a zen/spa/clothing-optional experience, visit Wilbur Hot Springs. Phone: (530) 473-2306, website: www.wilburhotsprings.com.

For those looking for a bit of the big city in the country, there's the Cache Creek Casino Resort. Phone: (800) 452-8181, website: www.cachecreek.com.

Nearby Coast Range trails include the Blue Ridge Trail, the Cache Creek Ridge Trail, and the Redbud Trail.

Sierra Foothills Getaways

A favorite commercial campground for families and white-water rafters alike is Camp Lotus, on the banks of the South Fork American River in the Coloma-Lotus area. Phone: (530) 622-0103, website: www.camplotus.com.

The state operates the very rustic five-site Ruck-A-Chucky Campground on the Middle Fork American River in the Auburn State Recreation Area. Phone: (530) 885-4527, website: www.parks.ca.gov (use the site's search function to find the Auburn State Recreation Area page).

The BLM operates the South Yuba River Campground, which is one of the trailheads for the South Yuba River Trail. Phone: (916) 985-4474, website: www.blm.gov/ca/st/en/fo/folsom/yubacampground.

Check out the historic Sierra Nevada Inn in Coloma, which not only provides restful overnight accommodations but fine dining as well. Phone: (530)626-8096, website: www.sierranevadahouse.com.

Knowledgeable outdoors people recommend the Outside Inn in Nevada City. Phone: (530) 265-2233, website: www.outsideinn.com.

Nearby Sierra foothills trails include the Monroe Ridge–Monument Trail, Cronan Ranch Regional Park, Olmstead Loop Trail, American Canyon Loop, Western States-Riverview Trails, Codfish Falls Trail, Empire Mine Loop Trails, and Humbug–South Yuba River Trail.

Sierra Nevada Getaways

Public campgrounds abound in this region. Hikers visiting trails along Interstate 80 may want to camp at the 7400-foot-high Grouse Ridge Campground, near the trailhead for the Grouse Lakes Loop. Contact the Tahoe National Forest. Phone: (530) 288-3231, website: www.fs.fed.us/r5/

tahoe (click on Recreational Activities, Yuba River South District, Summer Fun for campsite and access info).

For Hwy 50 trails, try the centrally located Silver Fork Campground at the Caples Creek–Silver Fork Loop Trailhead. Contact the Eldorado National Forest. Phone: (530) 644-6048, website: www.fs.fed.us/r5/eldorado (click on Recreational Activities, Developed Campgrounds, Hwy 50 area south, Silver Fork Campground).

Woods Lake Campground is near the Winnemucca–Round Top Lakes Loop Trailhead and other Hwy 88 trailheads. Contact the Eldorado National Forest. Phone: (530) 644-6048, website: www.fs.fed.us/r5/eldorado (click on Recreational Activities, Developed Campgrounds, Hwy 50 area south, Woods Lake Campground).

All three campgrounds are first come, first served, and will likely fill quickly on summer weekends.

For overnight accommodations on I-80, check out the European-style Rainbow Lodge and its excellent restaurant, located in the Big Bend area. Phone: (800) 500-3871, website: www.royalgorge.com (click on Resort Info, Lodging, Rainbow Lodge).

For Hwy 50 trails, visit Strawberry Lodge on Hwy 50 in Kyburz. Phone: (530) 659-7200, website: www.strawberry-lodge.com.

There are several rustic resorts along Hwy 88 in the vicinity of Silver and Caples Lakes, but my favorite—Sorensen's Resort—is just over Carson Pass on Hwy 88 in Hope Valley. Phone: (800) 423-9949, website: www.sorensensresort.com.

Sierra Nevada trails adjacent to accommodations off Interstate 80 include the Grouse Lakes Loop, Salmon–Loch Leven Lakes Trail, Pacific Crest Trail to Castle Pass, and the Mount Judah Loop. Trails adjacent to accommodations along highways 50 and 88 include the Caples Creek–Silver Fork Loop, Horsetail Falls Trail, Twin Lakes Trail, Lyons Creek Trail, Winnemucca–Round Top Lakes Trail, Shealor Lake Trail, and Lake Margaret Trail.

Appendix 3

Governing Agencies

Tahoe National Forest (U.S. Forest Service)
Website: www.fs.fed.us/r5/tahoe
Supervisor's office: (530) 265-4531
Truckee Ranger District: (530) 587-3558
Yuba River Ranger District: (530) 288-3231
American River Ranger District: (530) 367-2224
Big Bend visitors center: (530) 426-3609

Eldorado National Forest (U.S. Forest Service)
Website: www.fs.fed.us/r5/eldorado
Supervisor's office: (530) 622-5061
Visitor information: (530) 644-6048
Amador Ranger District: (209) 295-4251
Placerville Ranger District: (530) 644-2324
Pacific Ranger District: (530) 644-2349

Bureau of Land Management Folsom Field Office
Website: www.blm.gov/ca/st/en/fo/folsom
Phone: (916) 985-4474

Bureau of Land Management Ukiah Field Office
Website: www.blm.gov/ca/st/en/fo/ukiah
Phone: (707) 468-4000

U.S. Fish and Wildlife Service—Stone Lakes National Wildlife Refuge
Website: www.fws.gov/stonelakes
Phone: (916) 775-4420

California State Department of Parks and Recreation

Website: www.parks.ca.gov (enter name of park in site's search function)
Auburn State Recreation Area: (530) 885-4527
Empire Mine State Historic Park: (530) 273-8522
Delta Meadows State Park: (916) 777-7701
Folsom State Recreation Area: (916) 988-0205
Malakoff Diggins State Historic Park: (530) 265-2740
Marshall Gold Discovery State Historic Park: (530) 622-3470
Old Sacramento State Historic Park: (916) 445-7387

California Department of Fish and Game

Gray Lodge State Wildlife Area
Website: www.dfg.ca.gov/lands/wa/region2/graylodge
Phone: (530) 846-7505
Spenceville Wildlife Area
Website: www.dfg.ca.gov/lands/wa/region2/spenceville
Phone: (530) 538-223

Sacramento County Department of Regional Parks

Website: www.sacparks.net/
Phone: (916) 875-6961

Yolo County Parks and Resources Management Division

Website: www.yolocounty.org/prm
Phone: (530) 666-8775

Sacramento Municipal Utility District—Rancho Seco Recreation Area

Website: www.smud.org/about/recreation
24-hour information line: (209) 748-2318,
camping reservations: (916) 732-4913

UC Davis Stebbins—Cold Canyon Reserve

Website: nrs.ucdavis.edu/stebbins
Phone: (530) 752-6949

Middle Mountain Foundation (Sutter Buttes)

Website: www.middlemountain.org
Phone: (530) 671-6116

Appendix 4

Major Organizations

American River Conservancy

A local group based in Coloma that acquires land to protect wildlife habitat and biodiversity. It also operates the American River Nature Center in Coloma, and features environmental education, stewardship programs, natural history, and outings programs.

Address: 348 Hwy 49, P.O. Box 562, Coloma, CA 95613
Phone: (530) 621-1224
Website: www.arconservancy.org

Auburn State Recreation Area Canyon Keepers (ASRACK)

Volunteers who conduct monthly hikes and meetings (open to the public) for those interested in learning more about the history and natural beauty of the American River Canyon. ASRACK also helps maintain and improve hiking trails in the area. Its website features more than 20 downloadable hiking guides.

Phone: (530) 885-3776
Website: http://members.psyber.com/asra//asrack.htm

California Wilderness Coalition

A statewide organization dedicated to protecting California's last wild places and native biodiversity. The CWC is active in developing public support for the protection of wild places statewide, including many of the areas that include trails featured in *Top Trails Sacramento*.

Address: 1212 Broadway, Suite 1700, Oakland, CA 94612
Phone: (510) 451-1450
Website: www.calwild.org

Cosumnes River Preserve

Managed as a joint project of The Nature Conservancy, the BLM, and several other government agencies and nonprofit groups. The Preserve offers many recreational, educational, and volunteer activities.

Address: 13501 Franklin Boulevard, Galt CA 95632
Phone: (916) 683-2142
Website: www.cosumnes.org

Effie Yeaw Nature Center

Has as its goal creating greater awareness, appreciation, and understanding of the natural and cultural resources of the Sacramento region. The Center offers a wide variety of activities and events for the general public and for school groups.

Address: 2850 San Lorenzo Way, P.O. Box 579, Carmichael, CA 95609
Phone: (916) 489-4918
Website: www.effieyeaw.org

Friends of the River

Statewide organization dedicated to the protection and restoration of California's rivers and watersheds, and to sustainable water use. Friends of the River has been particularly active in the protection of Sierra Nevada rivers, including the Yuba, American, and Mokelumne. It organizes annual events and operates a rafting program that trains volunteer white-water guides who lead educational raft trips for the public.

Address: 915 20th St., Sacramento, CA, 95814
Phone: (916) 442-3155
Website: www.friendsoftheriver.org

Mother Lode Chapter, Sierra Club

Local chapter of the Sierra Club, with 20,000 members and active local groups in Sacramento, Yolo, El Dorado, Placer, and Nevada counties. The chapter and its groups organize a variety of outings and programs and are actively involved in the conservation of local public lands, wildlife habitat, and other natural resources.

Address: 1414 K St., Suite 500, Sacramento, CA 95814
Phone: (916) 557-1100, Ext. 119
Website: www.motherlode-sierraclub.org

Protect American River Canyons

Local group based in Auburn that focuses on the protection of the North and Middle Forks of the American River. It organizes special events such as the annual Confluence Festival and seasonal outings.
    Address: P.O. Box 9312, Auburn, CA 95604
    Phone: (530) 885-8878
    Website: www.parc-auburn.org.

Sacramento Audubon Society

Local chapter of the Audubon Society, which promotes the protection, scientific study, enjoyment, and appreciation of wild birds, and provides proactive leadership in the conservation of open space in the Sacramento region. It owns and manages the Bobelaine Sanctuary and hosts weekly field trips that cover a wide variety of areas and birding experiences
    Address: P.O. Box 160694, Sacramento CA 95816
    Website: www.sacramentoaudubon.org

Sacramento Valley Conservancy

Local organization based in Sacramento and dedicated to the acquisition and preservation of open space. Among its many projects was the protection and acquisition of the Deer Creek Hills Reserve. The Conservancy leads outings in the Reserve and trains volunteer leaders and docents.
    Address: P.O. Box 163351, Sacramento, CA 95816
    Phone: (916) 216-2178
    Website: www.sacramentovalleyconservancy.org

Save the American River Association

Local group that spearheaded the establishment of the American River Parkway. Today SARA works to protect and enhance the Parkway's wildlife habitat, fishery, and recreational resources. A current focus is advocating for enhanced budgets and management of the parkway by Sacramento County.
    Address: P.O. Box 277638, Sacramento CA 95827
    Phone: (916) 387-1736
    Website: www.sarariverwatch.org

Sierra Forest Legacy

A coalition of groups working to ensure that the National Forests of the Sierra Nevada are managed in a way that protects and restores the forest ecosystem through the application of the best science, advocacy, and grassroots organizing.

Address: 915 20th St., Sacramento CA 95814
Phone: (916) 442-3155
Website: www.sierraforestlegacy.org

South Yuba River Citizens League

A local group based in Nevada City dedicated to the protection, preservation, and restoration of the entire Yuba River watershed. SYRCL is perhaps best known for the leading the campaign that designated the South Yuba a Wild & Scenic River. It hosts a variety of special events, raft trips, river cleanups, and monitorings.

Address: 216 Main St., Nevada City, CA 95959
Phone: (530) 265-5961
Website: www.syrcl.org

Stone Lakes National Wildlife Refuge Association

A nonprofit volunteer organization dedicated to supporting the refuge's mission of conserving, interpreting, and restoring the habitats and wildlife native to the Stones Lakes region.

Phone: (916) 775-4418
Website: www.stonelakes.org/nwr

Tuleyome

Takes its name from a Maidu word that means "Deep Home Place." Based in Yolo County, Tuleyome is dedicated to protecting the wild and agricultural heritage of the Putah and Cache Creek watersheds for existing and future generations. Among its many projects are Cache Creek Wild, which led the campaign that protected the Cache Creek Wild & Scenic River, and the Capay Valley Hiking Club, which schedules hikes on local trails in the Coast Range (visit www.yolohiker.org to view the current schedule).

Address: 607 North St., Woodland CA 95695
Phone: (530) 350-2599
Website: www.tuleyome.org

Appendix 5

Useful Resources

Books

Ambrose, Stephen E. *Nothing Like It in The World: The Men Who Built the Transcontinental Railroad, 1863–1869*. New York: Simon and Schuster, 2000.

Blackwell, Laird R. *Wildflowers of the Sierra Nevada and the Central Valley*. Edmonton, Canada: Lone Pine Publishing, 1999.

Hill, Mary. *Geology of the Sierra Nevada*. Berkeley and Los Angeles: University of California Press, 2006.

Protect American River Canyons (PARC). *Discover The American River Guide Book: North, Middle, and South Forks*. Auburn, CA, PARC. Website: www.parc-auburn.org/book.html.

Schaffer, Jeffrey P. *The Tahoe Sierra*, fourth ed. Berkeley, CA: Wilderness Press, 1998.

White, Mike. *Top Trails Lake Tahoe*. Berkeley, CA: Wilderness Press, 2004.

Websites

Boucher, Virginia. "Quail Ridge Reserve Geology," 2005, http://nrs.ucdavis.edu/Quail/Natural/geology.htm.

Moores, Eldridge M. and Judith E., "Geology of the Putah-Cache Region," 2001, http://bioregion.ucdavis.edu/book/geo_toc.html.

World Wildlife Fund, "Conservation Science: Terrestrial Ecosystems of the World," 2007, www.worldwildlife.org/science/ecoregions/terrestrial.cfm.

Appendix 6

Maps

Many people are using topo map programs that can be purchased at many outdoor stores. I used National Geographic's TOPO! Maps on CD-ROM to develop most of the base maps for this book. You can also print your own personalized maps using this program at REI for a fee. If you like maps, it's cheaper to buy the program and use it at home.

It is getting increasingly difficult to find stores or other walk-in outlets that carry and sell a decent selection of U.S. Geological Survey (USGS) 7.5 minute topographical quad maps. Fortunately, you can order USGS maps via the Internet from USGS and various online businesses. Visit www.topomaps.usgs.gov.

Most local National Forest recreation maps and wilderness maps published by the Forest Service can be found at outdoors stores. They are also available via the Internet by visiting www.fs.fed.us/recreation/nationalforeststore.

Outdoor clubs and organizations, trail enthusiasts, and local outdoor-related businesses offer a variety of maps via the Internet. Search for the name of the area or trail you are interested in and see what you get.

Maps for *Top Trails Sacramento*

Chapter 1: The Great Valley

Trail 1 **Bobelaine Sanctuary Trails:** Nicolaus 7.5 quad. Download a hand-drawn map of Sanctuary trails from the Sacramento Audubon Society at www.sacramentoaudubon.org.

Trail 2 **Riverwalk Trail, Cosumnes Preserve:** Bruceville 7.5 quad. Download a map from the Cosumnes River Preserve at www.cosumnes.org.

Trail 3 **Deer Creek Hills Preserve Trails:** Folsom SE 7.5 quad. Download a general-location map from the Sacramento Valley Conservancy at www.sacramentovalleyconservancy.org.

Trail 4 **Delta Meadows and Locke Trail:** Courtland 7.5 quad.

Trail 5 **Effie Yeaw Natural Area Trails:** Carmichael 7.5 quad. Download a simple trail system map from the Effie Yeaw Nature Center at www.effieyeaw.org.

Trail 6 **Gibson Ranch Trails:** Rio Linda 7.5 quad.

Trail 7 **Wetlands Discovery and Loop Trails, Gray Lodge:** Pennington 7.5 quad. Download simple trail maps of the Gray Lodge State Wildlife Area at www.dfg.ca.gov/lands/wa/region2/graylodge.

Trail 8 **Sutter Buttes Trails:** Sutter Buttes, Sutter, Pennington, and Meridian 7.5 quads. Download a simple location map at www.middlemountainfoundation.org.

Trail 9 **Howard Ranch Trail:** Goose Creek 7.5 quad. Download a simple trail map from SMUD at www.smud.org/about/recreation.

Trail 10 **Jedediah Smith Memorial Trail Loop:** Carmichael 7.5 quad. Download an American River Parkway map from Sacramento County Parks at www.sacparks.net.

Trail 11 **Lake Natoma Loop:** Folsom 7.5 quad. Download an American River Parkway map that includes the Natoma Unit of the Folsom Lake State Recreation Area at www.sacparks.net.

Trail 12 **Sacramento Northern Bikeway:** Sacramento East and Rio Linda 7.5 quads.

Trail 13 **Sacramento Waterfront Loop:** Sacramento East and West 7.5 quads.

Trail 14 **Wren Wetlands Trail, Stones Lakes Refuge:** Florin 7.5 quad. Download a map of the refuge from the U.S. Fish and Wildlife Service at www.fws.gov/stonelakes/refugemap.

Chapter 2: The Coast Range

Trail 15 **Blue Ridge Trail:** Glascock Mtn. 7.5 quad. Download a Blue Ridge Trail map at www.yolohiker.org.

Trail 16 **Cache Creek Ridge Trail:** Wilson Valley and Glascock Mtn. 7.5 quads. Download a Cache Creek Ridge Trail map at www.yolohiker.org.

Trail 17 **Redbud Trail:** Lower Lake 7.5 quad. Download a Redbud Trail map at www.yolohiker.org.

Trail 18 **Cold Canyon–Blue Ridge Loop:** Monticello Dam and Mt. Vaca 7.5 quads. Download a Cold Canyon Loop Trail map at www.yolohiker.org.

Chapter 3: Sierra Foothills

Trail 19 **North Yuba Trail:** Goodyears Bar 7.5 quad. Purchase the Forest Service's Tahoe National Forest map and National Geographic's Tahoe National Forest–Yuba & American Rivers map at outdoors stores.

Trail 20 **Humbug Creek–South Yuba Trails:** North Bloomfield 7.5 quad. Purchase the Forest Service's excellent South Yuba River Recreation Guide (map), as well as the Tahoe National Forest map and National Geographic's Tahoe National Forest–Yuba & American Rivers map at outdoors stores.

Trail 21 **Osborn and Hardrock Loops, Empire Mine State Park:** Grass Valley 7.5 quad. Download a simple trail map at www.empiremine.org/trails. Get detailed maps at the park's visitors center.

Trail 22 **Shingle Falls Trail:** Camp Far West and Wolf 7.5 quads. Download a simple trail map at www.dfg.ca.gov/lands/wa/region2/maps/spenceville.

Trail 23 **Stevens Trail:** Chicago Park, Dutch Flat, Colfax, and Foresthill 7.5 quads. Most of the trail (except for the trailhead) is on the Auburn State Recreation Area map by Sowarwe-Werher, which is available at REI. Download a simple brochure and trail map at www.psyber.com/~asra/tgsteven.pdf.

Trail 24 **Codfish Falls Trail:** Greenwood 7.5 quad. Purchase the excellent Auburn State Recreation Area Topographic Trail Map by Sowarwe-Werher at REI. Download a simple description and map of this trail at http://members.psyber.com/asra//guides.htm.

Trail 25 **American Canyon Trail:** Greenwood 7.5 quad. Purchase the excellent Auburn State Recreation Area Topographic Trail Map by Sowarwe-Werher at REI. Download a simple description and map of this trail at http://members.psyber.com/asra//guides.htm.

Trail 26 **Western States Trail–El Dorado Canyon:** Michigan Bluff 7.5 quad. Purchase the Forest Service's Tahoe National Forest map and National Geographic's Tahoe National Forest–Yuba & American Rivers map at outdoors stores.

Trail 27 **Western States Trail–Riverview Trails:** Auburn 7.5 quad. Purchase the excellent Auburn State Recreation Area Topographic Trail Map by Sowarwe-Werher at outdoors stores.

Trail 28 **Olmstead Loop Trail:** Auburn and Pilot Hill 7.5 quads. Purchase the excellent Auburn State Recreation Area Topographic Trail Map by Sowarwe-Werher at outdoors stores. Download a simple description and map of this trail at http://members.psyber.com/asra//guides.htm.

Trail 29 **Cronan Ranch Loop:** Coloma 7.5 quad. Download a good trails map from www.coloma.com/recreation/cronan-ranch-map.gif.

Trail 30 **Monroe Ridge–Monument Trails, Marshall Gold Discovery State Historic Park:** Garden Valley 7.5 quad. Pick up a trail map at the park's visitors center.

Chapter 4: Sierra Nevada

Trail 31 **Mount Judah Loop Trail:** Norden 7.5 quad. Purchase the Forest Service's Tahoe National Forest map and National Geographic's Tahoe National Forest–Sierra Buttes/Donner Pass map at outdoors stores.

Trail 32 **Pacific Crest Trail to Castle Peak:** Soda Springs, Norden 7.5 quads. Purchase the Forest Service's Tahoe National Forest map and National Geographic's Tahoe National Forest–Sierra Buttes/Donner Pass map at outdoors stores.

Trail 33 **Salmon Lake Trail to Loch Leven Lakes:** Soda Springs 7.5 quad. Purchase the Forest Service's Tahoe National Forest map and National Geographic's Tahoe National Forest–Yuba & American Rivers map at outdoors stores.

Trail 34 **Grouse Lakes Loop Trail:** Graniteville, English Mtn. 7.5 quads. Purchase the Forest Service's Tahoe National Forest map and National Geographic's Tahoe National Forest–Sierra Buttes/Donner Pass map at outdoors stores.

Trail 35 **Picayune Valley Trail:** Granite Chief 7.5 quad. Purchase the Forest Service's Tahoe National Forest map and National

Geographic's Tahoe National Forest–Yuba & American Rivers map at outdoors stores.

Trail 36 **Lake Margaret Trail:** Caples Lake 7.5 quad. Purchase the Forest Service's Eldorado National Forest map and Mokelumne Wilderness map (which includes this adjacent area) at outdoors stores.

Trail 37 **Granite and Hidden Lakes Loop:** Caples Lake 7.5 quad. Purchase the Forest Service's Eldorado National Forest map and Mokelumne Wilderness map (which includes this adjacent area) at outdoors stores.

Trail 38 **Shealor Lake Trail:** Tragedy Spring 7.5 quad. Purchase the Forest Service's Eldorado National Forest map and Mokelumne Wilderness map (which includes this adjacent area) at outdoors stores.

Trail 39 **Winnemucca–Round Top Lakes Loop:** Caples Lake and Carson Pass 7.5 quads. Purchase the Forest Service's Eldorado National Forest map and Mokelumne Wilderness map at outdoors stores.

Trail 40 **Caples Creek–Silver Fork Loop:** Tragedy Spring, Caples Lake 7.5 quads. Purchase the Forest Service's Eldorado National Forest map at outdoors stores.

Trail 41 **Horsetail Falls Trail:** Pyramid Peak, Echo Lake 7.5 quads. Purchase the Forest Service's Eldorado National Forest map and Desolation Wilderness map (which includes this adjacent area) at outdoors stores.

Trail 42 **Twin Lakes Trail:** Pyramid Peak 7.5 quad. Purchase the Forest Service's Eldorado National Forest map and Desolation Wilderness map (which includes this adjacent area) at outdoors stores.

Trail 43 **Lyons Creek Trail:** Pyramid Peak 7.5 quad. Purchase the Forest Service's Eldorado National Forest map and Desolation Wilderness map at outdoors stores.

Index

adobe lily 141
Alder Creek 93
Allen Camp Trail 296–297
Alumni Grove 87
American Canyon 201, 202
    American Canyon Creek 203–205
    American Canyon Trail 201–205
American River 53, 56, 77, 85, 88, 89, 94, 96, 102, 112
    American River canyons 221
    American River Conservancy 229
    American River, Middle Fork 201, 204–205, 282
    American River, North Fork 193–195, 197, 198, 199, 213
    American River, North Fork of the Middle Fork 210
    American River, Silver Fork 314
    American River, South Fork 229, 230, 231, 235, 236
    American River Parkway 4, 53, 56, 85, 86, 102, 107
Ancil Hoffman County Park 53
Aquatic Center 96, 97
Arcade Creek 103
Arguello, Don Luis 76
Auburn coffer dam 215, 218
Auburn Dam 213, 215, 216, 221
Auburn State Recreation Area 197, 201, 213, 221, 222, 226

Baton Flat 145
Baton Flat "badlands" 144
Beale Air Force Base 185
Beals Point 85, 88
Bear Creek 137, 139
Bear Flag Revolt 76
bears 12
Berryessa Peak 127

Berryessa Reservoir 147, 150, 151
Betsy Mine 182
Betty Adamson Observation Hide 69
Big Gun Diggings 208, 210
Bloodsucker Lake Trail 337
blue oak 5
Blue Ridge 127, 129, 130, 149, 150, 151
    Blue Ridge Trail 127–131
Bobelaine Audubon Sanctuary 29
Boomerang Lake 331
Bourne Jr., William Bowers 181
Bureau of Land Management (BLM) 35, 121, 133, 141, 143, 150, 191, 229
Bureau of Reclamation 221

Cache Creek 128, 133, 137, 138, 144, 145
    Cache Creek Canyon 130
    Cache Creek Natural Area 127, 133
    Cache Creek, North Fork 143
    Cache Creek Ridge Trail 133–139
    Cache Creek watershed 121
    Cache Creek Wild & Scenic River 127, 129, 141
    Cache Creek Wilderness 133, 135, 136, 138, 141
California Central Valley Grasslands Ecoregion 3–5
California Conservation Corps 79
California Department of Fish and Game 35, 65, 141, 143
California Department of Parks and Recreation 94
California State Railroad Museum 111
California State University, Sacramento 87
California Wild & Scenic Rivers System 127, 133
California Woodlands and Interior Chaparral Ecoregion 5–7, 121

Callumah 239
Canyon Creek, South Fork 275, 276, 278
Cape Horn 192
Caples Creek 288, 313, 314, 315, 316, 317, 318
  Caples Creek, North Fork 290
  Caples Creek Proposed Wilderness 287, 301, 302, 313
  Caples Creek, South Fork 288
  Caples Creek-Silver Fork Loop 313–319
Carson, Kit 76
Carson Pass Trail 309
Castle Creek 261, 262
Castle Pass 263
  Castle Pass Truck Road 262
Castle Peak 259, 263
Castle Peak Wilderness 259
Castle Valley 261, 263
Center Trail 30–31, 32, 33
Central Pacific Railroad 192
Central Park 104
chaparral 5, 7
Cherry Point Trail 270
Chicken Hawk Ridge 210
Chinese Taoist Temple 239
Coast Range 121–151
Codfish Canyon 199
Codfish Creek 199
Codfish Falls Trail 197–199
Coffer Dam Trail 224
Cold Canyon 151
  Cold Canyon-Blue Ridge Loop Trail 147–151
Cold Creek 148, 149
Coldstream Canyon 257
Coldstream Valley 255
Colfax 191
Coloma Valley 235, 236, 238
Conlon Mine Spur Trail 182
Cool 222, 224, 227
Cool quarry 217
Cosumnes River 35, 38
Crandall, Lake 30, 33
Crevis Creek 43
Cronan Ranch Loop 229–233
Cronan Ranch Regional Park 230
Cronan Ranch Regional Trails Park 229
Cronan Ranch Road 233

Crooked Lakes 277
  Crooked Lakes Trail 276
Crystal Range 296

Daisy Hill Mine 183
Dead Truck Trail 204
Deadwood mining camp 208, 211
Deer Creek 42
Deer Creek Hills Preserve 41–45
Del Paso Heights 99, 103
Delta King 108–109, 112
Delta Meadows State Park 47, 49
Delta smelt 48
Desolation Wilderness 313, 324, 327, 330, 333, 334, 336
Deterding Woods 56
Devil's Canyon Creek 165
Discovery Museum and History Center 111
Discovery Park 85, 88, 107, 112
  Discovery Park Bike Path 112
Discovery Trail 55, 57
Dolloy Museum 51
Donner Pass 253
Donner Peak 257
Down and Up Trail 230, 231
Downey Lake 275
Dry Creek 59–60, 63, 99, 104, 186, 188, 189
  Dry Creek Parkway 59, 104
  Dry Creek Trail 60–61, 63
Ducks Unlimited 35
Dunfield Flat 136, 137

East Ridge Trail 230, 231, 233
Edwards Crossing 175
Effie Yeaw Natural Area 53
Effie Yeaw Nature Center 53–57
El Dorado bed straw 6
El Dorado Canyon 207, 210–211
  El Dorado Canyon Creek 211
El Dorado mule-ear 6
Elverta 99
Elverta Road 61
Embassy Suites Hotel 108
Empire Mine State Historic Park Loop Trails 177–183

Empire St. 181
  Empire St. Trail 181
encephalitis 12
Esto Yamani 75

Fairbarn Water Intake Structure 87
Fairy Falls 185
Farallon Plate 2
Feather River 31, 32, 33
fire 8
Folsom-Auburn Bridge 94
Folsom, J.L. 96
Folsom Lake State Recreation Area 85, 88, 91, 94
Folsom Light Rail Station 95
Folsom-South Canal 94, 97
Foresthill Bridge 221
Forgotten Flat Trail 318
Fourth of July Lake Trail 310
Fremont, John C. 77
freshwater marsh 35

gabbro soils 6
Gibson Lake 59, 62
  Gibson Lake Loop 62
Gibson Ranch Regional Park 59
Glacier Meadow Interpretive Loop Trail 260
gold 1–2
  discovery of 8, 77, 229, 235
Gold Discovery Trail 239
Gold Rush 45, 91, 96, 155, 163, 169, 186, 201, 208, 229, 235
Gold Rush toll road 191
Goodyear's Bar 164, 165
Gopher Ridge volcanics 44
Government Meadow 314, 316
Granite and Hidden Lakes Loop 293–299
Granite Chief Wilderness 281, 282
Granite Lake Trail 295
Grasslands Trail 31
gravestone schist 223
Gray Lodge Wildlife Area 65
Great Ice Age 2
Great Valley 19–117
  grassland 79
  sequence 2

Greenwood Creek 231, 233
Grouse Lake 330
  basin 274
  outlet stream 330
Grouse Lakes Loop Trail 273–279
Grouse Ridge 279
  Grouse Ridge Campground 274
  Grouse Ridge Trail 274, 279
Guy West Bridge 87, 88

Hardrock Loop Trail 178–181
Harry Adamson Observation Hide 69
Hay Meadow Trail 17E51 315, 318
Hazel light rail station 93
Hell Hole Dam 218
Hidden Lake 296
Hidden Valley Cutoff Trail 233
Hoboken Creek 204
Horsetail Falls 321, 323
  Horsetail Falls Trail 321–325
Howard, Charles 79
Howard Ranch 81
  Howard Ranch Trail 79–83
Howe Avenue bridge 87, 88
Howe Avenue parking area 87
Hudson Bay Company 76
Humbug Creek (North Yuba River) 166–167
Humbug Creek (South Yuba River) 169–171
Humbug Creek-South Yuba Trails 169–175
Humbug Falls 172
Humbug Trail 169, 171

I Street Bridge 109–111, 112
Illinois Bar campsite 174
Illinoistown 194
Indian villages 5
Ione formation 44
Iowa Hill 194, 194
Island Lake 276, 331

Jake Schneider Meadow 315
Jedediah Smith Memorial Trail 85–89, 102

Joe Shoong School 51
Judge Davis Trail 135

Kadema Indian Village 88, 89
Kennebec Creek 175
    Kennebec Creek Trail 174–175
    mining road 175
Kiel, Eric 194
Knickerbocker Creek 224–225, 227
    Knickerbocker Creek Trail 221

La Grange 111
Lake Margaret Trail 287–291
Lake Natoma 91, 93
    Lake Natoma Inn 94
    Lake Natoma Loop 91–97
    Lake Natoma Unit 93, 97
Lake Tahoe 253
Last Chance mining camp 208
Leidesdorff, William 96
Little Wolf Creek 179, 180
Loch Leven Lakes 265
    High 271
    Loch Leven Lakes Trail 269–270
    Lower 269
    Middle 269–270
Locke 47, 50–51
Long Lake 276
Los Picachos 76
Lost Cabin Mine 310–311
Lotus Ditch 236
Lower Loop Trail 188
Lyme disease 12
Lyons Creek Trail 333–337
Lyons Lake Trail junction 337

Magpie Creek 103
Maidu Indians 75–76
Malakoff Diggins 173
Marsh Wren Wetland 117
Marshall Gold Discovery State Historic Park Loop 235–239
Marshall Monument 237, 238
marshlands 3–4
Marysville 185
Matthew McKinley 109

Maytag Rapid 167
McNabb cypress 6
Mediterranean climate 3
Mediterranean grasses 6
Merhoff, Ada 129
Michigan Bluff 208
Michigan City 208
Middle Lake 279
Middle Mountain Foundation 73
Middle Slough 37
Milk Lake 275, 276
    Milk Lake Spur Trail 275
mining history 177
Minkalo Trail 294, 298, 299
Mississippi Bar 96
mixed conifer forest 7
Mokelumne Wilderness 293, 296, 308, 313
Monroe Family homesite 236
Monroe Orchard 236
Monroe Ridge Trail 235, 236
Monument Trail 235
Moraga, Gabriel 76
mosquitoes 12
Mount Judah Loop Trail 253–257
mountain lions 12–13
Mountain Quarries (No Hands) Bridge 213, 218, 219
Mountain Quarries Railroad 213, 217
Muir, John 237

National Forest lands 237
National Forest System 8
National Register of Historic Places 191, 208–209, 219
National Wildlife Refuge System 115
Native Americans 8
native grasslands 5
Natomas East Main Drain Canal 102
Nature Conservancy, The 35, 79
Negro Bar 96
    Negro Bar Group Campground 94
Newark 109
Nimbus Dam 94, 96
Nimbus Fish Hatchery 97
Nisenan Indians 53, 88, 239
Noralto 99, 103
North American Plate 2

North Beach parking area 236
North Butte 75
North Canyon Creek 173–174
North Canyon Spur Trail 174
North Fork canyon 215, 217
North Trail 31, 32
North Valley Trail 187
North Yuba River Trail 163–167

Oak Forest loop 38
Oak Trail 30
oak woodlands 5
Observation Trail 55–57
old-growth forests 8
Old Sacramento 107, 108, 112
Old Silver Lake Trail 317
Olmstead Loop Trail 221–227
ophiolite 1
ophiolite basement 2
Osborn Crosscut Trail 182
Osborn Hill Loop Trail 179, 181–183
Osborn Hill Road 182
Otter Trail 30–31
Overlook Point picnic area 174

Pacific Crest Trail (PCT) 253, 254
Pacific Flyway 4, 65
Pacific Plate 2
Pan Ravine 171
Park Loop Trail 61
Payne Ranch 133
Penn Gate Trailhead 178, 181
Penner Lake 277
Pennsylvania Mine 178
perennial bunchgrasses 5–6
Perkins Creek 143
Perkins Ridge Trail 144
Picayune Falls 285
Picayune Valley 281, 283
    Picayune Valley Creek 284–285
    Picayune Valley Trail 281–285
Pine Hill flannelbrush 6
Plasse's Resort 297, 298
plate tectonics 1
poison oak 11–12
Pond, William B. 56
Ponderosa Bridge 198

Pony Express 110
Poor Man's Canyon Creek 210
Poverty Bar 205
Powerline Trail 182
Prescott Mine Loop Trail 181–182
purple martins 111
Putah Creek watershed 121, 147
Pyramid Creek 321–325
    Pyramid Creek Loop Trail 322, 325

Quarry Trail 223

Rancho Seco Lake 80, 83
Rancho Seco nuclear power plant 80, 83
Rancho Seco Park 79, 81
Range of Light 237
rattlesnakes 12
Rayhouse Road 128
Redbud Trail 141–145
red fir forests 7
Ringtail Bypass 33
Rio Linda 99, 104
    train station 104
Rio Linda-Elverta Community Center
        Park 104
riparian forests 4, 35
riparian habitat 30
riparian vegetation 6
riparian woodlands 3
River Walk 107, 109–110
    River Walk Loop 37
    River Walk Trail 35, 36–39
Riverview History Trail 55–57
Robbers Ravine 192, 194
Robie Point 216
Robla 99, 103
Robla Creek 103
Rock Lake Trail 277
Rocky Creek 145
Rocky Rest parking area 167
Roller Pass 255
Round Lake 275, 276
Round Top Lake 307, 308, 310
    Round Top Lake Trail 309
Round Top Peak 310

Sacramento County 99
Sacramento Municipal Utility District (SMUD) 79
Sacramento Northern Bikeway 99–105
Sacramento Northern Railroad 99, 100–101
Sacramento River 85, 88, 107, 110, 112
    Sacramento River Overlook 111, 112
    Sacramento River Promenade 107, 108
Sacramento-San Joaquin Delta 48
Sacramento splittail 48
Sacramento Valley Conservancy 41
Sacramento Waterfront Loop 107–113
Salmon Lake 268
    Salmon Lake Spur Trail 268
    Salmon Lake Trail to Loch Leven Lakes 265–271
Salt Creek 224
Salt Spring slate 44
Sand Ridge 279
    Sand Ridge Trail 275, 279
Sand Tailings 179
Sargeant's cypress 6
Sawmill Lake 278
Seabiscuit 79
Secret Ravine 195
Secret Ravine Creek 195
serpentine 6
Shealor Lake 301
    Lower 301, 303, 304
    Shealor Lake Trail 301–305
    Upper 301, 302, 303–304
Shingle Falls Trail 185–189
Shotgun Lake 278
Shotgun/Middle Lakes Trail 278
Sierra Foothills 155–239
Sierra Nevada 243–237
Sierra Nevada Ecoregion 7–8
Sierra uplift 2
Silver Fork 313, 317
Silver Fork Road trailhead 319
Silver Lake 296, 299, 302
Slaughter Ravine 192
Smith, Jedediah 76
Snow Mountain Wilderness 121, 136, 137
South Forty Trail 33
South Stone Lake 115
South Trail 32–33
Southern Pacific Railroad 48
Spenceville Mine 186
Spenceville Wildlife Area 185
Spirit of Sacramento 109
springhouse 238
Squaw Ridge 296, 297
St. Catherine Creek 166
Stanford, Leland 208
Stebbins Cold Canyon UC Reserve 147
Steelhead Creek 102
Stevens Trail 191–195
Stevens, Truman Allen 194
Still Gulch 129
Stockton Municipal Camp 298
Stone Lakes National Wildlife Refuge 115
Summit Lake Trail 260
Sutter Buttes 68, 73–77
Sutter's Mill 239
Sycamore Swale 33
Sylvia Lake 333, 337

Talbot Campground 282
tectonic movement 2
Tevis Cup Ride 213
Tevis Cup segment 205
The Jams 144
The Sisters 310
Thompson Canyon 135, 136
Thunder Mountain 294–296, 299, 302
ticks 12
Tihuechemne Slough 38
tombstone rocks 44
tombstones, natural rock 223
Tower Bridge 108–109, 111
Tragedy Creek 302
    drainage 302, 303
    incident 302
Trail 12E11 276
Trail 12E12 277
Trail 13E13 275, 279
Trail 13E28 278
Trail 17E20 314, 316–318
Trail 17E20/17E51 junction 319
Trail 17E51 314, 318
Trail 17E63 318
Trail 17E71 315, 317–318
Trail 17E72 298

Training Hill Trail 223
Troublemaker Rapid 236
Tuleyome 127
Twin Lakes 327
    Lower 327, 330, 331
    Twin Lakes Trail 327–331, 333
    Upper 331

Union Pacific Railroad 100, 111, 192
University of California 147
Upper Loop Trail 187–188

vernal pools 5

Watt Ave. bridge 89
Wendell Robie Trail 202
West Nile virus 12
West Ravine Trail 230
West Sacramento 109, 110
Western States Endurance Run 213
Western States-Riverview Trails 213–219
Western States Trail 205, 213, 215–219, 223
    El Dorado Canyon 207–211
    trailhead 209
    Wendell Robie segment 223
wetlands 3–4

Wetlands Discovery Trail 67–68
Wetlands Loop Trail 68–70
Wetlands Walk Trail 36
Willow Creek 94
Willow Slough 36
Wilson Valley 145
Winnemucca Lake 307
    Winnemucca Lake Trail 308, 309
Winnemucca-Round Top Lakes Loop 307–311
Woods Creek 308
Woods Lake Campground 311
Woods Lake Road 311
Work, John 76
Work Your Own Diggings (WYOD) Loop Trail 178–179
Wren Wetlands Trail 115–117
Wrights Lake 329
    inlet stream 328

Yeaw, Effie 56
Yolla Bolly Wilderness 121
Yuba River, North 163, 167
    canyon 164
Yuba River, South 169, 173
    South Yuba Trail 169, 173–175

Ziggurat Building 110

Author

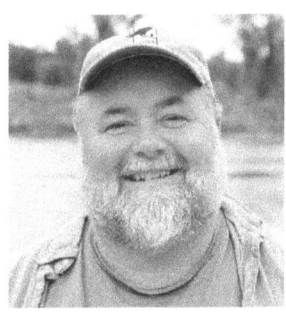

Steven L. Evans

Steve Evans was born and raised in the Mojave Desert near the typically dry Mojave River. When he moved up to Northern California in the 1970s for college, he discovered that most rivers actually had water and fish in them. He began exploring the wild places of the Sierra Nevada, and when he discovered that many of them were threatened by logging and other development, he became a full-time environmental activist as well as a hike leader for the Sierra Club. Steve has been hiking and backpacking Northern California trails and running its rivers for more than 30 years. As a resident of the Sacramento region for the last 20 years, he is familiar with the many trails in the valley, foothills, and mountains beloved by Sacramentans. It took Steve three years to hike the more than 235 miles of trails in *Top Trails Sacramento*, while continuing to work full time for Friends of the River (California's statewide river conservation organization). It's no coincidence that many of the trails lead to or follow some of the most scenic rivers and streams in the region. *Top Trails Sacramento* is Steve's first book for Wilderness Press.